P9-BYF-179

Introduction to Environmental Toxicology

Introduction to Environmental Toxicology

Edited by

Frank E. Guthrie and **Jerome J. Perry**

Interdepartmental Program in Toxicology
North Carolina State University, Raleigh, North Carolina

Elsevier · New York
New York · Oxford

Elsevier North Holland, Inc.
52 Vanderbilt Avenue, New York, N.Y. 10017

Distributors outside the United States and Canada:

Blackwell Scientific Publications
Osney Mead
Oxford, England OX2 0EL

Copyright 1980 by Elsevier North Holland, Inc.

Library of Congress Cataloging in Publication Data

Main entry under title:

Introduction to environmental toxicology.

    Bibliography: p.
    Includes index.
    1. Pollution—Environmental aspects. 2. Pollution—Toxicology.
    3. Environmental protection. I. Guthrie, Frank E. II. Perry, Jerome J.
QH545.A1I575   628.5   80-12853
ISBN 0-444-00359-2

Desk Editor   Gail Huggins
Design   Edmée Froment
Art Editor   Virginia Kudlak
Production Manager   Joanne Jay
Compositor   General Graphics Services, Inc.
Printer   Halliday Lithograph

Manufactured in the United States of America

Contents

Chapter 16. Pulp and Paper Industry   210
William T. McKean

Chapter 17. Case History: PCBs in the Hudson River   227
Lenore S. Clesceri

Chapter 18. Case History: Pollution of the Rhine River   236
G.M. Rand and G.T. Barthalmus

Preface

The origins of the activities that cumulatively are now known as environmental pollution can be traced to the advent of the Industrial Revolution in the latter part of the 19th century. The environmental deterioration associated with industrialization has been magnified in the 20th century by the Chemical Revolution. This century has also witnessed a worldwide population explosion, and the concomitant escalation in the human desire for material goods has brought civilization to the brink of environmental catastrophe. If we are to extricate ourselves from this plight we must delineate the causes and augment effective programs for alleviating contamination. A major aspect of investigations into problems associated with pollution is the study of environmental toxicology, which may be defined as the nature, distribution, and interaction of "foreign chemicals" that have become an integral part of the biosphere. In some cases the contaminant may be a naturally occurring material present in such quantity or under such physical conditions that it cannot be recycled.

Environmental pollution generally results from an unwillingness to accept the obvious fact that the world and its resources are finite. As the problem has been a product of humans and their activities, it must be solved by humans, and this can occur only through education. The process of finding a solution through education is fraught with problems, as world leaders may not fully comprehend the critical nature and consequences of environmental deterioration nor have the determination to reverse the pattern.

An exhaustive list of the factors associated with environmental pollution cannot be presented in this text, but an attempt has been made to present a representative cross-section of hard-core problems. Among the elements considered are the following:

1. Effects of overpopulation and the need for population stabilization.
2. Agriculture-related pollutants.
3. Pollutants of industrial origin.
4. Levels of contaminants in various aquatic environments.

5. Energy-related problems.
6. Effects of pollutants on plants and animals.

As will be repeatedly stressed throughout this book, an intelligent estimate of the potential dangers of very few chemicals is available at this time. An assessment of the actual (and growing) list of at least 20,000 chemicals and their possible interactions in the biosphere seems a hopeless task for the environmental toxicologist. The fact that the past one or two generations have experienced major exposure to many of these contaminants and apparently survived provides some hope for successful adaptation by the human population.

There is a considerable quantity of data on the acute (immediate) and subacute toxic effects of many chemicals. Determinations of the LD_{50} (amount of chemical required to kill 50% of an experimental group) of these substances and limited studies on growth and reproductive effects have been conducted mostly in mammals and, in a limited number of cases, in other vertebrates. Acute effects in invertebrate organisms are virtually unknown except for a small number of disease-causing organisms and agricultural pests.

The major fear associated with chemical contaminants is generally not related to the acute effects (although such measurements are valuable guides)—it is the chronic effects that are more important and less well defined. Adverse actions such as carcinogenicity, teratogenicity, and long-term reproductive and behavioral effects have received much attention but are not clearly understood. The information presently available pertains to higher organisms, and the effects on the other 99.9% plus species are not under investigation at the present time. Undoubtedly, the majority of species will not be adequately studied, but a critical number of organisms have to be included if environmental effects are to be estimated.

With this brief introduction in mind, it is obvious that more is not known than is known about environmental toxicology. This book may appear deficient in some areas of toxicology, but in many cases the data are insufficient to make adequate predictions. For example, much is known regarding the effects of pesticides in the terrestrial environment, but other contaminants have been largely ignored. Millions of dollars and considerable investigational resources are being expended to ascertain the effects on humans, and much less effort is directed toward the effects on other organisms. It is in regard to the latter consideration that substantial questions will be raised in the future.

This book is an outgrowth of a course taught at North Carolina State University for many years, primarily as a result of Training Grant ES-07046 from The National Institute of Environmental Health Sciences. The students in the course come from varied backgrounds, but a minimal understanding of ecology and chemistry is desirable. We have prepared the book for advanced undergraduates and beginning graduate students as a textbook, not as a sourcebook. Citations have purposefully been avoided to maximize readability, but a list of Suggested Reading is given at the end of each chapter. When assigned as a text for advanced students in toxicology, a more specific and comprehensive list of outside reading would be appropriate. These additional references might reflect the area of emphasis and priorities of the instructor.

A number of colleagues who were kind enough to review early drafts of these chapters are herewith acknowledged: Drs. W. M. Brooks, W. R. Davis, J. S. Doolittle, J. B. Evans, W. C. Griffith, P. B. Hamilton, J. W. Hardin, C. H. Hill,

D. B. Marsland, J. M. Miller, R. P. Patterson, T. L. Quay, H. E. Schaffer, P. V. Shah, E. C. Sisler, C. Smallwood, J. B. Weber, and G. T. Weekman of North Carolina State University; B. Fowler, H. Tilson, and D. Tuey of NIEHS; R. L. Baron of the Environmental Protection Agency; E. Kuenzler of the University of North Carolina at Chapel Hill; and D. P. Morgan of the University of Iowa. The expert typing and editorial assistance of Ms. Faye Lloyd and Ms. Nancy Stoddard are gratefully acknowledged.

Frank E. Guthrie
Jerome J. Perry

Contributors

CHARLES E. ANDERSON
Department of Botany, North Carolina State University, Raleigh, North Carolina

NEAL E. ARMSTRONG
Department of Civil Engineering, University of Texas, Austin, Texas

GEORGE T. BARTHALMUS
Department of Zoology, North Carolina State University, Raleigh, North Carolina

JOHN R. BEND
Laboratory of Pharmacology, National Institute of Environmental Health Sciences,
Research Triangle Park, North Carolina

W.T. BLEVINS
Department of Botany and Microbiology, Auburn University, Auburn, Alabama

J.R. BRADLEY, Jr.
Department of Entomology, North Carolina State University, Raleigh, North Carolina

STEVEN H. CADLE
Environmental Sciences Department, General Motors Research Laboratories,
Warren, Michigan

LENORE S. CLESCERI
Department of Biology, Rensselaer Polytechnic Institute, Troy, New York

B.J. COPELAND
Sea Grant Program, North Carolina State University, Raleigh, North Carolina

W.C. DAUTERMAN
Department of Entomology, North Carolina State University, Raleigh, North Carolina

E.D. ERMENC
Southwestern Ohio Air Pollution Control Agency, Cincinnati, Ohio

A.F. GAUDY, Jr.
Department of Civil Engineering, University of Delaware, Newark, Delaware

D.S. GROSCH
Department of Genetics, North Carolina State University, Raleigh, North Carolina

FRANK E. GUTHRIE
Department of Entomology, North Carolina State University, Raleigh, North Carolina

WALTER W. HECK
Agricultural Research, United States Department of Agriculture, and Department of
Botany, North Carolina State University, Raleigh, North Carolina

JOHN E. HOBBIE
Marine Biological Laboratory, Woods Hole, Massachusetts

E. HODGSON
Department of Entomology, North Carolina State University, Raleigh, North Carolina

DONALD HUISINGH
University Studies, North Carolina State University, Raleigh, North Carolina

MARGARET O. JAMES
Laboratory of Pharmacology, National Institute of Environmental Health Sciences,
Research Triangle Park, North Carolina

R.B. LEIDY
Pesticide Residue Research Laboratory, North Carolina State University, Raleigh,
North Carolina

PATRICIA E. McDONALD
School of Law, University of North Carolina, Chapel Hill, North Carolina

WILLIAM T. McKEAN
College of Forest Resources, University of Washington, Seattle, Washington

RICHARD B. MAILMAN
Departments of Psychiatry and Pharmacology, University of North Carolina School of
Medicine, Chapel Hill, North Carolina

DAVID H. MARTIN
Department of Physics, North Carolina State University, Raleigh, North Carolina

MICHAEL J. MATTESON
School of Chemical Engineering, Georgia Institute of Technology, Atlanta, Georgia

GEORGE J. NEBEL
Environmental Sciences Department, General Motors Research Laboratories,
Warren, Michigan

JEROME J. PERRY
Department of Microbiology, North Carolina State University, Raleigh, North Carolina

JOHN B. PRITCHARD
Laboratory of Pharmacology, National Institute of Environmental Health Sciences,
Research Triangle Park, North Carolina

GARY M. RAND
Corporate Health Department, Hooker Chemical Company, Niagara Falls, New York

ROBERT J. REIMOLD
Georgia Department of Natural Resources, Brunswick, Georgia

THOMAS J. SCHOENBAUM
School of Law, University of North Carolina, Chapel Hill, North Carolina

T.J. SHEETS
Pesticide Residue Research Laboratory, North Carolina State University, Raleigh, North Carolina

JUDY A. SIDDEN
Helix Associates, Chapel Hill, North Carolina

LYNNE A. STIRLING
Papanicolau Cancer Research Institute, Miami, Florida

J. ROBIE VESTAL
Department of Biological Sciences, University of Cincinnati, Cincinnati, Ohio

ROGER D. WYATT
Department of Poultry Science, University of Georgia, Athens, Georgia

Frank E. Guthrie

1

Nonagricultural Pollutants

1.1. Introduction

Although not limited to highly developed nations, environmental contamination is primarily a problem of the minority population presently utilizing the majority of world resources. It must certainly be a major goal of enlightened leadership to devise methods for the control of pollution before the less affluent nations are able to enjoy the "technological benefits" now limited to the minority. This, of course, is a thesis that will not be met with acclaim by the less developed nations, but it is nonetheless true that should the majority of the world reach the capacity of the highly industrialized societies, environmental contamination would likely be a major constraint on further progress. The consequences of unrestricted development are just now being realized, and it seems imperative that steps be taken to ensure that the world does not go beyond reasonable biological constraints if catastrophic ones are to be avoided. The thousands of chemicals that have been introduced into the environment must be sufficiently evaluated in terms of human and environmental consequences to ensure at least minimal compatibility of these xenobiotics with their various substrates. Such assurances are not presently available, and in a growth economy they will not be attained without sacrifice from all segments of the population.

This chapter is devoted to a brief examination of nonagricultural pollutants. The more specialized cases of heavy metals and radioactive substances will be discussed in Chapters 3 and 4, respectively.

Upon release into the environment, a contaminant may appear in air, water, or soil. There is interchange among these pathways, and it seems most appropriate to consider the sources of pollution from the viewpoint of air and water contamination, assuming that the pollutants going into soil will become problems only when transportable. This approach is a great simplification, especially since it ignores the biological transport of pollutants, but reading of the subsequent chapters devoted to specific problems will clarify the need for an introductory approach at this point.

1.2. Air Pollutants

Air-borne contaminants are normally retained in the lower stratosphere and eventually interact with terrestrial organisms or are dissolved in water. Despite the ultrahygienic environment our population believes to be necessary—ranging from sterile hospitals to air-conditioned houses and cars—the industrialized world has not the slightest qualm about releasing hundreds of thousands of pounds of gaseous pollutants into the air each day. For the most part, these particles are not or are only briefly seen and they can be easily ignored until the often insidious consequences are manifested by illness or major environmental damage.

Any process producing energy releases "something" into the environment, usually in a gaseous or air-borne form. Thus, the vast energy-producing component of our society is the greatest contributor to gaseous contamination. The petroleum and chemical industries (directly and indirectly) produce the second greatest portion and certainly contribute the most "species" of air pollutants. Some natural contamination occurs from volcanos, forest fires, and microbial actions, but the necessity for control has not yet become apparent, in contrast to the man-made contamination. A partial list of air pollutants and some of their threshold values are shown in Table 1.1. To produce a manageable list, the sources of the pollutants are frequently combined into broad categories. It must be stressed that most of the information on thresholds has been obtained from industrial exposures, and chronic effects of air pollutants are inadequately known except in rare instances.

1.2.1. Energy-Related Sources

Because of the magnitude of their release into air, five air pollutants have been selected for primary consideration—sulfur oxides (SO_x), nitrogen oxides (NO_x), hydrocarbons (HC), carbon monoxide (CO), and particulates. Table 1.2 compares the magnitude of these emissions and the sources from which they were derived in 1940, 1970, and 1976. One notes the great increase in certain of these pollutants since 1940 and the changes in magnitude as fuel sources were altered (coal to petroleum to natural gas to coal) and technology developed. The last line of Table 1.2 indicates that significant decreases in some emissions have been evident in recent years.

The burning of coal results in high concentrations of SO_x (especially from the use of high-sulfur coal), NO_x (a high-temperature combustion product), and particulates. Particulates are especially evident in industrial areas; however, a substantial part of the particulate problem is not caused directly by coal. As the United States moves into an economy based on coal-derived energy, the problem of these pollutants will become more important. The use of petroleum leads to high concentrations of NO_x (which do not derive primarily from the nitrogen in petroleum per se but from the oxidation of nitrogen in air-associated combustion).

The HC problem is primarily a result of transportation, but certain industrial processes involving the use of petroleum and chemicals also contribute significant quantities of HC, as does the miscellaneous use of organic solvents. Both NO_x and HC further contribute to the problem of photochemical oxidants.

Table 1.1 Atmospheric Emissions of Selected Gaseous Pollutants (United States, 1972, ktons/year) and Some Threshold Values

Material	Man-made sources								Natural sources (worldwide)	Threshold values[a]	
	Transport	Energy	Mining	Processing	Manufacture	Waste disposal	Use	Total		ppm[b]	mg/m³[c]
Arsenic		0.73		4.6	0.84	0.30	3.01	9.48			0.5
Asbestos			5.81		0.49		0.41	6.71			20
Barium		3.76	0.10	3.7	0.06		0.18	7.80			0.5
Benzo[a]pyrene	0.03	0.27		0.11	0.02	2.72		3.15			0.002
Beryllium		316		21	0.06	0.54		337.6			
Boron		4.52		2.4			0.02	6.94		1	10
Cadmium				1.7	0.01	0.01		1.71			0.1
Carbon monoxide	76,129	13,266		3,959	13,854	5,445	10.3	112,654	100,000	50	55
Chlorine	21	351		47.3	1.82	3.06	56.1	477		1	3
Chromium		1.9		8.3				13.2			0.5
Copper		0.17	0.15	9.7				10			0.1
Fluoride		20.1		80.9	17.1	1.04	3.30	122			2.5
Hydrocarbon	15,932	443		225	2,952	1,834	3,884	25,270			
Iron		251		168	0.46	1.82		421			1
Lead (including gasoline)	224	17.4	0.06	10	3.19	5.01		260			0.15
Magnesium		50.6	8.48	11.4	38.7			110			10
Manganese		1.97		14.9	0.48	0.18		17.5			
Mercury		0.11		0.05		0.01	0.3	0.5			0.05
Molybdenum		0.68	0.16	0.18				1.0			5
Nickel		3.73	0.14	0.63	0.06	0.04		4.6			1
Nitrogen oxides	8,508	12,715		117	516	194	21	22,071	500,000	5	9
Particulates	760	7,488		6,228	1,062	1,039	258	16,385			
Phosphorus		22.5	0.31	13.4	21.7	0.08	0.02	58			0.1
Selenium		0.7		0.08	0.2			1.0			0.2
Silver		0.05		0.11	0.01	0.02	0.02	0.2			0.01
Sulfur oxides	622	23,836		39.55	2,172	75.6	33.2	30,694	11,000	5	13
Titanium		42.7	0.26	3.29	3.07			51.1			
Vanadium		4.7	0.07	0.17				4.9			0.1
Zinc		4.9	0.05	92.8			2.50	100			5

Source: Data from Lee, D. H. K. (Ed.). Section 9: Reaction to Environmental Agents. In *Handbook of Physiology.* Baltimore: Waverly Press, 1977; and International Labor Organization (UN). *Encyclopedia of Occupational Health and Safety.* New York: McGraw-Hill, 1972.

[a] 8-hr work day, 40 hr/week. [b] ppm: part of material per million parts of air by volume. [c] mg/m³: milligrams of material per cubic meter of air.

Table 1.2 Comparison of Nation-Wide Emission Estimates, 1940–1976 (10^6 tons/year)

Source	Sulfur oxides			Particulates			Carbon monoxide			Hydrocarbons			Nitrogen oxides		
	1940	1970	1976	1940	1970	1976	1940	1970	1976	1940	1970	1976	1940	1970	1976
Transportation	0.6	0.7	0.8	0.3	1.1	1.2	34.9	79.2	69.7	7.5	12.6	10.8	3.2	8.4	10.1
Highway vehicles		0.3	0.4		0.7	0.8		69.7	61.4		11.1	9.3		6.3	7.8
Non-highway vehicles		0.4	0.4		0.4	0.4		9.5	8.3		1.5	1.5		2.1	2.3
Stationary fuel combustion	16.8	22.3	21.9	9.5	7.1	4.6	6.3	1.2	1.2	1.4	1.5	1.4	3.5	10.9	11.8
Electric utilities		15.7	17.6		4.1	3.2		0.2	0.3		0.1	0.1		5.1	6.6
Industrial		4.6	2.6		2.6	1.1		0.5	0.5		1.3	1.2		5.1	4.5
Residential–commercial		2.0	1.7		0.4	0.3		0.5	0.4		0.1	0.1		0.7	0.7
Industrial processes	3.8	5.9	4.1	10.3	12.4	6.3	22.5	8.0	7.8	5.4	8.5	9.4	0.2	0.6	0.7
Chemicals		0.5	0.3		0.3	0.3		3.0	2.4		1.5	1.6		0.2	0.3
Petroleum refineries		0.6	0.7		0.1	0.1		0.2	2.4		0.7	0.9		0.3	0.3
Metals		4.1	2.4		2.1	1.3		2.1	1.9		0.2	0.2		<0.1	<0.1
Mineral products		0.5	0.5		7.7	3.2		<0.1	<0.1		<0.1	<0.1		0.1	0.1
Oil and gas production		0.1	0.1		<0.1	<0.1		<0.1	<0.1		2.7	3.0		<0.1	<0.1
Organic solvent use		<0.1	<0.1		<0.1	<0.1		<0.1	<0.1		2.7	2.9		<0.1	<0.1
Other processes		0.1	0.1		2.2	1.4		0.9	1.1		0.7	0.8		<0.1	<0.1
Solid waste	0.4	0.1	<0.1	0.5	1.1	0.4	1.8	6.1	2.8	0.7	1.7	0.8	0.1	0.3	0.1
Miscellaneous	0.2	0.1	0.1	6.4	0.9	0.9	19.0	5.3	5.7	4.5	5.4	5.5	0.7	0.2	0.3
Wildfire and managed fires		<0.1	<0.1		0.5	0.6		3.5	4.8		0.7	0.8		0.1	0.2
Agricultural burning		<0.1	<0.1		0.3	0.1		1.4	0.5		0.3	0.1		<0.1	<0.1
Coal refuse burning		0.1	0.1		0.1	0.1		0.3	0.3		0.1	0.1		0.1	0.1
Structural fires		<0.1	<0.1		<0.1	0.1		0.1	0.1		<0.1	<0.1		<0.1	<0.1
Organic solvents		0.1	0.1		<0.1	<0.1		<0.1	<0.1		4.3	4.5		<0.1	<0.1
Total	21.5	29.1	26.9	27.1	22.6	13.4	85.4	99.8	87.2	19.1	29.7	27.9	7.9	20.4	23.0
Percent change, 1970–1975[a]		-4			-33			-15			-9			+7	

Source: Environmental Protection Agency. Air Pollution Emission Trends 1940–70, 1976.

[a] Estimates are determined from newly calculated sets of data and will lack continuity with 1970 data, but percent change is actual comparative compilation. Although total particulates have decreased, fine particulates may be increasing.

Carbon monoxide pollution is primarily a result of the incomplete combustion of petroleum in the internal combustion engine, but substantial quantities are also produced by other incomplete combustion processes.

When these gaseous pollutants are considered from the viewpoint of the total health problem, the hazards are not necessarily proportional to the quantity of the pollutant. Table 1.3 provides an estimate of the potential health hazard of these pollutants and the percentage produced by various sources. Whereas CO is the primary pollutant in terms of total emission, it is considered the least hazardous to health, in part because the symptoms of CO poisoning are rapidly reversible when animals are removed from the source of contamination. Particulates, comprising a smaller percentage of total air pollution according to 1976 estimates, are considered to be a major health hazard, largely because certain carcinogenic products of combustion (such as benzo[a]pyrenes) tend to be absorbed onto such particles. Sulfur oxides are presently believed to be the greatest overall health hazard. Thus, stationary fuel consumption and industrial processing, which are the sources of both the SO_x and particulate problems, produce nearly 70% of the total health hazard, far greater than the hazard from transportation, even though emissions from that source are over 50% of the total.

These "Big Five" pollutants are presently considered to be of the greatest concern in air pollution, and a brief discussion of the individual components follows; the problem of air-borne lead is considered in Chapter 3. The definition of two common terms regarding air pollutants is necessary at this point. A threshold value is the minimum concentration of a pollutant necessary to induce injury in a population in a specified time. The National Ambient Air Quality Standard (NAAQS) is a legal standard prescribing the exposure (concentration and duration) that a political jurisdiction determines should not be exceeded in a specific geographical area. It is usually lower than the threshold value.

Table 1.3 Relative Health Hazard of Air Pollutants and Sources of Pollution

| | Percent contribution | |
Category	Total emissions	Health significance
Pollutant		
SO_x	12.9	34.6
Particulates	9.7	27.9
NO_x	8.6	18.6
HC	13.1	17.7
CO	55.7	1.2
Source		
Stationary fuel consumption	16.9	43.0
Transportation	54.5	22.2
Solid waste disposal	4.2	3.0
Industrial processing	15.3	25.7
Agricultural burning	7.3	4.4
Miscellaneous	1.8	1.7

Source: Murdoch, W. W. Environment. Sunderland, Mass.: Sinauer Associates, 1975.

1.2.1.a. Sulfur Oxides

In addition to important health effects, SO_x have an insidious feature that affects the environment. These gases, a primary combustion product of coal, are converted to acids in the atmosphere ($SO_2 \rightarrow SO_3 \rightarrow SO_4$). When these acids are returned to the earth in the form of rain, pH changes may occur in both soil and water. These changes may have a drastic effect on plants and animals that are not tolerant to marked acidity. The problem is further compounded as appreciable amounts of SO_x are transported in air by prevailing wind currents. For example, Scandinavian scientists have accumulated strong evidence that SO_x emitted from Germany, England, and other northern European countries are borne by wind across the Baltic Sea, eventually to be returned to the earth in acid form. The acidity of rainfall in that area has changed from nearly neutral to, in some cases, pH 4 over the past 20 years. Similar trends are appearing in the highly industrialized northeastern United States, a problem that will require careful monitoring as this country moves to a coal economy. In addition to the possible effects of intolerable pH levels on living organisms, stone statuary, buildings, and any material affected by long-term acid oxidation are being seriously and irreversibly disfigured. Disintegration of the vast treasury of stone statuary in Venice is but one dramatic example of the effects of acid rains.

The precise mode of action in humans is not yet known, but there is general agreement that the acid per se causes adverse effects on the lungs. Sulfurous acid aerosol (SO_3^{2-}) is able to penetrate deep into lung tissues, primarily as an adherent to fine particulates. The effects of SO_x are particularly important in persons with respiratory problems. The NAAQS for SO_2 has been set at 0.03 ppm (60 μg/m^3) on an average annual basis and 0.14 ppm for 24 hr. Many epidemiological studies have shown that the incidence of a number of diseases, including cancers, is highly correlated with city pollution. The data presented in Table 1.4 illustrate the correlation of respiratory cancer with size and/or air pollution of metropolitan areas. The exact causative factor is unknown, but SO_x are considered to be among the primary suspects. Fortunately, SO_x are among the easiest air pollutants to clean up, as discussed in more detail in Chapter 31.

1.2.1.b. Particulates

These contaminants constitute a poorly defined group of particles, ranging from soots and fly ashes to mineral particles (gravel, dust, cement, sand, etc.), that are 0.1–100 μm in diameter. The majority of these particles primarily cause irritation, but those products resulting from incomplete combustion often contain polycyclic aromatic hydrocarbons, one of which is the carcinogen benzo[a]pyrene. Although it is well established that benzo[a]pyrene is a product of tobacco smoke, it is perhaps surprising to note (Table 1.5) that benzo[a]pyrene is inhaled in higher quantities in industrialized areas than in cigarette smoke. Particulate air pollution is primarily a city problem; the U.S. cities with the highest particulate concentrations are Chicago, Pittsburgh, and Philadelphia. The NAAQS for annual mean total suspended particles is 75 μg/m^3 and the 24-hr maximum is 260 μg/m^3. This problem can be largely eliminated through the installation of proper equipment, which is much in evidence in larger industrial

Table 1.4 Mortality Data for Respiratory System Cancer

Metropolitan area	Deaths per year				Mean deaths, 1961–1964	Death rate per 10^5 population
	1961	1962	1963	1964		
El Paso, Tex.	34	44	43	42	40.8	13.0
Denver, Colo.	152	177	188	195	178.0	19.2
Charlotte, N.C.	36	56	69	54	53.8	19.8
Atlanta, Ga.	208	198	237	254	224.3	22.1
Seattle, Wash.	265	269	281	276	272.8	24.6
Birmingham, Ala.	147	146	161	176	157.5	24.8
Las Vegas, Nev.	22	29	37	43	32.8	25.8
Los Angeles, Calif.	1704	1709	1919	1933	1816.3	26.9
Detroit, Mich.	928	1037	1082	1103	1037.5	27.6
San Francisco, Calif.	744	817	802	892	813.8	29.2
Chicago, Ill.	1757	1759	1904	1922	1835.5	29.5
Cleveland, Ohio	503	582	566	610	565.3	31.5
Philadelphia, Pa.	1247	1411	1357	1503	1379.5	31.8
New York, N.Y.	3415	3557	3624	3719	3578.8	33.5
Boston, Mass.	877	930	875	864	886.5	34.2

Source: Adapted from Hickey, R. et al. Ecological statistical studies concerning environmental pollution and chronic disease. I.E.E.E. Trans. Geosci. Electronics GE 8:186–202, 1970.

Table 1.5 Levels of 3, 4-Benzo[a]pyrene in Different Situations in England and Wales

Location or source	Air concentration (mg/km^3)	Yearly intake with air (mg)
North Wales	5–6	41
Liverpool	62	450
London (traffic)	1–68	7–475
2 packs/ day smoker	—	120

Source: Walker, C. Environmental Pollution by Chemicals. London: Hutchinson Educators, 1971.

plants. For economic reasons, it will not be easy to have expensive equipment installed in small plants.

A second important health effect of fine particulates is that they may act as a vector to carry sulfurous acid to deep lung recesses. Components of SO_x would ordinarily be detained and eliminated in the upper respiratory tract, but when absorbed (as SO_3^{2-}) onto fine particulates their hazard is increased as they can then penetrate to areas of greater sensitivity.

1.2.1.c. Nitrogen Oxides and Hydrocarbons

These contaminants are usually found together and are primarily produced by processes related to transportation (including the refining industry), although a substantial portion of NO_x also arises from stationary combustion. For many years their emission was considered to cause mainly a smog problem (discussed below), but there has been increasing concern in recent years that these gases (especially NO_x) contribute markedly to chronic health problems. The NAAQS for NO_2 is 0.05 ppm (100 $\mu g/m^3$) per year and 0.13 ppm for a 24-hr period. Public health scrutiny has recently increased because it has been discovered that NO_2 may affect lipid peroxidation and enzyme inhibition as well as have an ill-defined effect on lung ciliary action that would reduce lung clearance. Hydrocarbons affect health less than NO_x, and the NAAQS has been set at 0.24 ppm (160 $\mu g/m^3$) for a 3-hr period. The HC problem is produced by the use of petroleum for transportation and the use of any organic solvent in abundance.

Where there is very heavy traffic, the effects of NO_x and HC contribute to additional ozone (O_3), and ultimately peroxyacetyl nitrate (PAN), to cause the general problem of higher concentrations of photochemical oxidants. Sulfur oxides have recently been implicated in this combination of actions, and possible interactions among these compounds make it very difficult to identify single factors. Among the important reactions occurring in the lower stratosphere are the following (where hv is photooxidative energy):

$$NO_2 + hv \longrightarrow NO + O\cdot$$

$$O\cdot + O_2 \longrightarrow O_3 (ozone)$$

$$O_3 + NO \longrightarrow O_2 + NO_2$$

$$NO + HC \longrightarrow PAN + NO_2$$

The NAAQS for photooxidants is 0.08 ppm (160 $\mu g/m^3$) for a 1-hr period; a standard for O^3 apparently will be set at 0.1 ppm for that period. Until fairly recently, these pollutants were considered to be hazardous primarily to plants; however, the chronic effects are now considered to be an important human health problem. Photochemical oxidants have an acute effect as irritants of tender tissues (eyes, respiratory tissues, and skin). In addition, especially upon air inversion, photochemical oxidants can cause marked reduction in visibility. The main effort to reduce the production of photooxidants is aimed at upsetting the chemical sequence of events noted above by reducing HC emissions by the use of the catalytic converter in automobiles.

1.2.1.d. Carbon Monoxide

Until recently, the release of this pollutant was considered to be the most important problem associated with transportation emissions, primarily because it was formed in the greatest quantity. The NAAQS is 9 ppm (10 mg/m^3) for an 8-hr period and 35 ppm for a 1-hr period. These concentrations are occasionally experienced for short intervals by heavily exposed workers (tunnel police), and levels of 5 ppm are common in areas with much traffic. The mode of action is the combination of CO with blood hemoglobin (to form carboxyhemoglobin), which greatly decreases the capacity of blood for O_2 transport. However, the action of CO is rapidly reversible and this apparent nonchronic action makes it a much less important health hazard than it was previously held to be.

Many of the problems associated with these contaminants are amendable through government action, and cleanup legislation is discussed in Chapter 35.

1.2.2. Industrial Sources

Over 50 toxic gases whose 8-hr threshold limits are below 10 ppm may on occasion be discharged into the atmosphere (cyanides, chlorides, ammonia, hydrogen sulfide, hydrogen fluoride, formaldehyde, phosgene, vinyl chloride, etc.; see Table 1.1 for a partial list). The problem is generally believed to be one of occupational health hazards, and only on the relatively rare occasions of accidents are these gases a hazard outside the industrial area. Nonetheless, dozens of transportation accidents occur each year; over 10 deaths attributed to exposure of the public to toxic fumes resulted when railroad tank cars over-turned in 1978. Small quantities of potentially toxic gases are discharged from tall emission stacks so that they may be diluted by large volumes of air.

The problems associated with pollution resulting from industrial sources are only poorly understood because (a) our knowledge of the identity and magnitude of toxic gases from industrial effluents is very limited, and (b) the chronic effects of these gases have not received adequate scrutiny, primarily because the major effort is directed toward the study and control of the Big Five. Local episodes have occurred from time to time that may be important signals. For example, an area of some 20 miles^2 near Raleigh, North Carolina, has been denuded of pine trees by an unidentified gaseous pollutant released by an unidentified industrial plant, one of several small industries in the area. A local vinyl chloride incident in Ohio had more important direct health effects, but in this case both pollutant and source were identifiable.

1.2.3. Domestic Sources

A large number of potentially dangerous volatile chemicals are sold to the public each year. The average citizen has little understanding of the chronic toxicity of a variety of organic chemicals with appreciable vapor action that are used in large quantities—paints, thinners, solvents, pesticides, preservatives, and waxes. They are often carelessly used, and there may be important long-term conse-quences, especially for heavy users.

An example of an unforeseen problem caused by mass use of a chemical initially considered to involve little hazard is that resulting from the use of household aerosol bombs. When fluorocarbons were introduced as propellants for pesticides to protect troops in World War II, no one considered the possible side effects, nor did anyone predict the tremendous aerosol industry that ultimately resulted in hundreds of aerosol home products. Recent studies have shown that these gases accumulate in concentrations of 50–100 ppm in the rarified upper atmosphere, and their reactivity has caused a possible world-wide problem. A simplified scheme follows:

Fluorohydrocarbon   High-energy   Lower energy   Activated
(aerosol propellant)   free radical   intermediate   ozone
                       intermediate

The initial reaction causes destruction of one molecule of O_3, and the intermediate can be raised to a higher energy level for another O_3 interaction (much like an enzymic reaction), so that one aerosol molecule may destroy over 100,000 O_3 molecules. The O_3 layer in the stratosphere prevents the penetration of ultraviolet rays, and destruction of this protective layer could permit the penetration of potentially toxic amounts of this energy source, a known skin carcinogen. The calculated disappearance of 0.5% of the O_3 layer to date resulted in a recommendation by the Environmental Protection Agency (EPA) to ban aerosols of this type.

1.2.4. Other Potential Long-Term Hazards

A highly controversial problem is that of the long-term increase in atmospheric CO_2, a consequence of fossil fuel combustion. The large quantities of CO_2 produced appear to exceed the capabilities of the two sinks designed to recycle this gas—photosynthetic activity and dissolved CO_2 ($CaCO_3$) in the ocean. As a result, atmospheric CO_2 has risen from 315 to 330 ppm over the past 16 years. Surface thermal energy escaping from the earth can be radiated back to the earth, and concern has been expressed that the increase in CO_2 would be manifested by a long-term increase in temperature. The consequences of the relatively sudden 5% rise over the past few years cause some uneasiness because such an effect would be irreversible.

1.2.5. Effects on Nonmammalian Species

The environmental effects of air pollution on a great number of organisms have not been adequately addressed, nor is there any current attempt to do so, except for the relatively minor effort by plant scientists and small, grant-supported, basic research projects. The expensive technology required for scientific investigations has limited the availability of funds primarily to the study of health and agricultural production problems, and the rest of the environment lies in limbo; it is hoped that no irreversible damage is occurring.

1.3. Water Pollutants

Water pollution from nonagricultural sources results in two types of aquatic contamination: (a) highly enriched, overproductive biotic communities, such as occur in a lake or river enriched with nutrients from municipal sewers, (e.g., sewage, detergents, effluents of food processing, etc.); and (b) a body of water poisoned by a toxic chemical that eliminates many living organisms.

The first effect is well known and reasonably controllable; it is treated in depth in subsequent chapters. It is the second problem (toxic chemicals) that is of greatest importance as a potential hazard to both humans and their environment because there are so many "unknowns." Pollutants may derive from point sources and enter at a well-defined place (food processing, sewage, or chemical plant), or they may derive from a general (nonpoint) source (salt added to de-ice highways, ill-defined sources in the somewhat diffuse petroleum and refining industry, or agricultural runoff). The biota of streams are well adjusted to cleaning much of the man-made contamination, even when the oxygen deficiency temporarily excludes aerobic organisms; Figure 1.1 demonstrates some of

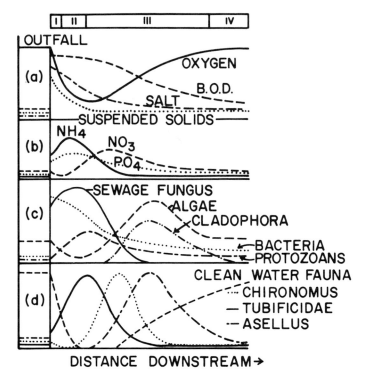

Figure 1.1 Changes in condition of a river below an outfall of sewage. Chemical changes are shown in (*a*) and (*b*), changes in microorganisms in (*c*), and changes in aquatic animals in (*d*). *Zone I* indicates mixing, *Zone II* is an area of active decomposition and may overwhelm cleansing activities, *Zone III* is a septic area where water is first deficient of organisms and then recovery is initiated, and *Zone IV* is the area where processes take place to change water to its original condition. (Modified from Federal Water Pollution Control Administration. The Cost of Clean Water. Washington, D.C.: Government Printing Office, 1968.)

these activities. However, if the effluent contains toxicants, or if the stream receives additional effluent from another source before it has completed cleanup of a problem immediately upstream, a nearly sterile body of water may result. There have been numerous examples of this situation (the Thames River until recently), and such episodes of neglect may no longer be tenable now that there is greater concern for governmental control by an environmentally conscious population. Fortunately, only isolated, local situations of this nature are presently in evidence in the United States.

1.3.1. Treatment of Effluents

Because most rivers are unable to clean up effluents in many instances, sewage systems are necessary. Four primary types are in use (discussed in greater detail in Chapter 33):

1. Primary treatment. Sewage is placed in an open tank where solid particles are allowed to settle and light particles are skimmed off. After a brief holding period, the effluent is delivered to a stream.

2. *Secondary treatment.* In addition to the above, the sewage is held for a longer period where optimal conditions for microbial growth are maintained. Ordinarily, over 75% of organic matter can be consumed before returning the water to a stream. This effluent may be enriched with inorganic materials that are not fully utilized.

3. *Tertiary treatment.* Sewage from secondary treatment is further subjected to physical and chemical processes that remove nitrates, phosphates, and some toxic constituents. However, this procedure is selective, and many toxic constituents may escape removal, especially if methods for their removal have not been perfected. This is a very expensive operation; less than 1% of wastes the United States are so treated.

4. *Storage.* When toxic or other undesirable compounds are not permitted to enter a waterway, they may be pumped into holding ponds for storage.

1.3.2. Specific Problems of Water Pollution

1.3.2.a. Toxic or Potentially Toxic Compounds

A large number of chemical plants are located along various types of waterways, such as the Rhine River (see Chapter 18) and the lower Mississippi River. Figure 1.2 shows the magnitude of the problem between Baton Rouge and New Orleans. Many industries introduce chemicals into the water, and the identity of most of them is not available to monitoring agencies. Some of the more than 350 organic chemicals in U.S. rivers and lakes have been identified and are usually present in levels below 1 ppb. Fewer than 5% of these compounds have been adequately examined for possible carcinogenicity. Among the compounds found in a 1977 study were methyl palmitate, methyl stearate, diethylhexyl phthalate, terpinol, methyl myristate, dibutyl phthalate, chloroform, trichloroethylene, tetrachloroethylene, 1,2-dichloromethane, toluene, and bromodichloromethane. Concentrations are normally quite low, but in some instances the effluent contains acutely toxic dose levels. Table 1.6 presents the acute toxicity to some common assay organisms of a number of compounds that are potential candidates for release into waterways.

1.3.2.b. Heat

In some industries (especially electricity-generating and steel plants), large quantities of water are required for either coolant purposes or conversion of one energy form to another. The release of large quantities of hot water causes problems for organisms living near the effluent because warmer water (even when the thermal effects are not adverse) is decreased in oxygen content, exacerbating the obvious physiological problem that metabolism (hence the need for additional O_2) is increased at higher temperatures. Some organisms are capable of remarkable adaptation to temperature changes and can withstand temperatures exceeding 90°F. The more desirable aquatic forms, however, are usually more susceptible to temperature changes, and in waters normally maintained at low temperatures (below 60°F) a rise of a few degrees may be adverse to those organisms. In controlled situations, heated waters are not introduced such that they increase the temperature of large bodies of water except within narrow limits. The heated effluent must be delivered at a rate that

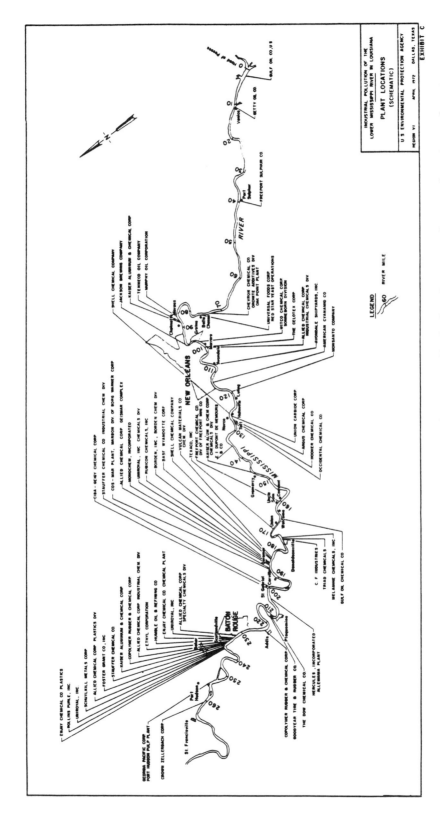

Figure 1.2 Industrial development along lower Mississippi River, where river affords abundant water for manufacturing and waste disposal. (Modified from EPA, Industrial Pollution of Lower Mississippi River, Dallas, Texas, April 1972.)

Table 1.6 Toxicity of Potential Pollutants to Fish

Substance	Fish tested	Lethal concentration (ppm)	Exposure time (hr)
Acetic acid	Goldfish	423	20
Aluminum potassium sulphate (alum)	Goldfish	100	12–96
Aluminum nitrate	Stickleback	0.1	144
Ammonia	Goldfish	2–2.5 NH_3	24–96
Amyl alcohol	Goldfish	1	161
Aniline	Minnow	200	48
Aniline	Brown trout	100	48
Sodium arsenite	Minnow	17.8 As	36
Sodium arsenate	Minnow	234 As	15
Barium chloride	Goldfish	5,000	12–17
	Salmon	158	?
Barium nitrate	Stickleback	500 Ba	180
Bromine	Goldfish	20	15–96
Butyl alcohol	Goldfish	250	7–20
Cadmium chloride	Goldfish	0.016	9–18
Calcium hydroxide	Goldfish	100 (pH 11.1)	?
Carbon dioxide	Various species	100–200	?
Carbon monoxide	Various species	1.5	1–10
Chloramine	Brown trout fry	0.06	?
Chlorine	Rainbow trout	0.03	?
Chromic acid	Goldfish	200	60–84
Citric acid	Goldfish	894	4–28
Cobalt chloride	Goldfish	10	168
Copper nitrate	Stickleback	0.02 Cu	192
	Rainbow trout	0.08 Cu	20
	Salmon	0.18	?
Copper sulphate	Stickleback	0.03 Cu	160
Cupric chloride	Goldfish	0.019	3–7
Cresylic acid	Goldfish	1	6–18
Cyanogen chloride	Rainbow trout	0.1	?
Ethanol	Goldfish	0.25 ml/liter	6–11
Ferric chloride	Stickleback	pH 4.8	144
Hydrochloric acid	Stickleback	pH 4.8	240
	Goldfish	pH 4.0	4–6
Hydrogen sulphide	Goldfish	10	96
Lactic acid	Goldfish	654	6–43
Lead nitrate	Minnow	0.33 Pb	?
	Stickleback	0.33 Pb	?
Lead sulphate	Goldfish	25 Pb	96
Magnesium nitrate	Stickleback	400 Mg	120
Mercuric chloride	Stickleback	0.01 Hg	204
Methanol	Goldfish	0.25 ml/liter	11–15
Naphthalene	Salmon	3.2	?
	Perch	20	1
Nickel chloride	Goldfish	10	200
Nickel nitrate	Stickleback	1 Ni	156
Nitric acid	Minnow	pH 5.0	?
Oxalic acid	Goldfish	1,000	1
Tartaric acid	Goldfish	100	200
Zinc sulphate	Stickleback	0.3 Zn	204
Detergents			
Entire packaged detergent	Fathead minnow	41–85 (soft)[a]	96
		15–37 (hard)[a]	96

Substance	Fish tested	Lethal concentration (ppm)	Exposure time (hr)
Surface-active agents			
Alkyl benzene sulphonates	Fathead minnow	4.5–23 (soft)	96
		3.5–12 (hard)	96
Polyoxyethylene ester	Fathead minnow	57(soft)	96
		38 (hard)	96
Sodium lauryl sulfate	Fathead minnow	5.1 (soft)	96
		5.9 (hard)	96
Sodium tetrapropylene			
benzene sulphonate	Rainbow trout	12	6
Builders			
Sodium perborate	Rainbow trout	320	24
Sodium pyrophosphate	Rainbow trout	1,120 PO_4	24
Sodium silicate	Rainbow trout	>250	24
Sodium sulfate	Rainbow trout	>700	24
		9,000 (soft)	96
		13,500 (hard)	96
Sodium tripolyphosphate	Rainbow trout	1,120 PO_4	24
	Fathead minnow	140 (soft)	96
	Fathead minnow	1,300 (hard)	96
Soaps			
Household soaps	Fathead minnow	29–42 (soft)	96
		920–1,800 (hard)	96
Pure sodium sterate	Fathead minnow	100 (soft)	96
		>1,800 (hard)	96
Herbicides			
Aminotriazole	Coho salmon	325	48
	Bluegill	10,000	48
Boron	Chinook salmon	2.3	48
	Largemouth bass	4.6	24
Diquat	Chinook salmon	28.5	48
	Rainbow trout	60	96
Endothal	Chinook salmon	136	48
Monuron	Coho salmon	110	48
	Various species	40	240
Simazine	Chinook salmon	6.6	48
Insecticides			
BHC	Goldfish	2.3	96
	Rainbow trout	3	96
Carbaryl	Fathead minnow	13	96
	Bluegill	5.6	96
Chlordane	Goldfish	0.082	96
	Rainbow trout	0.5	24
Chlorothion	Fathead minnow	3.2	96
DDT	Goldfish	0.027	96
	Rainbow trout	0.5	24
Dieldrin	Bluegill	0.008	96
	Rainbow trout	0.05	24
Guthion	Bluegill	0.005	96
	Fathead minnow	0.093	96
Malathion	Fathead minnow	12.5	96
Parathion	Fathead minnow	1.4–2.7	96
Toxaphene	Rainbow trout	0.05	24
	Goldfish	0.0056	96

(continued)

Table 1.6   Toxicity of Potential Pollutants to Fish *(continued)*

Substance	Fish tested	Lethal concentration (ppm)	Exposure time (hr)
Phenolic substances			
Orthocresol	Minnow	60	2
Paracresol	Minnow	50	2
	Rainbow trout	5	2
Phenol	Minnow	20	4
	Rainbow trout	6	3
Potassium chromate	Rainbow trout	75	60
	Largemouth bass	195 Cr	68
Potassium dichromate	Rainbow trout	57	72
Potassium cyanide	Goldfish	0.4 CN	118
Pyridine	Perch	1,000	1
Quinoline	Perch	30	1
Silver nitrate	Stickleback	0.004 Ag	180
Sodium chlorate	Goldfish	>1,000	120
Sodium fluoride	Goldfish	1,000	60–102
Sodium hydroxide	Goldfish	pH 10.6	168
Sodium sulphite	Goldfish	100	96
Strontium chloride	Goldfish	10,400 Sr	17–31
Strontium nitrate	Stickleback	1,500 Sr	164
Sulphuric acid	Goldfish	pH 3.9	5–6
Tannic acid	Goldfish	100	180
	Salmon	4.8	?

Source: Data from Klein, L. River Pollution. London: Butterworth, 1959–1966; and Henderson, C. et al. The toxicity of synthetic detergents and soaps to fish. Sewage Ind. Wastes 31:295–306, 1959.

[a]Lethal concentration in soft or hard water.

prevents shore-to-shore coverage of a moving stream, thus permitting migration of fish through the unheated area. Nuclear power is a particularly important source of heated water, and there is much concern for this problem in the future if large numbers of such plants are to be constructed along major waterways. A secondary effect of heat is increased microbial growth, which is generally advantageous in maximizing degradation, but in the case of maximizing conditions for disease organisms, it is disadvantageous.

Heated water has generally been considered to be of local importance. Where water temperature rises less than 5–10°F, the adverse effects are short range. The fact that many potentially adverse situations have been monitored for years is encouraging in that no long-range problems seem evident; that is, when properly regulated, warm effluent has thus far resulted in only temporary, point problems. Nonetheless, local problems cannot be completely ignored, and the proposed increase in steel production and nuclear power facilities will require careful monitoring for possible large-scale effects. One area where large-scale effects are becoming critical is the Rhine River Basin (Chapter 18).

1.3.2.c. pH Changes

Apart from the previously mentioned problem associated with SO_x, the primary source of pH alteration is the mining industry. Other industries also contribute by releasing acids and bases, but these are of less importance and are more frequently controlled. Mining effluents usually cause problems of a local nature, and the factors of dilution and buffer capacity prevent major problems. Nonetheless, in certain situations, many miles of a stream may be deprived of normal biota by mining effluents as a result of the joint contribution of pH change and toxic elements. In such situations, the effluents must be channeled to holding reservoirs. When the pH is less than 5 or greater than 9, few organisms are able to adapt.

1.3.2.d. Suspended Solids

Many industries and services contribute suspended materials. The steel industry has local problems along the Great Lakes with iron filings temporarily suspended in water plus manufacturing sludges, but the problem, albeit undesirable, has been contained to relatively small lakeside areas. The rapidly increasing number of food processing plants, among others, contribute much organic matter to water, resulting in increased biological oxygen demand (BOD, a test used to measure the amount of organic material in a water sample) contributing to eutrophication.

New technology has not always been compatible with the prevention of water contamination and indeed has drastically increased the magnitude of pollution (Table 1.7). Although plant efficiency in the steel industry has increased, it has been partly at the potential expense of increased water contamination. The newly proposed, rather stringent EPA standards should circumvent such a problem if environmental concerns continue to have a high priority in future planning.

Table 1.7   Comparison of Wastes (lb/day) Produced by Steel Industry with Older and Advanced Technologies

Substance	Old technology	Advanced technology
Suspended solids	198,514	1,513,610
Phenols	131	525
Cyanides	56	257
Fluorides	63	252
Ammonia	161	645
Lube oils	5,890	19,500
Sulfuric acid	5,810	23,240
Ferrous sulfate	21,640	86,450
Emulsions	637	9,630
Chromium		518
Zinc		21
Tin		132
Ferric chloride		17,290
Hydrochloric acid		4,660
Wastewater volume	19 million gallons/day	113 million gallons/day

Source: Abridged from WATER POLLUTION by Julian McCaull and Janice Crossland, © 1974 by Scientists' Institute for Public Information. Reprinted by permission of Harcourt Brace Jovanovich, Inc.

1.3.3. Sources of Pollution

The nonagricultural water pollution problems can be primarily charged to:

Steel industry (heat and sludges)

Chemical industry (toxic substances)

Food processing (BOD problems)

Mining (pH and toxic elements)

Municipal wastes (BOD and toxic substances).

Since problems related to the steel and mining industries have already been considered and food processing primarily causes oxygen deficiency problems, the two main sources to be addressed here are municipal wastes and the chemical industry.

1.3.3.a. Municipal Wastes

Two important facts regarding municipal wastes are not recognized by the average citizen: (a) nearly one-third of the households in the United States are not served by sewage services (wastes from 60 million persons enter waterways untreated) and (b) even the more advanced sewage systems are only 90% efficient. In the highly populated New York City area alone, for example, raw sewage of 100,000 persons enters the Hudson River each day. The main problem of the city per se is the BOD problem, which is compounded by the synthetic detergent industry. Although much unwanted waste is delivered to sewage drainage systems by citizens, hospitals, universities, and other organizations, these varied pollutants (pharmaceuticals, low-level radioactivity, solvents, etc.) are not a major problem. In many cities, one-half of all municipal waste is derived from nearby industries that contract with the city for waste disposal. Thus, the potential for a sizable quantity of low- and high-toxicity chemicals is manifest, and the identity of the compounds may be largely unknown. Such materials, containing toxic elements as part of the effluent, are often adverse to microorganisms and higher organisms that normally have a major role in the degradation of sewage.

The re-use of water is now commonplace and is a potential public health problem. Although the developed world has generally solved the problem of water-borne diseases, a large number of major population centers in the world contain disease organisms in their municipal water systems. For the most part, the native populations are immune to these organisms, but visitors to the area must exercise considerable caution. However, the removal of toxicants is much more difficult than the control of disease. Most drinking water in industrialized areas contains trace amounts of potentially toxic chemicals. In fact, some of the water treatment methods themselves require careful scrutiny. In Chicago, the use of Cl_2 for water treatment has increased 67% over a 20-year period. Whereas the chlorine content of Lake Michigan rose only 0.1 ppm during the three decades before 1940, over the past three decades it has risen 4–9 ppm. No specific problem has been identified, but the continued use of large quantities of this rather reactive chemical is worthy of attention.

Usually storm sewer effluents are not connected to sewage treatment facilities, and this run-off is delivered directly to streams. Although the problem of storm sewers is not a major one nationally, nearly anything imaginable could become part of such effluent. For example, there are 0.5 million dogs in New York City whose wastes are largely disposed of via storm sewers.

The problem of detergents has become a severe one for water systems over the past two decades. Well over 2 million pounds of detergents are used each day in the developed countries, around 90% of which are anionic synthetics. These compounds are long-chain, usually branched, hydrocarbons that may contain an aromatic ring and terminate in a negatively charged group. The compound below is illustrative:

$$CH_3-CH_2-CH_3-CH-CH_2-\overset{\overset{\textstyle CH_3}{|}}{CH}-CH_2-CH_2-\langle O\rangle\ \overset{\overset{\textstyle O}{\|}}{\underset{\underset{\textstyle O}{\|}}{S}}-O^-Na^+$$

$$\underset{\underset{\textstyle CH_3}{|}}{\overset{\overset{\textstyle |}{CH_2}}{}}$$

Alkyl-benzene sulfonate detergent

These compounds lower the surface tension of water and encourage water foaming. Most detergents also contain phosphorus (as a part of the "extra" ingredients), which permits dirt in suspension to be more easily washed away. Although the phosphorus may cause eutrophication problems at times, it is not normally of importance because sewage contains other eutrophic materials in abundance. The primary problems are associated with the difficulty of breaking down branched-chain detergents by microorganisms at a sufficiently rapid rate. In most sewage plants, about one-half of the detergents are released to streams before appreciable breakdown. This causes foaming, and as little as 1 ppm of detergent can significantly reduce aeration. Levels of detergents in waterways in the United States are frequently 5–10 ppm and Europe 3–5 ppm. The exclusion of aerobic organisms prevents biodegradation. Moreover, detergents have marked toxicity to a number of animals: 2–5 ppm have been shown to be toxic to water shrimp, water fleas, and pond weed, for example; fish are somewhat more resistant. Detergents of a more degradable nature were introduced several years ago as replacements but were not uniformly acceptable by housewives or the EPA. Although sufficient breakdown of branched-chain compounds can be effected by holding in sewage plants for extended periods, this adds consid-erably more to the cost of waste disposal, as would tertiary treatment.

1.3.3.b. Chemical Wastes

A large number of chemicals are possible candidates for release (accidentally or purposely) into the environment. Their importance as potential pollutants will depend upon their rate of release (related to production), lifetime in the environment, concentration in parts of the system (surface films, estuaries) or in organisms, and toxicity. In several subsequent chapters the potential effects of many chemical groups are discussed and a brief overview of example problems is presented to indicate the magnitude of the problem.

The U.S. production of 10 important chemicals is shown in Table 1.8. Although production would vary, a crude estimate suggests that U.S. production is approximately one-third of world production for these common chemicals.

The potential for initial water pollution by the chemicals depends upon such factors as direct or indirect release into water, solubility, vapor pressure, and use. The last item is of importance because a number of the chemicals listed in Table 1.8 are primarily used for synthesis of other chemicals, and these parent compounds are often so completely utilized that less than 1% is available for release into the environment. Following emission, chemicals may be chemically degraded in the environment or they may have volatility characteristics that cause their release from water, ultimately becoming atmospheric problems. The rates of degradation in a water and atmospheric medium may differ. The accumulation of materials in systems and organisms is primarily a function of water and lipid solubility, sedimentation, and binding to inorganic or organic substances. The toxicity of many industrial chemicals is partially known in humans largely because of potential exposure of the labor force, but the effects, especially chronic ones, are poorly known for the vast majority of organisms, both plant and animal, terrestrial and aquatic.

To illustrate one ramification of the problem, four low molecular weight HC will be briefly discussed. Pollution by other chemicals may have drastically different ramifications, as discussed for selected major pollutants in subsequent chapters.

The compounds selected for illustration (tetrachloroethylene, trichloroethane, dichloroethane, and dichloropropane) were chosen because a substantial amount of information is available concerning their properties. All of these compounds are fat soluble but have water solubilities ranging from 150 to 500 ppm. They have marked volatility and will readily partition from water into the atmosphere. Under nonphotochemical conditions they resist breakdown, but photochemical (primarily free radical) processes hasten degradation via formation of less toxic acid intermediates.

In humans they are moderately toxic; threshold limit values (TLV) range from 50 to 300 ppm for an 8-hr period. They act as narcotics, primarily by dissolving nerve lipids. These chlorohydrocarbons may be concentrated in the liver but are far less hazardous than other low molecular weight HC such as carbon tetrachloride.[1]

The primary uses of tetrachloroethylene and trichloroethane are as dry cleaning agents and degreasers. For this reason, these compounds are primarily discharged through drainage systems, although a large amount may volatilize before reaching a water medium. Dichloroethane and dichloropropane are used as chemical intermediates for a variety of chemical syntheses. Therefore, although their use is high, less than 2% of the amount used is released into the environment.

When introduced into water, the majority of each of these chemicals tends to vaporize; hence the problem is more atmospheric than terrestrial. Photochemical reactions appear to degrade these compounds rapidly; half-lives are usually measured in days and infrequently in weeks. Thus, their concentrations in ambient air are seldom at a measurable concentration (<1 ppb).

---

[1]Since the initial draft of this chapter was written, dichloroethane has been implicated as a carcinogen, which illustrates the need for an adequate appraisal of such important chemicals.

Table 1.8 Production of Some Low Molecular Weight Hydrocarbons and Aromatic Chemicals in the United States, 1971

Substance	Quantity (metric tons)
Hydrocarbons	
1,2-Dichloroethane	3423×10^3
Carbon tetrachloride	493×10^3
Chloroethylene	1963×10^3
Tetrachloroethylene	319×10^3
Ethyl chloride	281×10^3
Trichloroethylene	232×10^3
Methyl chloride	198×10^3
1,1,1-Trichloroethane	169×10^3
Aromatics	
Benzene	4×10^6
Toluene	2.8×10^6

Source: Data from U.S. Tariff Commission, 1973.

The portion of these chemicals remaining in water tends to be more resistant to degradation; half-lives of 6–12 months are frequently reported. For this reason, they may be detected in major water systems at concentrations ranging from 0.01 (more usually) to 0.2 ppm (occasionally).

The toxic concentration of these chemicals for a number of aquatic organisms has been determined to be approximately 2 ppm for the more susceptible species and several hundred ppm for the most resistant ones. The bioaccumulation ratios tend to be less than 100, a relatively low level. In addition, living organisms readily metabolize and/or eliminate these compounds when they are placed in uncontaminated water.

Thus, these specific examples (which may not necessarily be similar to other low molecular weight HC) do not present a current or immediately pending problem of water pollution, despite their appreciable production.

The other group of chemicals shown in Table 1.8, the aromatics (benzene and toluene), may present a different hazard. These compounds are fairly soluble, with water solubility over 500 ppm. Both are present as components of the light oil fraction of petroleum, and their main use is as chemical intermediates. The effects of these compounds on aquatic and terrestrial organisms are insufficiently known because they are often present in combination with other components of petroleum fractions. Although they do not appear to be highly hazardous compounds, they are considered to be more toxic than the lower molecular weight (LMW) compounds mentioned above. Their chronic toxicity to some aquatic organisms is on the order of 1–5 ppm. These compounds have a bioaccumulation factor about twice that of the LMW compounds, which is still fairly low. As with the LMW compounds, a substantial portion of these compounds is released into the air. Their photodegradation has not been fully elucidated, but they appear to be degraded much more slowly than the LMW compounds; the half-lives are usually measured in weeks or months. Concentrations in ambient air may be on the order of 10–30 ppm. Their fate in water is poorly understood, and although they may be degraded by a number of microorganisms, they appear to persist in small quantities for appreciable periods of time. Both compounds have been detected in municipal and river water throughout the United States and Europe, usually at concentrations of 0.2

ppb or less, but occasionally as high as 1 ppb. These compounds do not appear to be primary hazards themselves, but some of the chemicals made from these intermediates are important persistent and environmentally hazardous problems (polychlorinated biphenyls, hexachlorobenzene, chlorinated insecticides), as discussed in subsequent chapters.

Metallic wastes also present a potential environmental problem. The more toxic heavy metals are discussed in Chapter 3, but two metals appearing in water in large quantities warrant brief mention—copper (Cu) and iron (Fe). Both are important components of the earth's crust, have low water solubility, tend to chelate with organic and inorganic matter, and are of low toxicity. Their yearly effluence into water (ultimately ocean) has recently been estimated:

Iron		Copper	
Source	Yearly delivery to water (kg)	Source	Yearly delivery to water (kg)
Natural weathering	12×10^9	Copper industry	12×10^6
Iron and steel industry	3.7×10^9	Natural weathering	10×10^6
Coal combustion	2.9×10^9	Coal	4.3×10^6
Crushed stone	1.5×10^9		
Cement industry	0.4×10^9		

Natural weathering is a major factor for both metals, but far greater for iron. The average iron concentration in the Amazon River is 30 μg/liter and in the ocean 3 μg/liter. A number of industrial processes are also important contributors to water pollution; the combustion of coal is a common source of metal contamination. In water these compounds tend to absorb onto particles or to settle and become bottom sludge. They have bioconcentration factors approaching 1000, and an increase in these metals is beneficial to most organisms. On rare occasions at areas of very high concentration, however, these contaminants may constitute a toxicological problem. Although the concentrations are slowly increasing, their ultimate fate in the somewhat nonbiologically available bottom sludges has suggested no problem in several major studies. Obviously, any compound received by ocean waters in these high quantities will require careful, continuous monitoring.

Thus, the water pollution problems caused by the chemical industry may be largely the result of ignorance. Chemicals are not adequately identified as to quantity and quality. Furthermore, the chronic effects on both humans and the environment are largely unknown.

Suggested Reading

General

Walker, C. Environmental Pollution by Chemicals. London:Hutchinson Educators, 1971.

Air Pollution

National Air Quality and Emissions Trend Report, Vol. I. E.P.A.-450/1-76-002. Environmental Protection Agency. Research Triangle, N.C., 1976.

International Labor Organization (UN), Geneva. Encyclopedia of Occupational Health and Safety, Vols. 1 and 2. New York:McGraw-Hill, 1972.

Lee, D.H.K. (Ed.). Section 9: Reaction to Environmental Agents. In Handbook of Physiology. Baltimore:Waverly Press, 1977.

National Academy of Sciences. Halocarbons: Environmental Effects on Chlorofluromethane Release. Washington, D.C., 1977.

Stern, A.C. (Ed.). Air Pollution, Vols. 1–5. New York:Academic Press, 1962, 1968, 1976, 1977.

Water Pollution

Bartsch, A.F., Ingram, W.M. Stream life and the pollution environment. Public Works 90:104, 1959.

Klein, L. River Pollution, Vol. 1, Chemical Analysis, (1959). Vol. 2, Causes and Effects (1962); Vol. 3, Control (1966). London:Butterworth.

McCaull, J.M., Crossland, J. Water Pollution. New York: Harcourt Brace Jovanovich, 1974.

National Academy of Science. Assessing Potential Ocean Pollutants. Washington, D.C., 1975.

T. J. Sheets

2

Agricultural Pollutants

2.1. Introduction

Agriculture is a basic industry. People all around the world depend daily on this industry for sustenance, but in many underdeveloped countries productivity is too low to maintain adequate food supplies. As agriculture has evolved in the developed nations of Western Europe and North America, it has kept pace with the increase in population; in fact, the fruits of agricultural progress in these areas and a few others, such as Australia and New Zealand, help to maintain food supplies in areas where productivity is much lower.

The evolution of agriculture as an industry and a science has been highlighted by innovative developments of many types. Diverse and specialized machinery, knowledge of soils and climate, development and use of chemical fertilizers, discovery and use of pesticides, and development of productive strains of plants and animals are among the most noteworthy examples. As man has developed machinery and chemicals to sustain and to increase productivity, he has, at the same time, developed sources of environmental pollution that have had adverse effects on nontarget plants and animals, including humans. To arrive at the best decision for society as a whole on the question of the use of specific agricultural chemicals, the EPA must expand the concept of benefit–risk analysis and employ this procedure to draw its conclusions. In this chapter the pollutants that occur as a result of agricultural pursuits are examined. In-depth discussions of specific problems related to pesticides, fertilization, etc. are presented in Chapters 14, 22, and 23.

Agricultural activities are the source of several types of pollutants. Among these are pesticides (including herbicides, insecticides, fungicides, nematicides, growth regulators, defoliants, desiccants, rodenticides, and others), mineral nutrients, salts, radionuclides from fertilizers, wastes from polyethylene tarpaulin and petroleum mulches, and by-products of combustion of fossil fuels. Some of these are minor and of little toxicological significance; whereas others are of major importance.

2.2. Pesticides

Statistics on pesticide production in the United States reveal major changes in volume during the past 25 years (Figure 2.1). The production volume of insecticides (includes fumigants, rodenticides, and soil conditioners) and herbicides (includes growth regulators, defoliants, and desiccants) increased from the early years of use, peaked in 1975, and dropped in 1976. The decline in production in 1976 may indicate a leveling off of pesticide use or simply a temporary drop in supply and demand. Production of herbicides increased at a much faster rate in recent years than that of insecticides, and exceeded that for insecticides in 1975 and 1976. Production of herbicides in 1975, the peak year to date, amounted to 357×10^6 kg, exceeding production of insecticides by 58 million kilograms. The volume of fungicides produced peaked in 1960 and fluctuated between 1961 and 1976 at levels somewhat below peak production.

Figure 2.1 Production of pesticides in the United States, 1952–1976. Before 1960, fumigants were included with fungicides; and acyclic insecticides, rodenticides, and soil conditioners were included with herbicides. In 1960 and thereafter, soil fumigants, rodenticides, and soil conditioners were included with insecticides; and plant hormones were included with herbicides. (Data from Synthetic organic chemicals, U.S. Tariff Commission, 1952–1976.)

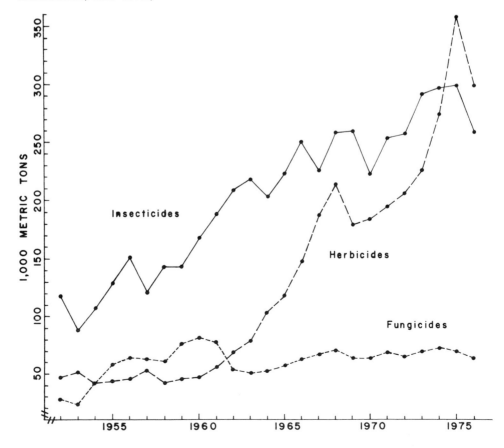

The volume of pesticide used differs from the production volume due to imports, exports, and carry-over. Estimates indicate that about 379×10^6 kg, exclusive of sulfur and petroleum, were used in 1971, 59% of which was used by farmers. The 41% nonagricultural use was attributed to industry, government, and homeowners.

Evaluation of the potential environmental hazards from pesticide use can be augmented by considering the areas treated with pesticides. Estimates in 1962 showed that approximately 5% of the total land area in the United States, excluding Alaska and Hawaii, was treated in an average year. Estimates for 1976 indicate that the total area treated may approach 10% of the land area in the 50 states.

Generally, herbicides are applied to many more hectares (ha) than are insecticides (Table 2.1). Fungicides, although very important to crop production, are used on a smaller number of hectares than insecticides. Insecticides and fungicides are often applied to the same fields several times during a single growing season; whereas herbicides are usually applied once, or at the most, twice. It is becoming common practice to mix herbicides or to use sequential treatments of different herbicides. Cotton is an example of an intensively treated crop. Before the development of pest management tactics, cotton usually received 10–20 applications of insecticides in a single growing season. The number of insecticide applications has been greatly reduced in recent years wherever the principles of pest management have been practiced.

Successful production of some crops requires frequent applications of insecticides and fungicides to maintain control of pests. Herbicides are applied to about 77×10^6 ha of croplands and ranges in the United States in a single year, whereas insecticides and related compounds are applied to about 27×10^6 ha. The intensity of usage of insecticides may account, at least in part, for the problems associated with insecticide use in former years.

There are several properties of pesticides that contribute to their behavior as pollutants in the environment. Among these are toxicity, stability, solubility, and adsorptivity. Different types of pesticide vary greatly in their toxicity to animals and plants. Herbicides, for example, are selected for their toxicity to plants; insecticides are selected for their effect on insects. Thus, as a general rule, insecticides tend to be more toxic to nontarget animals than herbicides, and herbicides tend to be more toxic to nontarget plants than insecticides. This rule, however, does not always hold true. For example, fungicides, which are selected

Table 2.1 Areas (10^6 ha) in the United States Treated with Pesticides in 1971 and 1976

Year	Total area in crops[a]	Area treated with			
		Herbicides	Insecticides	Fungicides	Other pesticides
1971	—	61.1	19.9	1.5	3.1
1976	335	76.6	26.8	2.3	3.7

Source: Data from Eichers, T.R., Andrilenas, P.A., Anderson, T.W. Farmer's use of pesticides in 1976. Agricultural Economic Report No. 418. Washington, D.C.: U.S. Department of Agriculture, 1978.

[a]Includes corn, cotton, wheat, sorghum, rice, oats, rye, barley, soybeans, tobacco, peanuts, alfalfa, other hay and forage, and pasture and rangeland.

for their activity against microscopic plants, are often toxic to warm-blooded animals. A grouping of pesticide toxicities is presented in Chapter 23 (Table 23.1).

Stability is an important characteristic related to the behavior of pesticides as pollutants. Pesticides that are rapidly degraded in the environment do not normally persist to cause significant problems, although exceptions to this generalization are known. The behavior of compounds such as DDT and other chlorinated hydrocarbons as pollutants can be attributed, at least in part, to their persistence in the environment. In contrast, biodegradable pesticides such as 2,4-dichlorophenoxyacetic acid (2,4-D) have not, as a general rule, caused problems even after widespread usage for many years.

Another characteristic of DDT that has contributed to its behavior as a pollutant is its solubility in lipids. This property, combined with its extreme stability, is a principal explanation for the accumulation of DDT and related compounds in the fat of many animals and for its movement from one trophic level to another in food chains. In contrast to the behavior of the lipid-soluble compounds, those that are soluble in water generally are excreted by animals and tend to remain in the aqueous phase of the environment as opposed to accumulating in animal fat. Hence, they are readily available to attack by microorganisms.

The adsorption or binding of a chemical to soil or other micellar components in the environment tends to reduce its availability to plants and animals, including microorganisms. Adsorption tends to reduce decomposition by microorganisms, and certain pesticides may be held, in large part, on soil colloids for extended periods. In this form they may be unavailable to plants and animals but may, at some future time, be released as changes in the environment occur that affect their adsorption. Much is known about the adsorption and desorption of many pesticide molecules, and predictions of their effects on plants and animals often can be made based on this knowledge.

There are now about 1850 basic chemicals that are active ingredients for about 33,600 pesticide products registered by the EPA. These products are manufactured and sold by about 4300 domestic and international companies. Of the total number of products, 49.3% are insecticides, 23.1% are diversified household and industrial pesticides, 15.4% are herbicides, 9.1% are fungicides, and 3.1% are rodenticides. Most of these chemicals cause no known problems and are not considered pollutants in nontarget areas of the environment. However, there have been several noteworthy exceptions, and these have tended to create an aura of fear and doubt over the many that are widely and safely used in agriculture and forestry and without which productivity could not be maintained at current levels.

Historically, the arsenical insecticides were the first chemicals used as pesticides that produced significant pollution problems. Distribution of the arsenicals was restricted almost entirely to the soil in which the treated crops were grown. In the early years of the 20th century, when lead and calcium arsenate were widely used in crops such as cotton and apples, it was a common practice for growers to use several applications of arsenates in a single year. With the use of arsenates (for example, in apple orchards) year after year, arsenic and, to a less extent, lead accumulated to relatively high levels in the soils. Levels of As_2O_3 as high as 580 ppm have been reported; the level of native arsenic usually ranges from about 4 to 15 ppm. The arsenic remained primarily in the surface layer of the soil and did not create a hazard to people eating apples because excessive residues did not appear in the fruit. Problems developed, however, when old orchards were renovated. The young trees planted in old orchard soils succumbed to the toxic effects of the arsenic. Similarly, in orchards that were cultivated after many years of use of the arsenicals, cover crops were injured by arsenic residues and could not be grown successfully. In cotton-growing areas arsenic accumulated in some soil to levels that were toxic to other crops; even today in some rice-growing areas of the Mississippi Valley, arsenic levels in soils from previous applications to cotton are such that the florets of rice plants abort, resulting in poor grain yields. A very small part of the arsenic presently causing rice florets to abort may be from the present-day use of organic arsenicals such as disodium methanearsonate (DSMA) and monosodium methanearsonate (MSMA) for weed control in cotton.

Some agricultural soils have been polluted with residues of other pesticides. The chlorinated hydrocarbons, DDT, tetrachlorodiphenylethane (TDE), aldrin, dieldrin, endrin, heptachlor, and others, are persistent. Residues remain in the soil for extended periods after application; when the amounts applied annually exceed the rates of degradation, residues accumulate. These chemicals are generally not very toxic to plants, and most common agricultural crops can be grown in such soil. Problems arise when such crop plants become contaminated from residues within the soil, either through absorption and translocation in plants or by splashing of contaminated soil onto plants. Most uses of the chlorinated hydrocarbons have been discontinued in response to concern about environmental pollution, effects on nontarget species, and suspected carcinogenicity in humans; although low levels can sometimes be detected with the ultrasensitive methods of analysis in use today, the residues are now of no known toxicological significance.

In the recent past, heavy metals were components of several pesticides; today, copper compounds are active ingredients in many important fungicides used to control leaf diseases of plants. Frequent use of pesticides containing heavy metals on the same fields, can cause the metals to accumulate in the same way as that described for lead and arsenic. Metals released into the soil as organometallic pesticides are degraded. These metals are not accumulating to levels that can cause major pollution problems under current agricultural practices; however, some minor, local problems have been observed.

The agricultural use of pesticides has led to pollution of water in many instances. Water has been contaminated with chlorinated hydrocarbons (e.g., DDT), leading to the uptake of such pesticides by aquatic organisms. The chlorinated hydrocarbons, because of their low solubility in water and adsorption to soil colloidal particles, are associated with sediment deposits in streams; organisms living or feeding in the sediment become exposed to residues of these pesticides where they occur. Surveys of major waterways during the years when these compounds were widely used showed their presence in most major rivers of the United States. The recent pollution of the James River with chlordecone (Kepone) cannot be attributed to agricultural use because the source of the contaminant was waste from a manufacturing plant.

Recent problems have been experienced with contaminants in pesticide formulations that have been used in animal shelters. Pentachlorophenol is a wood preservative widely used for many years to increase the life of wood in barns, animal pens, and fence posts. Formulations of this product, however, contained low concentrations of a highly toxic compound known as dioxin. Dioxins are extremely toxic to warm-blooded animals, the LD_{50} of many of them being less than 1 mg/kg; in contrast, the LD_{50} of pentachlorophenol is 50–150 mg/kg. Most pesticides used today have a much larger LD_{50} or are formulated or applied in such a way that exposure to humans and animals is minimal. In cases of dioxin poisoning in animal shelters, the animals apparently rubbed against walls and absorbed toxic amounts through their skin. Some dairy animals had to be killed to eliminate the potential source of dioxin in human food supplies.

Formulations of the herbicide, 2, 4, 5-trichlorophenoxyacetic acid (2, 4, 5-T) contain very low levels of 2, 3, 7, 8-tetrachlorodibenzo-p-dioxin. This impurity was present in greater concentrations (up to 40 ppm) in some formulations of 2, 4, 5-T applied to defoliate combat areas during the Vietnam war; reports on the effects of the dioxin on animals and people in that country have been contradictory. The concentration of dioxin is so low (less than 0.1 ppm) in the 2, 4, 5-T now marketed in the United States that there appears to be no substantial hazard to humans, domestic animals, or wildlife. In opposition to this view, held by many scientists, the EPA recently (March 1979) suspended several uses of 2, 4, 5-T, after purporting that a correlation had been found between the incidence of spontaneous abortion in women and the use of 2, 4, 5-T.

The air in the vicinity of spray operations often contains low levels of pesticides. Manufacturing and formulating plants are also potential sources of environmental pollution, but many safeguards in use today minimize the loss of pesticides to the surrounding area. In rare instances, where safeguards were not adequate, some damage to the immediate environment has occurred. The chlordecone (Kepone) incident in Hopewell, Virginia, is one example.

2.3. Nitrates and Phosphates in Fertilizers and Animal Wastes

Large quantities of mineral fertilizers are used annually in agricultural enterprises in the United States. The nutritional level of much of our soil has been depleted to the extent that production of crops is not economical without the use of copious amounts of mineral fertilizers. Without the use of fertilizer materials, the agricultural industry in the United States and other developed countries would not only be unable to contribute to the food supply of the underdeveloped nations, it would be incapable of producing sufficient food to feed indigenous populations. The benefits of such use are great; however, as with many other innovative developments in agriculture and in other industrial pursuits, undesirable side effects occur.

Nitrates and phosphates are the major mineral nutrients in fertilizers that have been implicated in water pollution problems. The consumption of nitrate and phosphate fertilizers has increased manyfold in the 20th century (Figure 2.2). In 1975, the total consumption of nitrogenous fertilizers, expressed as elemental nitrogen, was about 7.8×10^6 metric tons (t). Consumption of phosphorous amounted to about 4.1×10^6 t of available P_2O_5.

Another important source of nitrates in water is waste from farm animals. Animal feed lots have been recognized as major sources of nitrates found in water since the practice of confining animals in larger operating units has

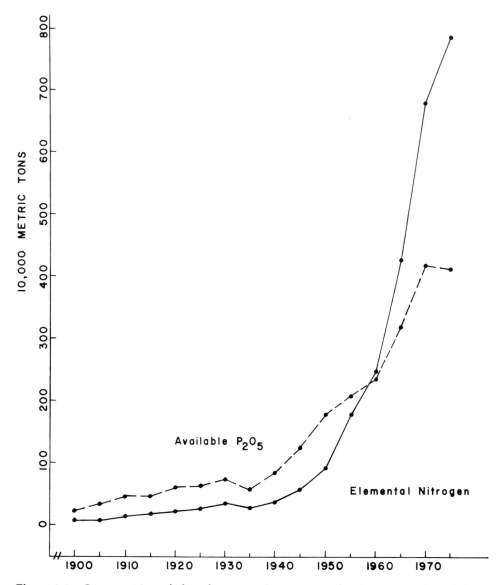

Figure 2.2 Consumption of phosphorous and nitrogen as fertilizer in the United States, 1900–1975. (Data from Consumption of Commercial Fertilizers, Primary Plant Nutrients, and Micronutrients. Bull. 472, Statistical Reporting Service, U.S. Department of Agriculture.)

increased. As this trend continues, the potential for ground and surface water contamination with nitrate will increase, especially in the vicinity of large feed lots. High levels of nitrate nitrogen (1100–2700 kg/ha) have been found in soil within 100 meters of old feed lots. Ground water in the same area contains relatively high levels of nitrates (up to about 70 ppm). Total animal wastes produced in the United States are estimated to equal the wastes from 2 billion people, or about 10 times the wastes produced by the human population.

Pollutants in water are often classified as point sources and nonpoint sources.

A point source is a concentrated source; in contrast, nonpoint sources are diffuse contributors of pollutants to water. Fertilizers are distributed at low levels over wide areas, and each field contributes a small amount to a drainage system. Animal feed lots are point sources of nitrates, whereas agricultural fields are nonpoint sources.

2.4. Heavy Metals from Fertilizers

Several heavy metals, including copper, manganese, and zinc, are essential for plant growth. They are required in very small amounts, and most soils contain sufficient concentrations to support normal plant growth. Deficiencies have, however, been encountered in some agricultural soils, usually in extremely sandy fields.

Such deficiencies occurred in Florida citrus orchards, and fertilizers containing copper were applied to bring production back to normal profitable levels. The fertilization practices were continued on a regular schedule. Without realizing it, however, after a few years the farmers were applying more copper than was needed to maintain production; in fact, levels accumulated to the point that symptoms of copper toxicity developed on the citrus trees.

The level of natural copper in soil usually ranges from around 3 to 15 kg/ha. During the time that overfertilization was occurring in Florida citrus orchards, the level of copper increased from the background or native level to 500–600 kg/ha in some soil. Analysis of the soil from such orchards revealed that the increase in the copper level was directly related to the application of fertilizers containing copper. Once the problem was recognized by agricultural scientists, fertilizer programs were altered to correct the problem created by overfertilization.

Superphosphate fertilizer contains cadmium at about the same levels present in the original rock. The concentration ranges up to about 50 ppm; thus, the amount of cadmium added to soil each year is very low. Cadmium is known to be absorbed by plant roots and transported to other plant parts. There appears to be no hazard to humans or animals from cadmium now present in agricultural soils. Some concern has been expressed that accumulation may occur with frequent application of phosphate fertilizer over many decades. A bone disease observed in some people of certain Oriental countries has been attributed to excessive cadmium in the diet. There is also potential for injury to soil microbes and higher plants.

In addition to copper and cadmium, heavy metals known to be present in fertilizers include chromium, manganese, nickel, and zinc; however, none of these is currently suspected to be a soil contaminant.

The toxic effects of heavy metals are covered in detail in Chapter 3.

2.5. Radionuclides in Phosphate Fertilizers

Several radionuclides are present naturally in soils, and mineral deposits that are sources of agricultural fertilizer similarly contain radioisotopes. The isotopes that are absorbed by plants are therefore toxicologically significant.

Potassium fertilizer is a source of the radionuclide, ^{40}K in agricultural soils. The most prevalent radioisotope of potassium, ^{40}K occurs naturally in soils at approximately 7000–8000 mCi/km^2. This isotope is absorbed readily by several forage plants. Therefore, ^{40}K is a source of radiation contamination in grazing animals.

Most superphosphate fertilizers in the United States have a ^{238}U content equivalent to that of the original rock. The estimated average U_3O_8 content of the rock is about 0.01% with a range of 0.001%–1.0%. Thus, the ^{238}U and any radioactive decay products from it are added to the agricultural soil in minute amounts with phosphate fertilizers.

Radioactive decay of ^{238}U yields, in succession, among other things, ^{226}Ra, and ^{210}Po. The properties of ^{226}Ra are similar to those of calcium and strontium; it is therefore absorbed and transported within plants. Based on the information available today, exposure to radionuclides from this source is minimal, and it is essentially at or slightly above background levels.

Long-term, heavy use of phosphate fertilizers, particularly those with relatively high levels of ^{238}U, may pose a problem in the future. If phosphate fertilizer containing 0.01% ^{238}U, the average for phosphate rock, is applied annually at a rate of 1000 kg/ha for 100 years, calculations show that about 10 kg ^{238}U would be deposited upon the treated hectare. Radioactive decay of the ^{238}U in this 100-year period still would produce about 4×10^{-6} kg ^{226}Ra/ha. This amounts to 394 mCi ^{226}Ra/km^2 over 100 years. The natural abundance of ^{226}Ra/km^2 of the earth's surface is equivalent to about the same amount; therefore, the 100-year application of phosphate fertilizer would approximately double the natural or background level of ^{226}Ra.

In evaluating the potential hazard of this deposition to humans, one must keep in mind that a high percentage of the natural ^{226}Ra present in the earth's surface is fixed in basic minerals and is therefore not readily available for uptake by plants. Moreover, a significant portion of the ^{226}Ra resulting from the application of ^{238}U in fertilizer would be fixed in an unavailable form within the soil minerals.

Refinement techniques are known by which ^{238}U can be removed from phosphate fertilizers. Such refining would increase the cost of the fertilizer, and at the present time, the hazard does not seem sufficient to justify the additional cost. If the risk becomes greater in the future, refinement techniques could be adopted to solve the problem.

2.6. Salts Associated with Irrigation

Salts associated with irrigation sometimes become serious problems, especially in heavily irrigated regions such as those in the southwestern United States. Salinity is or has been a problem in the interior valleys of California, the Great Basin, the Colorado and Rio Grande River drainage areas, parts of the Columbia River Basin, and localized areas in the Great Plains. Potential problems exist in coastal areas of humid regions if water with high salt content is used for irrigation.

Heavy irrigation has been used as a method to reclaim land containing excessive salt. The process involves leaching the salt out of the soil profile, or at least to depths below which roots of crop plants do not penetrate. However, with prolonged irrigation some of the salts that are leached out of the soils may return to the river and increase the salt content of the river water. Similarly, irrigation practices often return so-called tailings to rivers, and the tailings at the end of the irrigation runs frequently contain more salt than the water coming into the field. When the salt content of the river goes up, the next farmer downstream who pumps water out of the river for irrigation is forced to use water with a higher salt content than those upstream.

By using irrigation practices that alter the salt content of soil and river water, we are simply redistributing salt that nature provided in the first place. Thus, the problem is man made and results from our efforts to utilize lands in low rainfall areas for agriculture. Much is known about the problem. In recent years management practices have been developed that greatly reduce the return of salts to river waters. A need exists, however, for better control and management of the salt content of water in the western United States to minimize the problems associated with it.

Suggested Reading

Brady, N.C. Agriculture and the Quality of Our Environment. AAAS Publication 35. Washington, D.C.: American Academy for the Advancement of Science, 1967.

Brown, A.W.A. Ecology of Pesticides. New York: Wiley, 1978.

Eichers, T.R., Andrilenas, P.A., Anderson, T.W. Farmer's use of pesticides in 1976. Agricultural Economic Report No. 418 Washington, D.C.: U.S. Department of Agriculture, 1978.

Lewis, R.G., Lee, R.E., Jr. Air pollution from pesticides: Sources, occurrences, and dispersion. In Lee, R.E. (Ed.). Air Pollution from Pesticides and Agricultural Processes. Cleveland: CRC Press, 1976, pp. 5–50.

Richard B. Mailman

3

Heavy Metals

3.1. Introduction

Living organisms require not only preformed organic compounds such as carbohydrates, lipids, amino acids, and vitamins, but also quantities of certain elemental materials. These elements include sodium, potassium, and various anions as well as magnesium, manganese, copper, cobalt, molybdenum, zinc, calcium, selenium, and iron. One important role of the polyvalent elements is to perform structural or catalytic functions in vivo as a result of their ability to form coordinate covalent bonds. There are, however, other transition elements having similar chemical characteristics that may also interact with biological tissues, possibly resulting in toxic sequelae when present at sufficient concentrations. These elements are commonly called "heavy metals" because they are metals or metalloids that have higher atomic weights than do the essential elemental metals. Some heavy metals may actually have essential physiological roles, although at very low concentrations.

3.2. General Factors Affecting Heavy Metal Toxicity

3.2.1. Effective Concentration

There is ample evidence that either excesses or deficiencies of trace metals may result in severe physiological consequences. The dietary balance between several of these agents is also critical to proper functioning. Thus, since both concentration and balance are key considerations in evaluating essential nutrients, they are also significant factors to consider when assessing the impact of heavy metals on the environment and on members of the ecological community. For this reason, a major portion of this chapter is concerned with events that alter the effective concentrations of heavy metals in the environment through a variety of direct and indirect mechanisms.

3.2.1.a. Techniques for Measuring Heavy Metals

Heavy metals cause significant biological effects when present in relatively low concentrations. Normal gravimetric or colorimetric techniques are therefore virtually useless for quantitating these elements, and instead other methods that depend on the physical characteristics of these elements have been utilized. The most common is atomic absorption spectrophotometry, which depends on the ability of atoms both to absorb and to emit characteristic, narrow bands of visible and/or ultraviolet energy. In making atomic absorption measurements, the major difficulties are the elimination of background absorption and preparation of the sample in a usable form. Special procedures are necessary in order to prepare the metal in a form and concentration suitable for atomization.

Another method used to identify and to quantify heavy metals is mass spectroscopy. This technique provides information that allows determination not only of the metal of interest but also of the form of the molecule in which it occurs (unlike atomic absorption, which will only quantitate the metal). However, this technique is limited by several factors: there must be careful preparation to ensure a purified sample or mixture suitable for gas chromatography, and the equipment is expensive and more difficult to operate than atomic absorption spectrophotometers. Neutron activation analysis, which depends on the absorption of neutrons by the elements of interest, and the subsequent emission of appropriate energies of electromagnetic radiation, is also used to quantitate or localize particular elements. The major drawbacks of this method are the need for a neutron source, such as a nuclear reactor, and the inability to distinguish among different forms of the element by this technique.

The refinement of these and other analytical methodologies has created a problem in interpreting data about residues of heavy metals. If using current methods, significant residues of heavy metals are found, it may be difficult to assess whether these findings reflect changing concentrations due to environmental contamination and mobilization or merely reflect advances in analytical techniques. This dilemma was clearly illustrated during the past decade when there was increasing concern about the levels of mercury that were found in certain marine fish, as these findings suggested a serious environmental problem. However, examination of tissues from fish that had been caught and preserved decades earlier (before the major mobilization of mercury resulting from industrial causes) revealed significant mercury concentrations. Although this does not minimize the environmental importance of heavy metal contamination, nor justify the release of these materials into the environment, it does provide evidence that "zero tolerance" may be neither an achievable goal, nor one that is necessary to protect human health.

3.2.1.b. Persistence, Interconversion, and Effective Concentrations

One factor that results in increased scientific and public awareness about the effects of an environmental contaminant is its persistence. Since the heavy metals are elements they cannot be degraded once released. Despite this, heavy metals are not environmentally "constant" when released, but rather may be affected in several ways. First, biological and physical forces in the environment can change the chemical form of the heavy metal. Specific examples are discussed in detail in following sections, but generally, this means interconversion between organic and inorganic forms of the metal, or changes in the organic forms. These changes may produce marked differences in the reactivity of the heavy metal with biological and nonbiological sites in the environment, resulting in one of the major uncertainties for scientists and regulatory officials in assessing the environmental consequences of increases in the heavy metal burden.

The effects of heavy metals on the environment depend on the concentration of the heavy metal and its chemical form(s). For a single element, the concentration of direct importance may be that fraction of the total which is available to be mobilized by physical forces such as water, wind, or soil, and the partition of this form among the physical and biological constituents of the environment. Factors that alter the concentration of a single form of a heavy metal (such as chemical interconversions) may also contribute to significant changes in the concentration of the metal in a given locale. There are many documented examples of this. For instance, there is some unavoidable mobilization of heavy metals which results from leaching of ores by rain or running water, and, in fact, this leaching probably accounts for much of the background (nonindustrial) level of heavy metals. Some natural recycling occurs through animals and plants; e.g., pea plants and pine seedlings have been shown to release lead into the air as a function of metal concentrations at the roots.

A more important source of increased heavy metal concentrations is, however, the by-products of modern society. For example, it has been estimated that some 160 million pounds of mercury alone may have been released into the environment in the United States during the past 50 years through a variety of channels. Fossil fuel combustion, the dumping and burial of industrial wastes, and the use of leaded gasoline are but a few examples of ways in which modern society may alter the environment. Table 3.1 summarizes some of the various sources of heavy metals that increase the environmental levels or contamination. The fact that heavy metals have been present in some part of the environment for millennia is recognized; however, they were often concentrated in beds of ore, or immobilized in some other fashion, making them reasonably inert to environmental dispersal. The change in environmental concentration actually occurs by means of translocation, which permits interactions with biological components of the environment, including humans.

3.2.2. Assessment of Effects

Within the limitations of these and other analytical and theoretical considerations, scientists and politicians are faced with the problem of determining and quantitating (or approximating) the hazards associated with altered heavy metal levels in the environment. One important step is determining the most sensitive environmental target, since assessment of the critical level of a heavy metal is usually related to the most sensitive phase of life of the most sensitive organism. Therefore, if the germination of an important plant is inhibited at levels of a heavy metal far below those at which there is an effect on animal health, relatively low levels of environmental contamination with this element may be unacceptable. However, humans are generally regarded as the most sensitive as

Table 3.1   Some Aspects of the Environmental Toxicology of Heavy Metals

Metal	Sources and comments
Elements of primary concern	
Mercury	Chlorine-alkali manufacturing; released from coal combustion; accidental poisoning from organic mercurial fungicides
Lead	Battery manufacturing; chemical additive in gasoline and other products; formerly used in paints
Elements of possible concern	
Cadmium	Metallurgical industries, by-product of zinc production
Nickel	Metallurgical by-product; $Ni(CO)_4$ highly toxic; some nickel compounds may be carcinogenic
Gold, platinum, silver	High cost encourages conservation; chemical inertness of metal or salts decreases toxic effects
Bismuth	Relatively low toxicity because of poor absorption
Arsenic	Relatively high environmental levels exist naturally; many organic forms known
Selenium	Spares mercury toxicity and may spare carcinogenic effects of other heavy metals
Vanadium	Trace quantities in fly ash; not believed to be highly toxic
Chromium	Trace quantities in fly ash; metallurgical by-product; environmental hazards unknown
Thallium	Highly toxic; environmental impact may be influenced by biomethylation

well as the most important target species. The evaluation of the risk to humans exposed to heavy metal contamination involves numerous factors, including whether greatest risk occurs after exposures in utero, in the perinatal state, or in adults. Determination of the site(s) toxicity and evaluation of physiological changes that may not be manifested until the target organism receives either a physical or chemical challenge are also problems. Presently, these issues represent the most important aspects of research in environmental toxicology. The examination and development of new test procedures will have a marked impact on the regulation of the dispersal of these materials. Unfortunately, the question of risk assessment is not directly amenable to strictly scientific analyses. It is ultimately a public policy question incorporating not only scientific data and evaluations, but also cost–benefit relationships and the political strength or importance of affected parties.

3.3. Specific Heavy Metals

3.3.1. Mercury

Although elemental mercury is frequently found in ore deposits in concentrations as high as 500 ppb, it accounts for only 50–80 ppb of the earth's crust. Through natural cyclic processes, mercury deposits may be washed or leached into rivers, streams, or oceans. Available mercury concentration is affected by many factors, including geographical location (99% of the mercury ores that are mined are located in belts that correspond to the earth's mobile zones of dislocation); temperature (mercury is relatively volatile at ambient temperatures); and various soil conditions, including pH. Inorganic mercury is relatively insoluble and is not usually a threat to the human food chain. Nevertheless, concern about elevated mercury levels in tuna and swordfish led to banning of the latter as a food fish in the United States.

Most of the mercury produced is utilized by the chlorine–alkali industry to make chlorine and caustic soda, although other applications include battery cells, fluorescent bulbs, switches, paints, agricultural uses, dental preparations, slimicides for the pulp and paper industry, pharmaceuticals, and other consumer items. Man-made alterations in environmental levels of mercury are primarily a result of the dumping of used industrial materials containing high concentrations of mercury. In the past, dumping frequently occurred in various bodies of water and was tolerated because the inorganic forms of the metal did not cause noticeable environmental or health effects. However, when concerns about mercury concentrations were raised, some water supplies were found to have unacceptable levels. For example, waters near a battery plant in Michigan had concentrations of 1000 ppm; the permissable level for drinking water is only 5 ppb. A single incident nearly 20 years ago triggered increased awareness about the problem of mercury and other heavy metals. A major plastics plant in Japan located at the head of Minamata Bay increased the production of its main product, vinyl chloride, the production of which requires mercuric chloride as a catalyst. The mercuric chloride was dumped into the bay as a waste product with the plant's effluent. Unexpectedly, an outbreak of poisoning with central nervous system symptoms occurred, in which more than 100 people were disabled and dozens of others died as a result of mercury poisoning. This incident demonstrates the difficulty of predicting the consequences of environmental contamination.

Historically, toxicity resulting from exposure to inorganic mercury has been well documented. For several centuries miners of mercury in Europe had been reported to suffer ill effects from exposure, and the Mad Hatter in Lewis Carroll's *Alice in Wonderland*, exhibited symptoms typical of those seen in milliners who were exposed to inorganic mercury. However, despite these industrial exposures, mercury contamination of the environment was not considered a major risk since widespread distribution of mercury apparently did not occur. The poisonings at Minamata focused attention on previously unknown mechanisms that result in the mobilization of mercury in the environment. As shown in Figure 3.1, elemental or inorganic mercury dumped into bodies of water can be methylated by both enzymatic and non-enzymatic mechanisms, the latter presumably involving cobalamin coenzymes. This conversion of inorganic mercury to the methyl or dimethyl forms is favored by anaerobic environments, such as that at the bottom of Minamata Bay, where bacteria converted inorganic mercury to methylated forms. Methylated mercuries penetrate biological membranes much more readily than inorganic forms, accentuating the biomagnification of this element. Consumption of fish with excessive methyl mercury burdens introduced the mercury into the human gastrointestinal tract.

Methylated mercuries pass the gut, blood-brain, and placental barriers more easily than inorganic forms. After penetration into target tissues such as the brain, it is believed that demethylation occurs, permitting inorganic mercury to bind to sulfhydryl groups of sensitive enzymes. Because the effects of initial exposure to methyl mercury may cause symptoms that appear to be "psychological" in origin, diagnosis and cessation of exposure may be delayed. For example, the symptoms of inorganic mercury poisoning are commonly experi-

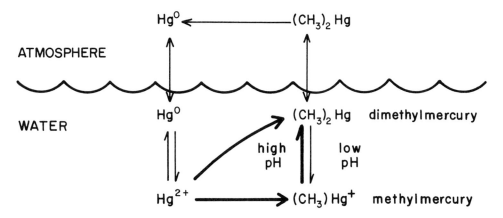

Figure 3.1 Environmental cycles of mercury. *Heavy arrows*: biomethylation processes.

enced in various combinations on a rather frequent basis. Some of the symptoms of this poisoning include appetite loss, headache, irritability, and fatigue, and later, visual impairment, deafness, impaired physical coordination and/or paralysis, vomiting, and fever. There are marked age differences in human sensitivity to methylmercury poisoning. In Minamata, symptom-free mothers gave birth to infants with permanent, cerebral palsy-like symptoms. Although differential sensitivity is not entirely understood, it is known that fetal red blood cells concentrate methylmercury 30% more than do adult red blood cells. When symptoms of mercury poisoning appear, it is usually impossible to prevent permanent damage. Chelation therapy prevents further damage but does not remove the mercury bound to sensitive sites, such as those in brain.

Awareness of the ability of methylmercuries to traverse biological membranes more easily has escalated concern about the dangers of increased environmental levels of mercury. Other major epidemics of mercury poisoning had occurred in Iraq (1956, 1961), Pakistan (1961), and Guatemala (1965), but the causes were primarily accidental exposure. Recent reports noting increases in the acidity of rainwater suggest that there may be concomitant increases in the natural leaching of ores that bear mercury or other heavy metals. The incidents cited above, as well as other accidental mercury poisonings (such as through consumption of grain treated with mercurial fungicides), have not answered any questions about the effects of mercury contamination on other aspects of the environment. It is possible that subtle but extremely important changes may occur in plants if environmental mercury levels are permitted to increase. Because many of the consequences of contamination are difficult to foresee, incidents such as the outbreak of Minamata disease should encourage a conservative viewpoint.

3.3.2. Lead

Lead is a naturally occurring constituent of plant and animal life and low background levels are present in the biosphere. The primary examples of lead poisoning have resulted from industrial uses of the metal, with toxicity noted among both workers and their children. Children are often exposed via dust transported from work when careful sanitation procedures are not followed.

Historically, several interesting lead poisoning epidemics have occurred. The roots of the decline and fall of the Roman empire now appear to be rather different than had been previously believed. Lead pipes were used to carry water to the homes of the wealthy, and undoubtedly large quantities of lead were ingested by those families. In addition, the use of certain lead-containing pottery glazes permitted lead to be leached into foods of moderate or high acidity, contributing to a chronic intake of lead. This probably caused low-grade neurological symptoms, although not death; this hypothesis is supported by the detection of high skeletal lead levels in the bones of individuals from the nobility of that time. In recent years, the use of inexpensive Mexican pottery as a container for acid foods has resulted in several instances of lead poisoning in the United States.

In animals, less than 10% of dietary lead is absorbed, and 90% of the retained lead resides in the skeleton. Lead is eliminated through perspiration, hair, urine, and the bile. Long-term exposure to low levels of lead may present an additional health hazard when physiological stresses that result in abnormally high calcium metabolism (e.g., prolonged high fever or corticosteroid therapy) cause the mobilization of bone lead and consequent increases in circulating lead levels. Blood, kidneys, and the nervous system are all sensitive to elevated levels of soluble lead. When lead exposure is known to have occurred, chelating agents such as ethylenediaminetetraacetic acid (EDTA), 2, 3-dimercaptopropanol, or D-penicillamine are somewhat useful in treatment.

An important aspect of lead toxicity is the exposure of children. One avenue for this has been the transmission of dust from industries such as battery manufacturing, via the worker's clothing, to the home. Another results from past use of paints containing high levels of lead. Pica (ingestion by children of foreign substances such as dirt or paint chips) may lead to the consumption of lead-contaminated materials such as peeling paint. Since a 1 cm² paint chip may contain as much as 50–100 mg lead, a few chips a day may cause the intake of unacceptable doses of lead. It has been estimated that 50,000 children have suffered from lead poisoning. Although physical recovery from this poisoning is possible, permanent damage and mental retardation may result because children are most commonly exposed during the first 5 years of life, which are critical for brain growth and development. Some evidence indicates that exposure to lead at levels below those causing any physical symptoms may result in permanent intellectual or behavioral deficits. Because lead appears to be the most common heavy metal contaminant, the resolution of this problem is important. The exposure of children accounts for the major known health hazard of lead, other than acute poisoning in industrial workers.

Many studies have recently been conducted on environmental release of tetraethyl lead used as an antiknock agent in gasoline. At the high operating temperatures of the internal combustion engines, the lead salts are volatized and expelled with the exhaust gases. Some evidence suggests that areas near roadways have a higher than average exposure to such salts. For example, studies in Maryland indicate that earthworms found near a major roadway have significantly higher lead accumulations than those found farther away (Table 3.2). The magnitude of this problem will decrease as the use of unleaded automotive fuels increases.

Other sources have contributed to increased lead burdens in the environment. The disposal of used lead sulfate automotive batteries provides a constant source

Table 3.2 Effects of Automotive Emissions on Localized[a] Environmental Lead Levels

Distance from roadway (ft)	Lead content in soil (ppm, dry weight basis)	Lead content in earthworms (ppm, dry weight basis)
10	700	300
20	200	170
40	90	100
80	60	50

Source: Data from Gish, C.D., Christensen, R.E. Reprinted with permission from Environ. Sci. Tech. 7:1058, 1973. Copyright by the American Chemical Society.

[a]Test conducted along Baltimore–Washington Expressway.

of the heavy metal from those batteries that are not recycled. In addition to appearing as a component of industrial effluents, lead arsenate has been used as an agricultural pesticide (with over 4 million pounds used in the United States as recently as 1971). The application of higher than recommended levels of this compound is believed to be responsible for the occurrence of the nearly sterile apple orchards in some areas of the Pacific northwest, although this agent has not been utilized in recent years.

3.3.3. Cadmium

Cadmium occurs at very low concentrations in the biosphere, and the incidence of cadmium toxicity, as well as increased environmental levels of the metal, is believed to result from industrial activities. Although cadmium may form covalent organic complexes under laboratory conditions, the toxic properties of the element are due solely to the biochemical actions of the divalent cadmium ion. Cadmium can enter the human body via water, food, or respiration of cadmium dust or fumes. The metal is rapidly absorbed in the form of soluble salts; the kidney and liver are the most sensitive tissues, however, pulmonary edema and permanent lung damage can also occur after exposure to high levels. Unlike many other heavy metals, there is no known role for cadmium in biological processes, and because cadmium has an extremely long biological half-life (10–30 years in humans), toxicity may be cumulative. However, toxicity resulting from exposure to low levels of cadmium may be minimized when the diet contains sufficient quantities of zinc; conversely, in zinc deficiency, there is a greater sensitivity to cadmium.

Cadmium has numerous industrial uses. It is used as an anticorrosive agent for steel, iron, copper, brass, and other alloys. Other products in which it is used include paint and other pigments, batteries, and plastics, in which it is used as a stabilizer. Despite this list of applications, total world production of cadmiun has recently been only 10,000–20,000 metric tons (t)/year. In nature, cadmium is generally found in association with zinc-containing ores and is therefore a by-product of production of that metal. Economically important deposits of cadmium usually occur in association with lead- and copper-bearing ores.

Because biomethylation or other activating processes for cadmium have not been described, at present the major hazards of cadmium would appear to be those resulting from exposure to dust or fumes containing high concentrations of the metal, or from foods contaminated through the use of cadmium-plated food preparation equipment, which was previously common. A condition known as Itai-Itai disease, found in Japanese living near the Jintsu River, was traced to cadmium toxicity. Cadmium has also been implicated as the cause of pulmonary cancers in cadmium smelters. At present, despite the toxicity of cadmium, it has not been demonstrated to be as great an environmental problem as lead or mercury, since both the level and scope of its contamination of the environment are smaller.

3.4. Other Heavy Metals

The emphasis in this chapter on mercury, lead, and cadmium is a result of the attention that these heavy metals have received in the past, but they are not the only causes for concern. Studies resulting from the outbreak of Minamata disease have investigated the possibilities that other metals may be biomethylated by mechanisms similar to that affecting mercury. Cadmium, as cited earlier, does not readily form these stable complexes, but it is known that tin, platinum, gold, paladium, tellurium, and thallium, as well as mercury and lead, may be methylated by reactions involving methylcobalamin. It has also been known for some time that arsenic and selenium are subject to these reactions. The chemical conditions necessary for these reactions are somewhat different for each of the metals, but fundamental studies of these problems may provide a prospective mechanism for avoiding major problems of environmental toxicity.

For example, tin is not usually considered to pose a major problem as a heavy metal contaminant. Recent studies have shown that under reducing conditions tin may be methylated, and these conditions are similar to those that occur at soil–water interfaces. This model was shown to have validity when a *Pseudomonas* bacteria that could methylate tin under conditions predicted by laboratory research was found in Chesapeake Bay. Alkyl tin compounds are known to be central nervous system poisons. These data suggest two areas of future concern: first, the increasing use of organotin compounds (e.g., as miticides) can result in a bioaccumulation of these agents that may become a local problem; and second, the dumping of waste containing large quantities of inorganic tin may result in the formation of methylated tins.

The biomethylation of heavy metals results in forms of the heavy metals that have increased toxicity and a greater chance of biomagnification. It also may mobilize relatively inert deposits of inorganic forms of the metals, thus increasing their "environmental levels" (i.e., their ability to interact with flora and fauna). Environmental toxicity resulting from heavy metals is therefore not one solely due to increased distribution of heavy metals throughout the environment by the activities of humans. It is also affected by alterations in the biological condition of bodies of water, the pH of rain, and other factors that may not as yet be known. Because these toxicants are elements and are not subject to chemical destruction, societal activities that cause translocation of significant quantities of heavy metals should be closely scrutinized.

3.5. Summary

Specific heavy metals and important mechanisms related to them, and perhaps other elements, have been emphasized in this chapter. Societal activities that mobilize these elements from their geological locations and changes in heavy metal speciation and resulting alterations in environmental distribution and availability are probably the factors of greatest environmental concern. The health implications of heavy metal exposure have been reviewed in numerous publications (several of which are listed under Suggested Reading), but there are also other important environmental considerations. For example, sewage sludge has been proposed as an excellent source of nutrient material for agricultural uses; this application would also provide a way to dispose of the large quantities of sludge accumulated by urban sewage processing plants. However, the microorganisms that digest the sludge bioaccumulate heavy metals that may be present in low concentrations in the sewage feedstock. Thus, when the sludge is harvested, it may contain much higher concentrations of heavy metals, which will become available for uptake by plants that grow on the fertilized fields. Since exposure to low levels of heavy metals may have important health effects, and since the form of the ingested heavy metals may not be known, the presence of these elements in the residual sludge restricts this usage.

Environmental toxicologists may make important contributions by being able to anticipate and evaluate these types of problems either before the initiation of new industrial activities or before health consequences are evident. The many putative or purported health sequelae of heavy metal exposure make it necessary to consider these potential hazards among the most important scientific and technological problems.

Suggested Reading

Friberg, L., Piscator, M., Nordberg, G. Cadmium in the Environment. Cleveland: Chemical Rubber Company Press, 1974.

Gilfillan, S. C. Lead poisoning and the fall of Rome. J. Occup. Med. 7: 53–60, 1965.

Goldwater, L. J. Mercury in the environment. Sci. Am. 224: 15–21, 1971.

Pharmacology and toxicology of heavy metals (several review articles). Pharmacol. Ther. 1: (Part A), 1976.

Weiss, B. The behavioral toxicology of metals. Fed. Proc. 37:22-28, 1978.

Wessel, M.A., Dominski, A. Our children's daily lead. Am. Sci. 65:294-298, 1977.

Wood, J.M., Cheh, A., Dizikes, L.J., et al. Mechanisms for the biomethylation of metals and metalloids. Fed. Proc. 37:16-21, 1978.

D. S. Grosch

4

Radiations and Radioisotopes

4.1. Introduction

This chapter is concerned with the ionizing types of radiation, relatively small amounts of which can cause damage to structure or disturbance of function in biological systems. Radioisotopes may be ingested, inhaled, or injected, similar to any other poisonous substance, but their toxicity is associated not with molecular structure but with emanations from unstable atomic nuclei. An additional feature of radioisotopes not characteristic of other toxicants is the ability of a source outside the organism, not even in contact with the surface, to supply penetrating radiations that cause damage inside the organism. With the best intentions, concerned mothers of New York City once marched on the mayor's office to demand action on the radiostrontium content of milk, but at the same time they insisted on diagnostic X-rays for their children from machines that were typically uncalibrated. They were associating the radiation threat only with something taken internally.

Most people limit their worries to the radiation damage in humans, although the entire ecological balance is at risk. Space limitations will not permit a comprehensive treatment of radioecology. Instead, selected examples are presented after the radiations and their origins are defined and explained. The nature of damage to higher plants and animals receives particular attention.

The quantity of radiation present in the environment is an important consideration. At one end of the scale is nuclear warfare, which could render our planet uninhabitable; at the other end of the scale is the irreducible minimum of natural background radiation. Biological damage from radiation can be detected after modest doses only slightly above background levels. The favored unit of measurement is the rad, defined as the unit of absorbed dose equal to 100 ergs/g tissue. The earliest unit of dosage used, the roentgen (R), is based on the quantity of ionization in air produced by X- or gamma rays; it serves as a measure of exposure dose. For soft tissue, a crude approximation is that a dose of approximately 1 rad will result from exposure to 1 R. The amount of energy is approximately that required to lift a common postage stamp 1.5 mm. However, only a couple hundred rads can kill a man, mouse, or pine tree. This destruction really requires only a minute amount of energy when one considers that 42×10^6 ergs are required to raise 1 g water 1°C. More important than the consideration of quantity, however, is where and how the energy from radiations is delivered. A derived unit, the rem, is defined as the absorbed dose that has the same biologic effect as 1 rad of "hard" X-rays.

Ionizing radiations are the dangerous penetrating types. By definition, an ionizing radiation dissipates its energy in passing through matter by ejecting electrons from atoms in its path. The "ionized" atoms are active and eager to participate in molecular changes. Even the genetically important DNA structures deep inside the cell nucleus can be reached directly by ionizing radiation. The delivery of energy in this manner is far more potent than the routes by which chemical agents function. Damage can result from direct ionization of a biologically important molecule, or indirectly from ionization of nearby molecules. Water is usually the most abundant compound present, and its radiolysis gives rise to peroxides responsible for much of the indirect action.

The main concern regarding many toxic agents is the damage that they can cause in the present generation, but an agent with mutagenic ability—and ionizing radiation is the prime example—can also influence the next generation or even all future generations (see Section 4.6).

The problem is to avoid adding too much radiation to the natural background, which comes from two sources: cosmic rays from outer space and radioactive rocks and soils in the earth's crust.

4.2. Atomic Considerations

4.2.1. Isotopes

A radioisotope, or more technically a radionuclide, is an element that has the property of emitting alpha, beta, or gamma rays from its unstable nucleus. In some instances, nuclear capture of an extranuclear electron from the K level results in a release of energy in the X-ray wavelength when an electron from a higher energy level fills the vacant position. Chemically, the behavior of a radionuclide is similar to that of the stable form of the element because the pattern of orbital electrons is the same. The vertical columns on the periodic table of the elements present their chemical similarities determined by the configuration of outer electrons. As such, the table is an important guide to where an isotope will go in an organism and how it will be used. In other words, congenic elements act similarly. For example, strontium and radium are utilized in the same way as calcium.

4.2.2. Rays

Both the particulate and nonparticulate transmission of energy is included under the loose designation "rays." X-rays and gamma rays have neither mass nor charge. Their wavelengths range downward from the ultraviolet band of the electromagnetic spectrum. Historically, X-rays were usually produced from man-made equipment, arising from outside the atomic nucleus. Gamma rays have even shorter wavelengths and emanate from unstable atomic nuclei. The shorter X-rays and gamma rays can penetrate completely through large organisms.

Particulate rays are emitted spontaneously by atomic nuclei of radioactive materials. An alpha ray is a stream of relatively heavy particles (two protons and two neutrons) with low penetration. The maximum penetration of 100 μm in tissue is the thickness of only about two cell layers. Beta rays are streams of electrons able to penetrate up to 8 cm, which is sufficient to traverse the width of most organs.

Neutrons are uncharged particles that are emitted by a few manufactured radionuclides. The most common source for biological experiments has been uranium fission in nuclear reactors. Since neutrons have no charge, no electromagnetic field is associated with their movement and they do not ionize atoms directly. On the other hand, they are not repelled by positively charged nuclei and impacts are common. Hydrogen nuclei are prevalent in living matter. When the hydrogen nucleus is struck by a fast neutron, energy is transferred so that it flys away from its orbital electrons. This moving, charged particle causes atomic ionization.

Irradiation may occur from either an external or internal source; that is, the rays may emanate from the surrounding environment or from material that has entered the organism. The latter ordinarily occurs via either the digestive tract or the respiratory tract. Under special circumstances, a wound or injection can be the route of entry.

4.3. Biologically Important Isotopes and Pathways

The naturally occurring nuclides are conveniently classified into those occurring singly and those that are components of one of three distinct chains of radioactive elements: (a) the uranium series that originates with ^{238}U, (b) the thorium series from ^{232}Th, and (c) the actinium series from ^{235}U.

The most important nuclide of those occurring singly is the beta emitter ^{40}K, which is found in rocks and soils; granite is especially rich in ^{40}K. Most of the potassium in animals is located in the muscles and reflects the occurrence of ^{40}K as about 0.01% of natural potassium. Uranium occurs in certain rocks and soils and is particularly high in the Florida phosphate deposits. Igneous rocks have the highest radium content. This product of the actinic series is an alpha emitter that gives rise to gamma-emitting descendents.

Uranium fission yields about 15 radioactive atoms of medium atomic weight grouped around strontium and cesium plus 6 rare earths. Those of greatest concern are shown on Table 4.1. Because there are no physiological transport mechanisms for the rare earths, they are not easily absorbed into plants and animals and serve primarily as a source of external radiation.

Strontium is an alkaline earth element concentrated in the bones of vertebrates and the calcareous shells of invertebrates; therefore, most of it is not passed along from meat eater to meat eater. The food chain from vegetables, grains, and dairy products is short. A discrimination factor [(^{90}Sr/Ca diet)/(^{90}Sr/Ca body)] of 2–4 functions in dairy cattle but not in plants. On the other hand, milling processes can reduce the dietary amount from grains. In this way, the refined diet of developed countries reduces the strontium uptake. The tissue of concern is the bone marrow cells, where beta rays damage the stem cells needed to give rise to the cells of peripheral circulation.

Table 4.1 Radionuclides of Particular Biological Concern

Nuclide	Half-life	Principle radiation[a]	Source
^{3}H	12.4 years	β	Induced in air
^{14}C	5730 years	β	Induced in air
^{32}P	14.3 days	β	Induced in soil
^{40}K	1.3×10^9 years	β, γ with EC	Soil, rock
^{55}Fe	2.7 years	EC	Induced in soil
^{65}Zn	245 days	β,γ	Induced in soil
^{90}Sr	28.9 years	β	Fission product
^{131}I	8.1 days	β,γ	Fission product
^{137}Cs	30.2 years	β, ^{137}Ba γ	Fission product
^{226}Ra	1622 years	α,γ	Soil, rock
^{232}Th	1.4×10^{10} years	α	Soil, rock
^{238}U	4.5×10^9 years	α	Soil, rock

[a]The radiations from various isotopes differ in energies (MeV) and ability to penetrate living tissues. Health physics texts should be consulted for additional information. EC indicates K-level orbital electron capture.

Cesium is a univalent cation like K^+ and Na^+, which, in large quantities, are essential constituents of cells and serum. Cesium has a wide distribution in body soft tissues and is passed through the food chain of meat eaters:

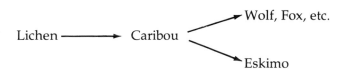

Radiocesium tends to be tightly bound to the soil and is not readily incorporated by way of plant roots, but it does enter the food chain by foliar absorption. Lichen, for example, have a particularly large surface area for absorption. Another route starts with aquatic plants. The gamma rays it gives rise to penetrate the entire organism.

Iodine-131 is of special concern in mammalian radiobiology because it concentrates in the thyroid gland, where it is incorporated into hormones. The children subjected to fallout on Rongelap Island showed thyroid insufficiency with attendant stunting of growth. This was alleviated by hormone supplementation.

Other radionuclides are induced in the soil by thermonuclear explosions. Phophorus-32 and isotopes of important trace elements such as magnesium, iron, cobalt, zinc, and a number of others arise in this fashion. The activation of elements can also occur in coolant water run through nuclear reactors. Accumulations of ^{65}Zn have been reported in prostate glands; one dietary source is shellfish. Oysters in Pacific Ocean beds were concentrating ^{65}Zn 300 miles downstream from Hanford, Washington, when the operation of the plant was at its peak. Iron isotopes are built into hemoglobin. Other trace minerals are important cofactors in enzyme action.

The isotopes considered above are of major concern to the health of the present generation. Apprehension about the radioactivity of some other elements is expressed because of their potential association with the DNA molecule. The problem is not merely that of mutations induced by the radiation, but also one of localized chemical toxicity when the decay product appears in place of the element originally incorporated.

4.4. Ecological Cycles

4.4.1. The Planet as a Closed System

Except for cosmic rays and cosmic debris, the planet earth is a closed system. Historically, the impression of the earth's vastness fostered a tradition of little concern about the release of wastes, but in recent years the failure of waste to dissipate has become an obvious problem. Some materials do not degrade fast enough, and the dilution of pollutants to trace levels is no guarantee of safety. Initially, from 1948 through the 1950s, radioactive fallout forced attention to the situation. In the 1960s DDT and other persistent pesticides attracted more attention. Both isotopes and pesticides are concentrated by living organisms. Indeed, any nuclide, radioactive or not, will be distributed according to its metabolic behavior in the various components of the food chain through which it passes. Each element has its particular molecular associations and its own path through the food chains. To demonstrate concentration factors,[1] Table 4.2 presents data pertaining to the radioactive food of a female muskrat captured because of an obvious cancerous growth on its leg. Although all other female muskrats in the region were pregnant, she was not. Conceivably, infecundity as well as the sarcoma could have been induced by radiation.

In 1954 two incidents associated with the Project Bravo bomb tests at Bikini triggered world-wide concern. Fallout spread by wind and water contaminated several thousand square miles, including the inhabited island of Rongelap and a Japanese fishing vessel, the Fukuryu Maru (Lucky Dragon). On a broader scale, radioisotopes passed through the tiny plants to small marine organisms to fish and into tuna, which is a staple of the Japanese diet. Subsequently, a large international research program was organized to investigate the movements of

Table 4.2 Radioactivity of Food Plants and Bone of a Muskrat with a Large Tumor on the Right Hindleg (from the X-10 Area of the Oak Ridge, Tennessee, Reservation)

Sample	Radioactivity (cpm/g wet weight)
Water	16,200
Wild lettuce heart	21,100
Curly dock stem	56,500
Curly dock heart	231,000
Muskrat femur	2,666,000

Source: Data from Krumholz, L.A., Rust, J.H. A.M.A. Arch. Pathol. 57:270–278, 1959. Copyright 1959, American Medical Association. Used with permission.

Note: Although radiostrontium accounted for only 40% of the water radioactivity, it amounted to about 68% of the vegetation's content.

---

[1]See Polikarpov, G.G. Radioecology of Aquatic Organisms. New York: Reinhold, 1966, for concentration factors of aquatic organisms.

the air-borne radioactive materials, their return to the surface, and their movements in ecological systems.

4.4.2. Consequences of Bomb Tests

A rise to the peak atmospheric burden occurred from 1948 to 1963, when an agreement to ban atmospheric testing of nuclear weapons was reached by the major nuclear powers. Since that time two nonsigners, France and China, have exploded a number of devices that have maintained a plateau of atmospheric isotopes.

The particles released from airbursts range from less than 1 μm in diameter to a few larger than 20 μm. Near-surface detonations suck up surface materials, which contribute particles of large size; 300-μm flakes fell on the Lucky Dragon. The heavier particles fall in the immediate vicinity of an explosion. In the Marshall Islands this amounted to about one-third of the total radioactive material. Some particles are injected into the trophosphere, but most of them are suspended in the stratosphere, where they remain for months or years. Our planetary closed system retains the material; it does not go away. Radionuclides with long half-lives fall while they are still radioactive. Due to meteorological factors, the midlatitudes of the Northern Hemisphere get most of the fallout, and much of it goes into the ocean, which comprises 61% of the earth's surface area.

In addition to bomb testing, mining, reactor operations, and fuel reprocessing add radioisotopes to our environment. These matters and the management of radioactive wastes are discussed in Chapter 6.

4.5. Damage to Exposed Organisms

4.5.1. Developmental Stages

A fundamental principle of radiation biology is the sensitivity of proliferating cells in contrast to the tolerance of differentiated nondividing cells. During division cell death is induced at much lower doses of radiation than those required to kill the same type of cell in interphase.

In early stages of development, when all the cells are dividing, the organism is more radiosensitive than at any other time in its life. Fish embryos that have an LD_{50} of only 50 R during cleavage may tolerate 800–900 R later in life. Frogs, birds, and mice show equally impressive differences between the dose lethal to early embryos and that which kills the mature individuals. Even more impressive than the vertebrate results is the increase in LD_{50} from 100 R for embryos to 100,000 R for adult homometabolous insects. The imago of a highly evolved insect is comprised of nerve, muscle, metabolic tissues, and integument—all mitotically inactive.

Irradiation during the middle stages of development causes morphological abnormalities at birth instead of prenatal mortality. In mice, small eyes, snout malformations, skeletal defects, and misshapen appendages are common. The failure to complete skull closure or abdominal closure results in protrusion of the brain or viscera, respectively. Anomalies such as these can result in neonatal death. The period for the production of a specific defect is short. For doses of 200 R, critical periods of only 1 day have been identified in the mouse 21-day gestation period. The sensitive period is correlated with cell proliferation and the first morphogenetic evidence of the structure's differentiation. An increased radiation dose increases the incidence of the malformation and often lengthens the period of sensitivity. In any event, a pattern of radiosensitive periods is demonstrable during the period of major organogenesis.

Similarities between the responses of mice and men have emerged. Every human anomaly suspected to be caused by radiation has been produced in mice, and confirmatory spot checks have been made in monkeys. Fortunately, medical radiology has not provided examples of gross human anomalies in recent decades.

Immediately before and after birth, radiation damage tends to be functional rather than structural. In particular, neurological and behavioral studies of mice and rats indicate induced damage to the nervous system not obvious on histological examination. In Japan, the Atom Bomb Casualty Commission examined over 200 children exposed in utero to the Hiroshima explosions. Six were retarded in intelligence and possessed heads smaller than normal in circumference. This incidence was significantly higher than that of the general population.

The terata of mammals are paralleled by appendage and body segment anomalies in invertebrates and malformations in plant seedlings. In insects the imaginal discs are mitotically active in late larvae and during the pupal stage. Plants have vulnerable growth centers known as meristems, which are the sites of cell proliferation.

In adolescent mammals, growth in bone length continues until the epiphyseal bone has joined the shaft bone. This occurs at about 20 years of age in humans. Before this time it is important to shield epiphyses during radiological exposures to avoid stunting of an appendage or digit.

4.5.2. Adult Structures

4.5.2.a. Plants

The best evidence of the significance of the chromosome aberrations in the structure and fate of the exposed generation of organisms was provided by plant investigations of the damage from gamma-ray sources erected in fields and forests. These experiments demonstrated that radiation causes a reduction in the number of cells per meristem, and this reduction varies directly with the number of cells showing chromosome damage. In turn, chromosomal size and DNA content proved to be important in determining the amount of energy absorbed at lethal and stunting doses.

Table 4.3 summarizes the results of exposure of the mixed vegetation of a Long Island forest to gamma rays for over a decade. The vulnerability of conifers and the radiotolerance of grasses is striking. In a crude sense, the exposure to radiation reversed the ecological succession, i.e., the progressive changes in vegetation and in animals which culminates in the ecological climax. However, the animals did not wait around to be killed. With the exception of insects that live inside dead trees, the animals left the denuded areas. Outbreaks of leaf-eating insects completed the demise of damaged oak trees. Large populations of bark insects and wood borers developed, partly due to an absence of predators but also in response to an abundance of food and habitat.

Table 4.3   Damage to the Major Types of Vegetation in a Long Island Forest Subjected to
Chronic Gamma Irradiation for Every Growing Season for 12 Years
Subsequent to the Installation of a Source Containing 9500 Ci^{137}Cs

Distance from source (m)	Dose (R/day)	Response
150	1	Pine needles shorter; tree diameter reduced
125	2	Scraggy stunted pines
115	5	No pines survive
85–80	10	No oaks survive
75	20	Blueberry bushes dying
20	160	Sedges and grass phasing out
0	3000	Some lichens and green algae in shadow of the pole

Source: Adapted from Woodwell, G.M. Radiation and the pattern of nature. Science, Vol. 156, pp. 461–470, Fig. 12,
28 April 1967.

Doses required for similar damage during one season of growth were about 10 times as high: 23 R/day was required to stunt pine trees and about 60 R/day for oaks; shrubs survived exposures of up to 150 R/day. However, a long-lived gamma source is not an exact simulation of exposure to fallout. Because many short-lived isotopes decay, the exposure rate in a fallout area diminishes rapidly. The sustained level of radiation in the gamma source experiments provides a maximum effect from a more serious chronic exposure.

In other gamma source experiments, abandoned fields provided examples of weeds that survived months of exposure to 100–300 R/day. Furthermore, grasslands are relatively tolerant of radiation and field crops only slightly more sensitive. Therefore, in most agricultural ecosystems the most sensitive organism is man. If the area is safe for man, pastures and crops will survive, although productivity will be reduced. It is most important, however, to realize that the ultimate source of all food and the maintenance of our atmosphere is the photosynthetic plants.

4.5.2.b. Vertebrates

Ever since 1906, when Bergonie and Tribondeau published their conclusion that the radiosensitivity of a tissue is directly proportional to the mitotic activity of its cells, a mass of presumptive evidence has accumulated that points to chromosome damage as a main cause of cell death. Recent advances in cultured cell techniques have made possible the determination of transmission and survival parameters for specific aberrations. The clear correlation between defective chromosomes and cell death can explain most of the in vivo tissue damage induced in irradiated vertebrates.

Much of the research effort has been concentrated on mammals, a type of organism that depends upon the integrity of a number of progenitive tissues for its healthy functioning. These tissues include blood-forming centers, skin, gastrointestinal tract linings, and vascular endothelium. Pathological tissue changes are related to the death of stem cells or their daughters, the maturation time of replacement cells, and the normal duration of mature cells. Table 4.4 summarizes some of these responses to radiation. For example, a blood deficiency in lymphocytes becomes evident within 2 days, while an obvious

Table 4.4 Consequences of Damage to Proliferating Cells on Which Adult Mammalian Tissues Depend for the Maintenance of Functional Capability

Cell type	Maturation time	Life span of mature cells	Consequences of irradiation
Skin	2 weeks	days[a]	Dermatitis, ulceration
Intestinal lining	2 days	2 days	Denudation, nausea, vomiting, diarrhea
Vascular epithelium	?	?	Leakage from blood vessels, fibrosis; or clot formation, blockage
Lymphocyte	4 days	1 day	Decreased immunity
Neutrophil	4 days	7 days	Reduced phagocytosis
Platelet	4 days	7 days	Blood clotting difficulty
Erythrocyte	4 days	100 days	Reduced O_2 transport
Eye lens	0.5–3 years	?	Cataract
Sperm	3–4 weeks	Days to weeks[a]	Temporary or permanent sterility

[a]Life span of mature cells depends upon activities of the individual.

reduction of the erythrocyte count is delayed until 2–3 weeks after a dose of 250 rads whole-body X-irradiation.

At Bikini, test animals that received high doses of over 1000 rads vomited and had diarrhea and soon became moribund. Those irradiated in the 100–500 rads range showed blood changes. The supply of new white and red cells was reduced by the gamma irradiation, and the situation was complicated by clotting failure and endothelial damage.

The classification of early deaths from acute doses of radiation is based upon a pattern of "leading organ" mortality. In order of increasing absorbed dose these are hematopoietic tissue (600–1000 rads), intestinal syndrome (1000–5000 rads), and central nervous system (> 5000 rads) modes of death. The central nervous system damage, characterized by tremor, convulsions, and lethargy, is associated with the prognosis of "hopeless." The individual who died shortly after the 1968 Yugoslavian critical assembly accident is believed to have experienced an exposure over 1000 rads. In addition to vomiting and diarrhea, he complained of headache and insomnia. Whole-body exposures such as this are expected only in warfare, nuclear energy accidents, or solar flare incidents during space flight. Some humans vomit after only 200 rads nonlethal whole-body exposures.

A more common industrial accident is partial body irradiation, especially of the hands and forearms. Skin reddening develops during the first day, but then a latent period of about 1 week intervenes before the onset of more serious symptoms. Progressive deterioration over 4 months after 6000 rads resulted in loss of a technician's hands in a much publicized 1967 case in western Pennsylvania.[2] During the early decades of this century many more examples resulted from the cumulative effect of repeated small exposure of the hands of radiologists and dentists. Although the skin reddening (erythema) from each exposure faded away, the consequences of the accumulated dose were more permanent. Ultimately, chronic dermatitis and fibrous scar tissue resulted, complicated by ulcerations and skin cancer in the most serious cases. Even a loss of fingers was not uncommon. Relatively few similar injuries have been traced to

[2]See Newsweek, March 18, 1968, pp. 94–95.

the handling of radioisotopes, except for a few instances of technicians handling radioactive material with a torn glove. Incidentally, both Pierre and Marie Curie received skin burns from the radium they were investigating.

In addition to skin damage, changes in the peripheral blood follow regional exposures to 100 rads or more. Shielding of the spleen or regions containing bone marrow is particularly effective in protecting experimental animals from the lethal consequences of ionizing radiations.

Modern diagnostic radiology does *not* feature doses at the levels considered above. For example, chest X-ray examinations can be obtained at only 10–20 mR (measured at skin) at Oak Ridge, Tennessee, while the average for the rest of the country is 45 mR.

4.5.3. Delayed Death

Chronic irradiation from external sources and internal isotopes may cause deleterious effects expressed late in the life of the organism. To some extent acute doses may also contribute to effects delayed as long as 30 months in mice and 30 years in man. These effects fall into three categories: cancer, degenerative disease, and shortened life span.

4.5.3.a. Cancer

The statistical evidence of the carcinogenic effects of radiation is convincing, although more than 20 years had to elapse before the extent of the problem became evident in the populations of Nagasaki and Hiroshima. Meanwhile, in many experiments, samples of laboratory mammals were exposed to a variety of external sources, including the bomb tests. Consistently dose-related shifts of the mortality curves resulted, in which the major cause of death was some type of cancer. Undecided issues are (a) the existence of a threshold dose and (b) the validity of extrapolating a line into the low dose and low dose rate ranges.

Historically, since medieval times, the miners of radioactive ores in Central Europe have suffered from *Bergkrankheit*, or mountain sickness, that had nothing to do with the altitude. Finally, in this century the fatal lung disease has been diagnosed as lung cancer. Now a clear association between the incidence of lung cancer in U.S. uranium miners and exposure to the radon chain of decay has been established. A source of environmental contamination of concern to the general public is the millions of tons of tailings from uranium processing. In the 1960s steps were taken to reduce the leachable radium content of the Animas River in southwestern Colorado. In Grand Junction, Colorado, mill tailings, until banned, were used in building construction. Within the metropolitan area of Salt Lake City, Utah, are 2×10^6 tons of fine granular wastes left from the operation of an abandoned uranium mill. Its decay products and radioactive dust are a threat to the health of thousands of people.

Since the late 1920s the accumulating number of cases of osteosarcomas, from the radium incorporated into the bodies of employees who painted luminous digits on clocks, has convinced forensic pathologists that burdens of radioactive bone-seeking elements have serious consequences. Added to this evidence over the decades has been the death toll of personnel of the Fondation Curie, where radioactive materials were used without precautions in the days of discovery of polonium and radium. Dr. R. Latarget, the recent director of the Fondation Curie, stated,

> We've paid our toll in this institute for that information. Madame Curie died from radiation-induced leukemia. Her daughter Irène died from radiation-induced leukemia. Her son-in-law Frédéric Joliot died of a polonium-induced cirrhosis of the liver. I came here in 1941 as a researcher, and of the total staff at that time only two still survive. Of those that died, only one died from something other than radiation.

In Hiroshima the latent period for leukemia was not as long as that for other types of cancer. Children less than 10 years old were most susceptible to its induction; by 1961 its incidence among them was three times as high as that of the general population in Japan. The increase was found not only for people present at the time of the detonation but also occurred in people entering the radioactive area within 3 days afterward. The incidence of other cancers rose over 25 years. In terms of cases per million people per year per rad the incidence now approaches 1.2 for thyroid, 2.1 for breast, and 2.0 for lung cancers.

4.5.3.b. *Other Causes of Death*

In the irradiated samples of mice that escape cancer, senescent changes such as nephrosclerosis and general organ fibroatrophy occur more frequently and earlier than usual. A decreased functional effectiveness of blood circulation due to induced arteriocapillary fibrosis has been advanced as an important consideration.

Finally, after individuals exhibiting cancers and degenerative changes have been subtracted from the sample, it appears that irradiation shortens the life span for the remainder. This has not been demonstrable in all experiments, possibly because the remainder is often a small sample. On the other hand, in adult insects evidence for radiation-induced shorter life spans is unequivocal; but in this form of life the circulatory system does not feature vessels and capillaries and somatic cancers are not a factor. The most important finding in insect experiments is that radiation-induced alteration in life span cannot be equated to postulated radiation-altered aging processes.

4.6. Damage to Future Generations

4.6.1. Dominant Lethality and Inactivated Gametes

By definition, a mutation is a heritable change. In the broad sense this definition includes microscopically visible chromosome aberrations induced in the sperm or eggs. Many of these are so drastic that they cause the death in early embryogenesis of the zygote they helped to form. In oviparous organisms this reveals itself as a decrease in the number of eggs that hatch. When the radiation exposure is high enough to yield a preponderance of dominant lethals in gametes, the ecological consequences are drastic. The successful eradication of the screwworm fly in the southeastern United States was accomplished by the release of an overwhelming number of irradiated males that carried a dominant lethal in every sperm.

In mammals the result is failure of implantation with an attendant decrease in size of the litter. For an experimental demonstration, the standard approach is to mate treated males with untreated females, and then the problem is to distinguish between failure in spermatogenesis and true dominant lethality. The simplest decisive experiments are performed in insects, in which both fertilized and unfertilized eggs will develop without difficulty. The proportion of offspring from unfertilized eggs increased after the males were exposed to doses of thousands of rads. These results, plus those from the irradiation of sperm samples used in artificial insemination of animals from oysters to domestic animals, show that mature spermatozoa are less sensitive to cell killing than cells in the immature stages of spermatogenesis.

4.6.2. Point Mutation

4.6.2.a. Methods of Detection

In the narrow sense, the term mutation refers to a change in the genetic code that can be localized to as small a change as a single nucleotide of the base sequence of a DNA molecule. These base sequences specify the amino acid arrangements of the structural and functional proteins, which in turn determine the activities of cells and the characteristics of the organism.

In diploid organisms the great majority of induced point mutations studied to date are recessive. This means that they are expressed only if both chromosomal homologs carry the mutation, or if there is no dominant gene to mask the recessive characteristic. Accordingly, inbreeding schemes are employed for their detection, or X-borne genes are assessed in the hemizygous sex. If a mutation at a particular locus is already available, a homozygous recessive parent can be used in a test cross to determine the mutation rate at the specific locus.

During recent years biochemical techniques have developed to a degree that enables the identification of altered proteins isolated from organisms. By this approach, which determines molecular phenotypes, many codominant examples have been identified. Codominance is a term used for two different alleles that are both expressed in heterozygote. The human hemoglobins and blood proteins are well-investigated examples which suggest that often the problem of detecting mutations can be solved by increasing the precision of the methods for recognizing the chemical products of gene action.

4.6.2.b. Results

Between 1928 and 1950, studies on *Drosophila* dominated the mutational literature. These studies featured Muller's experimental design, in which adult male flies were irradiated and mutations were induced in mature sperm. No threshold dose was demonstrable, and with increasing dose the mutation frequency increased linearly. Furthermore, neither low dose rates nor fractioned dose regimens altered the mutation yield from a particular total amount of radiation. These results are not presented merely for their historical interest. Many recent debates have been predicated on premises suggested by fly experiments that have limited quantitative application to mammals.

By 1950 a comprehensive program to determine mutation rates in mice at specific loci was under way. Within a few years W. L. Russell demonstrated that some of the conclusions from fly sperm irradiation experiments did not apply to irradiated gonial cells in male mice. Mice and other mammals carry a limited supply of sperm. Most of their offspring come from cells that were spermatogonia at the time of irradiation.

The dose–response curve Russell obtained was not linear (Figure 4.1). This may have been due to differential killing of different stages of the gonial series or it may have indicated the action of DNA repair processes. A dose-rate effect suggests some sort of amelioration of molecular damage. The number of mutations produced by a particular dose delivered at 90 rads/min is about twice that obtained from the same gamma-ray dose delivered at 0.8 rads/min. Reduction in dose rate to 0.009 R/min or to 0.001 rads/min did not further lower the incidence of mutations. An even greater dose-rate effect was found for the oocytes of female mice. At 0.009 R/min the frequency of mutation did not differ significantly from the spontaneous rate.

In experiments with both flies and mice, within each species, mutation rates at the various loci irradiated in sperm are about the same, but differences between loci are found when gonial cells are irradiated. Nearly a 30-fold difference occurred among seven loci tested at Oak Ridge, and the spectrum of mutation rates was different for irradiated oocytes. In England other loci were tested by other investigators who found other gonial mutation rates. Therefore, with the use of the specific locus approach the question arises as to whether the loci tested are representative of the entire genome.

Figure 4.1 Mean number of mutations per locus per gamete $\times 10^5$ plotted against radiation dose. *Solid line,* dose rate 80 R/min; *broken line,* dose rate 90 R/week. (Data from Russell, W.L. Nucleonics 23:53–56, Jan. 1965.)

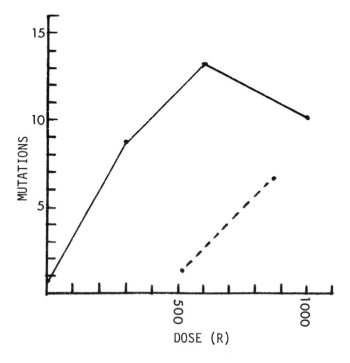

4.6.2.c. Consequences

Data are not available on induced mutation rates for humans. To date even the Nagasaki and Hiroshima surveys are negative, but presumably not enough time has elapsed for an increase to be demonstrable in an outbreeding population. However, population studies in lower organisms have caused concern among geneticists. The mutations present in a population are of three sources: (a) those from past generations, (b) those appearing "spontaneously" in the present generation, and (c) those induced in the present generation. Most new mutations are less desirable than those that have been selected over geological time periods for a particular habitat. In a large, freely interbreeding population, harmful recessives at all the various loci are expected to accumulate until each reaches an equilibrium frequency, the frequency at which mutant genes are eliminated as fast as they arise anew in each generation by mutation. The genes leave the population only by death or nonreproduction of individuals suffering from the disability caused by their presence in double dose. In other words, the frequency of the alleles of the various loci is established in a population by opposing tendencies: the alleles are formed by mutation and eliminated by selection.

For example, consider a single pair of alleles A and a among the 100 or more that make up a single chromosome. Figure 4.2 shows a conventional diagram of the offspring from matings of $Aa \times Aa$. If each kind of sperm has an equal opportunity to fertilize each kind of egg, offspring are expected in the classic genotypic ratio of 1/4:2/4:1/4. In contrast to this mendelian genetic scheme,

Figure 4.2 Contrast between the F_1 progeny from a mendelian monohybrid cross and the results of reproduction in a population containing genes of unequal frequency. The symbol p represents the frequency of gene A, and q the frequency of its allele a. (For application of similar diagrams to more complex situations, see Wallace and Dobzhansky. Radiation, Genes, and Man. New York: Holt, 1959.)

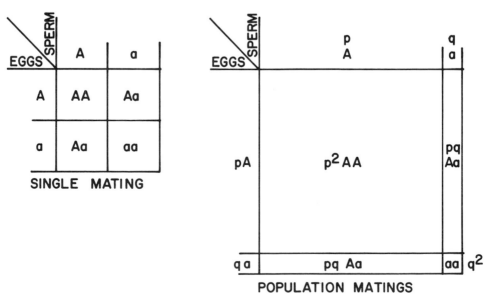

Figure 4.2 also shows that in the population genetics of deleterious mutants the gene frequencies of *A* and *a* are unequal. This distribution is represented by the displacement off center of the dividing lines in the square. *AA* individuals comprise most of the population, but some of each sex are *Aa*. The latter carry the *a* allele in the hidden heterozygous condition down through the generations. Time and time again *Aa* × *Aa* produces a defective heterozygote, *aa*.

The population's composition is represented by p² *AA*:2pq *Aa*:q² *aa*. When more *A* genes mutate to *a*, the frequency of q is increased and proportionately more *aa* offspring occur. Unfortunately, back mutation (*a* to *A*) is so rare in higher organisms that it can be disregarded. Indeed, gene damage from ionizing radiations is so severe that many geneticists completely discount reversion of this type of lesion. Once formed, the *a* gene is likely to persist for centuries except in the genotype selected against. In the simplest case, *aa* determines a fatal condition, and the population may already contain some *a* alleles from past generations. When a recently induced *a* mutation meets an *a* gene from past generations it is removed from the population by the death of the *aa* individual before reproduction occurs.

Somewhat different from the example just discussed is the case of an induced recessive mutation that has never before appeared spontaneously. This mutation must wait around for generations until it can meet up with itself before it can be expressed. As a recessive gene it can hide in the outbreeding human gene pool for many generations, slowly increasing in frequency if the lineage is a prolific one. Finally, after two or more centuries, distant relatives unaware of their consanguinity mate (*Dd* × *Dd*), and the trait expresses itself in one-fourth of their children (the *dd* genotype). With *d* concerned with defect or death, this serves to illustrate the concept that people exposed to environmental radiation today could be participating in a sort of time bomb experiment. The explosion would be one of mutant phenotypes in a population of a future age.

The *A* and *D* symbols used represent genes at only 2 of the 100,000 or more loci in a set of human chromosomes. Perhaps not every gene at each locus can be altered to a lethal condition, but nearly all of the 2000 mutations so far identified are deleterious to some degree. This large number of genetic disorders already present at various frequencies in the human gene pool may come as an unpleasant surprise to a layman, but physicians are currently taught to think of mutation as a specific etiological mechanism that results in a specific disease entity.

The situation is complicated not only on a numerical basis, but also genetically. Although gene-determined enzyme deficiencies tend to be recessive, mutational changes in nonenzymic proteins are usually inherited in a codominant fashion. This means that a new mutation may not be completely recessive, but function as a subvital gene in heterozygotes. Figure 4.2 shows the far larger fraction of the population that is *Aa* when only a few *aa* individuals appear. An incompletely recessive gene can debilitate a high number of descendents over many generations. Moreover, in experimental animals there are examples of heterozygous combinations that are lethal only in the presence of certain other genes, i.e., in a particular genetic background.

Furthermore, the accumulation in a population of mutations deleterious when homozygous does not necessarily result in a generation-by-generation decline in the viability of heterozygous individuals. In some irradiated fly populations deleterious genes are retained by virtue of their characteristics in heterozygous individuals. Consistent with this is Mukai's optimum heterozygosity theory. A related topic is the heterosis principle or hybrid vigor approach applied so successfully by corn breeders.

Many types of organisms have experienced irradiation from the radiation environments of bomb test sites and waste disposal areas, but only a few have been studied from the standpoint of genetics. The Marshall Island populations of *Drosophila ananassae* persisted despite the series of bomb tests. Over a period of 161 generations the Bikini population purged itself of an increase in detrimental mutations. This took only 4 years for the flies, but would require 3000–4000 years for an equivalent number of human generations. In order to return to a normal level of mutations carried in the population, *D. ananassae* paid a price in death and nonreproduction, but this is a price easily paid by an insect that produces 100 or more fertilized eggs per pair of parents. Similarly, the cotton rats of the White Oak Lake disposal area in Oak Ridge paid a price evident in decreased litter size. The size of the rat populations remained constant. However, humans are not as prolific as flies and rats.

Although some unique mutations were recovered, the mutational load of "visibles" from the Bikini test area was no greater than that from control areas. This was attributed to the masking effect of selection against lethals and sterility mutants induced on the same chromosomes with mutations that could alter the visible phenotype. Salivary gland chromosome analysis demonstrated that the number of previously undescribed rearrangements was low, but this evaluation was limited to the rearrangements that are successfully transmitted after irradiation. Numerous rearrangements were probably induced but subsequently eliminated by selection against them.

A unique opportunity for studying chromosomal damage was provided by the *Chironomus* larvae that live in the sediments of a creek that drains the White Oak Lake disposal area in Oak Ridge. For over 20 years the population has received at least 230 rads/year, about 1000 times background. Nevertheless, no quantitative difference in chromosomal morphology was demonstrable, but again qualitative differences appeared. Nine unique inversions appeared once, and one new inversion was found five times in the irradiated population.

4.7. Occupational Permissible Dose Versus General Population Exposure

There are several ways to assess the risks to humans from radiation and to regulate exposures.

4.7.1. Permissible Dose

The concept of permissible dose implies that there is an acceptable occupational risk to workers in atomic industries. This is expressed as that amount of radiation which, in the light of present knowledge, is not expected to cause appreciable injury to a person during his lifetime. It is based upon experimental and epidemiological evidence of tissue and organ damage. The maximum permissible dose (MPD) of radiation to the most critical organ is 5 rems multiplied by the number of years over age 18: MPD = 5 rems $(N - 18)$. A further qualification is that the dose in any 13 consecutive weeks shall not exceed 3 rems; 30 years of occupational exposure at this level would amount to 150 rems above background.

In 1972 a National Academy of Science Panel commissioned by the Federal Radiation Council (since absorbed by the EPA) decided that the maximum exposure for members of the general population should be only 170 mrems of man-made radiation each year exclusive of medical sources. This value can be compared with the estimates shown in Table 4.5.

The use of radiation in the practice of medicine is recognized as the largest component of radiation dose to the U.S. population. These applications include diagnostic radiology, radiation therapy, and the clinical use of radioisotopes. The main contributor (90%) is diagnostic X-irradiation. Indeed, the population of the United States receives more X-ray examinations than that of any other developed country. Fear of malpractice suits in the event of a missed diagnosis contributes to this widespread use.

In these matters, absolute safety does not exist. Standards are a compromise between calculated benefits and incalculable risks. Guidelines are set at levels at which biological damage is difficult to measure. The experts that set the standards accept the risk for the public.

4.7.2. Genetic Approaches

Two methods of quantifying doses of genetic import have been widely used. The first, known as the doubling dose, is the amount of radiation required to produce a mutation rate equal to that which occurs spontaneously. If mouse

Table 4.5   Average Annual U.S. Whole-Body Dose Rates for U.S. Population

Source	Whole-body exposure (mrems/year)
Natural radiation	
Cosmic radiation	44
Radionuclides in the body	18
External gamma radiation	40
Total	102
Man-made radiation	
Fallout	4
Occupational exposure	0.8
Nuclear power (1970)[a]	0.003
Total	4.803
Medical and dental	73

Source: NAC/NRC Report of the Advisory Committee on the Biological Effects of Ionizing Radiations, "BEIR Report," Washington, D.C., 1972.

Note: The Radiation Protection Guide (Federal Radiation Council) recommends a maximum exposure for the general population of 170 mrems/year (exclusive of medical radiation, for which no limit has been stated).

[a]By the year 2000, nuclear power is expected to account for 1 mrem/year. It is hoped that the contribution from fallout will decline.

mutation rates apply to man, the doubling dose is between 30 and 80 R, perhaps 40 R, for acute exposure. The doubling dose for chronic exposure may be a value four times larger. The total of 5 rems as a 30-year limit proposed in 1956 by the Federal Radiation Council approaches one-tenth of the presumptive doubling dose. However, even the mutation rate for mice has not been determined with absolute certainty, and any calculated values depend primarily upon assumptions favored by the calculator.

The genetically significant dose (GSD) is the gonadal dose that, if received by every member of the population, would be expected to provide the same total genetic effect on the population as the sum of the individual doses actually received. This is not a forecast of predictable adverse effects on any individual or unborn child. Instead, it is an index of the radiation received by the genetic pool. The gonad dose received by an individual is multiplied by the expected number of offspring and summed by age group for all irradiated members of the population:

$$\text{GSD} = \frac{\Sigma D_i \hat{N}_i P_i}{\Sigma N_i P_i}$$

where D_i is the average gonad dose to persons of age i, $\hat{N}_i$ is the number of persons who receive X-ray examinations, P_i is the expected number of children for a person of age i, and N_i is the number of persons in the population of age i.

Several different GSD evaluations have been published for identical years. Most accepted is the 1976 calculation for the year 1970: 20 ± 8 mrads at the 95% confidence level. Regardless of the GSD and the low probability of mutation, prudence demands continued effort to lower the amount of any potentially deleterious agent to which millions of people are exposed.

Suggested Reading

Arena, V. Ionizing Radiation and Life. St. Louis: Mosby, 1971.

Carrano, A.V. Chromosome aberrations and radiation-induced cell death. Mutat. Res. 17:341–353, 1973.

Casarett, A.P. Radiation Biology. Englewood Cliffs, N.J.: Prentice-Hall, 1968.

Eisenbud, M. Environmental Radioactivity, second edition. New York: Academic Press, 1973.

Environmental Protection Agency. Radiological Quality of the Environment, EPA-520/1-76-010. Washington, D.C., 1976.

Grosch, D.S., Hopwood, L.E. Biological Effects of Radiations. New York: Academic Press, 1979.

Hines, N.O. Proving Ground. Seattle: University of Washington Press, 1962.

Lapp, R.E. The Voyage of the Lucky Dragon. New York: Harper & Row, 1958.

Muller, H.J. Radiation damage to genetic material. Am. Sci., 38:33–59, 399–425, 1950.

Polikarpov, G.G. Radioecology of Aquatic Organisms. New York: Reinhold, 1966.

Searle, A.G. Mutation induction in mice. Adv. Radia. Biol. 4:131–209, 1974.

Zavidkovski, J. The Enterprise Wisconsin Radiation Forest, TID-26113-P2. Oak Ridge, Tenn.: ERDA Technical Information Center, 1977.

Frank E. Guthrie

5

The Energy Crisis

5.1. Introduction

The twin problems of a nearly geometrical decline in the availability of fossil fuels plus a generally increased demand for energy as nations strive for increased affluence have caused availability and use of energy as a world-wide resource to become a major, perhaps *the* major, constraint on economic growth of modern civilization. The 1973 and 1977 crises in the United States should have made this clear. It is a sad condemnation that man's superior intellect has been directed toward establishing a civilization dependent upon an energy source that seems likely to disappear within a few hundred years. A combination of increases in population and energy requirements leads experts to predict that the demand for fossil fuel will triple by the year 2000, if available. Modern civilization is dependent for its continued existence upon an as yet undiscovered technology! Whereas the wealthier countries may be able to afford high-priced energy while awaiting this development, the problem becomes extremely serious in the developing nations.

The dilemma began with the advent of the Industrial Revolution in the mid-19th century, when the world shifted from the use of renewable energy sources (wood and wastes) to fossil fuels. First coal, and then the more readily usable and versatile petroleum were sought as the necessary cheap energy sources to power the early stages of that revolution. Although over 200 million years of evolution were needed to produce fossil fuels, it may require but 300 years to deplete them.

The next 25 years will be extremely critical in meeting the energy problem. There is high hope, especially among environmentalists, that a major break-through in one or more alternative energy-producing methods will have occurred within that period. Therefore, a major goal will be to maintain the world economy during that time without serious disruption of standards of living or fragile governments. A significant part of this crucial effort will be conservation and reduced energy use. The big users of energy are the most unlikely to practice conservation, and the most wasteful country in the world, the United States, must assume a key role in such an undertaking if this period is to be successfully passed. As recent public opinion polls have shown that over 40% of the American public does not believe there is an energy problem, the magnitude of the task seems obvious. It is difficult to excite people about the energy situation as long as they can get all the gasoline and oil they want—at a price. Rocks and Runyon, in their book *The Energy Crisis* (Crown, 1972) have presented a perhaps too pessimistic overview for the average American: "we have no plans that close the energy gap in time to avert a complete shutdown of American industry and, with that, a collapse of our way of life and our national independence." The necessary education programs should not be aimed at the poorly educated, less affluent public who play but a minor role in energy use. Instead they must be directed to the educated, well-to-do public and its leaders. A decrease in energy growth is perhaps more controversial because world leadership is still wedded to the 18th century philosophy of problem solving. Intellectually, such leadership can only consider growth as the answer to economic problems.

The most frequently mentioned alternatives are nuclear and solar energy sources, and mankind is rapidly approaching the time when a choice must be made. Both have the desirable characteristic of being a "limitless" resource (at the highest promised level of technology). Although nuclear energy has some highly questionable environmental effects, most leaders are electing this source as the main solution to the shortage. On the other hand, much of the world, including many scientists, is opposed to that alternative and is convinced that the long-term answer must not include a source that has the drawbacks that nuclear power does and prefer solar sources.

5.2. Energy Consumption

Energy consumption is correlated with affluence. A comparison of energy consumption among five of the more "advanced" nations and three "emerging" ones is shown in Table 5.1. The United States, with 6% of the world's

Table 5.1 Comparison of Energy Consumption Among Nations

	Per capita daily energy consumption (kcal × 10³)	Percent of world energy consumption	Percent of world population
United States	224	35	6
East Germany	124	5	1.5
United Kingdom	109	6	1.5
USSR	90	16	7
Japan	64	3	3
Mexico	25	1	1
Brazil	11	1	3
India	4	2	15

Source: United Nations Demographic Yearbook, 1970.

population, consumes about 35% of the world's energy, whereas India, with 15% of the world's population, consumes but 2% of this resource. Even among relatively affluent countries there is a marked disparity in consumption: the United States uses approximately twice the energy used by European countries (per capita) and nearly four times that of Japan. A recent study that compared United States energy consumption with that of West Germany (two highly educated populations with similar per capita incomes and similar cultures) showed that the United States used approximately twice as much energy on a per capita basis.

Although this chapter is primarily devoted to an examination of the United States' energy problem, of direct interest to us is the growth of the world energy problem. It has been estimated from United Nations sources that during the period 1970–2000 the demand on energy will multiply the following number of times for the indicated geographical areas:

North America   2.5 times

Western Europe   3   times

Japan   3.5 times

USSR and Eastern Europe   3.5 times

Developing countries   · 8.5 times

Using these projections, one can construct a box illustration of these world demands:

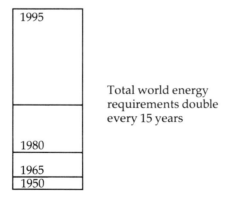

Even though the percentage increase in energy demand by the United States and other developed countries is projected to be slower, the total demand will be appreciably increased in these countries. The larger demand for increased energy will come from developing countries; although they will have a much lower per capita consumption, the overall increase is projected to be enormous, for these larger populations have had an extremely low per capita rate of energy consumption. Just where the necessary energy is to be derived from is a problem that as yet has defied solution.

5.2.1. Distribution of Energy

The distribution of energy sources is a function of availability of resources within a country and the ability to purchase fossil fuel. Hydropower is a major source of energy in the Scandinavian countries and New Zealand but is negligible in much of Western Europe. Organic matter is a major source of total energy in India (wood and animal wastes supply nearly one-half of all energy there). Fossil fuels are the main energy sources but are distributed unequally.

For purposes of illustration, the situation in the United States, a country with both resources and purchase capabilities, is selected, but the figures may even be drastically different from those in countries with similar affluence. If one breaks down energy use among the major U.S. consumers of energy (and products), the proportionate demands for 1990 are estimated at:

Nonenergy (synthetic chemical industry)	9%
Industry	32%
Transportation	22%
Residential and commercial	37%

Although there is some variation between estimates of energy consumption, use, and longevity, over the course of a decade, it really makes little difference which of the many informed estimates are chosen. Adjusting all energy to oil equivalents, the United States used nearly 30 million barrels per day in 1960 and is projected to use over 50×10^6 barrels per day by 1990, even though energy demand is predicted to decrease from a growth rate of approximately 4% (1960–1970) to slightly over 2.5% (1980–1990).

The projected demand represents a substantial reduction in the rate of energy growth in the United States as a result of anticipated conservation, but total energy requirements are nearly double those of 1960. The world-wide increase in energy demand is slightly higher than that of the United States on a per capita basis, but to keep pace with the population, this implies a tripling of the world-wide use of energy. Such an estimate would be drastically affected by an increase in affluence of any highly populous country. Even the optimistic estimates must project an inability of the world to realize supply at its projected rate of energy consumption.

Through the year 1960, the major sources of energy in the United States were hydroelectric power (5%), coal (22%), gas (29%), and petroleum (44%). Projected consumption in 1990 will include larger demands on the nuclear and coal industries while gas will rapidly decline in use; the approximate estimates are hydroelectric (plus geothermal and solar) 3%, nuclear 11%, coal 25%, gas 18%, and oil 43%.

5.2.2. Energy Constraint: Second Law of Thermodynamics

The Second Law of Thermodynamics governs efficiency on use of energy. Simplified, it states that energy proceeds to a maximum state of disorder, which means the inevitable degradation of energy from the usable to the nonusable. From a potential of 100% utilization, some energy is lost at each step of conversion. That is, at each transformation in dissipation of heat, only a portion of the energy released is utilizable. This principle is illustrated by the efficiency of machinery. On the average, most heat mechanical apparatuses are perhaps 40% efficient, this is, 60% of the energy is wasted. One example is a power generator (ignoring temperature loads and energy flexes):

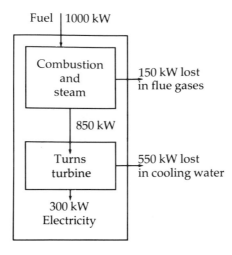

Obviously, more efficient machines may be designed, and notable advances in efficiency have occurred over the past 50 years. Important advances will continue to be made to some as yet undefined maximum. There also are possibilities of using the "waste" energy, and adequate consideration will undoubtedly be given in the energy-poor period we are approaching. Finally, the figure illustrates that much efficiency is lost in conversion, which might be circumvented: direct use of energy for heating (around 80% efficiency) would be far more economical than conversion to electrical energy for heating.

5.2.3. Sociological Considerations

The sociological aspects of the problem are often overlooked in the evaluation of energy in the United States. If one compares major energy utilization with financial resources some surprising trends are noticed (Table 5.2). The affluent use slightly more natural gas than the poor, about twice as much electricity, and

Table 5.2 Percentage of Family Income Spent on Energy as a Function of Income

Income level	Average income ($)	Energy per household (Btu × 10⁶)	Annual cost per household ($)	Percent income spent on energy
Poor	2,500			
Natural gas		118	147	5.9
Electricity		55	131	5.2
Gasoline		34	101	4.0
Total		207	379	15.2
Affluent	24,500			
Natural gas		174	200	0.8
Electricity		124	261	1.1
Gasoline		180	533	2.2
Total		478	994	4.1

Source: A TIME TO CHOOSE. Copyright 1974, The Ford Foundation. Reprinted with permission from Ballinger Publishing Company.

over five times as much petroleum. The poor, however, spend a sizable percentage of their income (over 10%) for heat and electricity—essential needs—whereas the affluent spend but a fraction of their income for these basic requirements.

5.3. Energy Supply

In the face of predictions that supplies of natural gas will essentially be exhausted by the year 2000, uranium (of acceptable price) by 2010, oil by 2050, and coal by 2400, it is apparent that drastic changes in world economy and standards of living will be inevitable within the next few decades unless some startling energy breakthrough is made. It is a habit of critics to attack any estimate vigorously. The important feature of the above estimates is not absolute accuracy, for they may well be in error by 10 or even 100 years. The indisputable fact is that resources are finite and world demand insatiable.

The estimated supplies of some major fuel sources in selected countries are listed in Table 5.3. The disproportionality of resources is highly apparent in Western Europe and Japan (which imports over 90% of its industrial energy) among the developed countries, and among the developing countries the energy supply and population boom seems designed to create major problems in India and Pakistan, most of South America, and Africa (except Nigeria) south of the Sahara Desert before the year 2000. Of course, the two latter land masses have not been adequately examined regarding energy resources. It is of special interest to note that communist countries and other nondemocratic governments are blessed with the bulk of the world's energy resources. The international political and economic characteristics of this imbalance seem obvious and, although beyond the scope of this chapter, must be recognized.

Table 5.3 Fossil Fuel Reserves (Oil Equivalents in Barrels $\times$ 10^9) of Selected Nations

Nation	Petroleum	Natural gas	Coal
Arab Persian Gulf nations	348	343	—
North African nations	84	141	—
Indonesia	10	6	—
Venezuela	14	35	—
Canada	10	55	600
USSR	75	635	4310
Republic of China	20	12	670
United States	37	271	1486
North Sea nations	8	163	250[a]
Australia and New Zealand	2	53	—
South America (excluding Venezuela)	16	33	—
Other Western European nations	4	16	127
Central America	—[b]	—[b]	—

Source: Lenihan, J., Fletcher, W.W. Energy Resources and the Environment. Glasgow: Blackie and Son Limited, 1976.

[a]Recent discovery of a very large coal resource in Kent, England, may be the largest coal deposit yet found in England.

[b]The most extravagent estimate of the recently discovered oil resources of Mexico is that they are comparable with those of Saudi Arabia.

5.3.1. Major Sources of Energy

The toxicological impact from the sources to be listed is discussed in greater detail in Chapter 1. The primary contributors to the toxicological problems will be merely listed under each energy source.

5.3.1.a. Nuclear Reactors

This source will be discussed in detail in Chapter 6. Most governmental and industrial leaders consider it as a major energy source for the immediate future. Although there are some extremely attractive features of nuclear energy, there are some disconcerting, long-term problems that require consideration, and an error in judgment at this time could result in unacceptable consequences. The factors involved in the use of nuclear energy that can be sources of health and environmental problems include the mining of uranium, delivery, thermal pollution, possible genetic and carcinogenic effects of radiation from accidents, and disposal.

5.3.1.b. Hydroelectric Power

This is a clean, source of renewable energy with respect to human health, but there are environmental effects as well as economic ones. Among the environmental effects of artifical reservoirs are the submergence of arable lands and homes, prevention of annual soil replenishment, dam failures, creation of new ecological situations for disease vectors, and loss of nutrient supply. The economic effect can be measured in terms of the cost of the land to be inundated, especially critical in areas where land is expensive. Although this is an important source of power in technologically advanced countries endowed with the expertise and capital to exploit such energy (such as Switzerland, Norway, and New Zealand), in other countries endowed with ample water natural resources the use of hydropower is complicated by the need for capital and the necessary engineering skills and equipment. The greatest potential for new sources of hydropower is in Africa, South America, and parts of Asia—areas not presently equipped to take advantage of this desirable resource. Greater use of small hydropower facilities has not received the attention in the United States that it has in Europe. There is a potential for additional hydropower in the United States equal to over 1×10^6 barrels of oil per day. The philosophy of the engineering profession and business world, which gives less consideration to the environment than to efficiency and monetary gain, is, in part, responsible for the neglect of this energy source. There is little interest in the minor contribution of small hydroelectric facilities. However, greater input into increased use of hydroelectric power in the United States (presently the equivalent of approximately 1.5×10^6 barrels of oil per day) could conceivably double present output.

5.3.1.c. Coal

Health and environmental problems associated with the use of coal include those related to mining (accidents and miners' health), the release of sulfur oxides (effects on health, pH changes, and building-defacing qualities) and substantial quantities of metals (including mercury, lead, arsenic, cadmium, and radionuclides), and the defacing of large areas by surface mining.

The United States government anticipates that coal will supply a sizable portion of industrial energy, especially electricity, for the next several hundred years, and some authorities believe that the increased release of SO_2 and heavy metals will create greater health and environmental problems than those envisioned from the proposed use of nuclear energy. Although the United States, Canada, the USSR, and China have sizable coal resources, Europe has essentially depleted its supply, and most other countries appear to lack appreciable reserves.

Coal is a unique resource in that it can be gasified and liquified—hence its versatility for several kinds of technology. However, conversion requires large quantities of heat, and many potentially toxic breakdown products may then be released into the air or waterways. Release of organic derivatives such as hexanes, thiophenes, pyrimidines, cresols, benzofurans, etc. would contribute significantly to an already critical environmental health problem.

The oil shale (and tar sand in Canada) from reserves in the Rocky Mountain states is a potential alternative source of fuel. Ten to 100 gal oil can be extracted per ton of shale, and the quantities are estimated to be sufficient to supply adequate oil for the United States for perhaps 100 years. This potential source has not been adequately evaluated, and there is much concern over possible land disfigurement on a gigantic scale from such a mining enterprise. Furthermore, vast quantities of water would probably be required, and, unless produced in situ, this amount of water would have to be transported to water-scarce regions.

5.3.1.d. *Petroleum and Natural Gas*

Environmental hazards associated with the use of these resources are those resulting from the gases formed during combustion (carbon monoxide, nitrogen oxides, hydrocarbons, and, indirectly, ozone and PAN), a number of toxic metals released in trace quantities (arsenic, cadmium, mercury, and selenium, and lead, both directly and from gasoline additives), the refining industry, the transport of oil (particularly ocean spills) and the purposeful release of oil by the shipping industries. Another problem which has been keenly felt in recent years, is that the supply of oil is subject to the vagaries of international politics (Table 5.3). This has been a particular problem for industrialized societies such as those in Japan, Europe, and the United States. The United States is in the unique position of being among the major producers of oil, but it uses such a tremendous amount that it must import large quantities. A country such as India is especially constrained by oil prices, for it has the capacity to develop but not the necessary purchasing power to obtain the energy sources to do so.

One aspect of the petroleum shortage that is often overlooked is the reliance of the chemical industry on this source of raw material. Although less than 10% of total petroleum is utilized for raw materials, the chemical industry is presently dependent upon this relatively cheap resource.

Some authorities have expressed the viewpoint that a rapid decrease in the use of oil for transportation and other less critical enterprises is clearly mandated; steps have already been taken to conserve fuel by requiring more efficient (and smaller) automobiles. However, the world-wide increased demand cannot be expected to be supplied very far into the next century, even though many optimists feel that untapped sources will continue to circumvent the problem well beyond the next century.

The environmental, problems created by the use of natural gas are of relatively minor consequence; natural gas, however, appears to be in the unenviable position of being the first fossil fuel source to become exhausted—most will be gone by the year 2000.

5.3.2. Minor and Alternative Sources of Energy
5.3.2.a. Organic Matter

The environmental and health hazards of burning organic matter are similar to those of burning coal: both gases and metals are released (in somewhat reduced concentrations). The use of organic matter as a source of energy may not require burning, and in these cases (microbial decomposition) the waste products problem would be largely that of organic wastes in water, i.e., high BOD levels. Organic material can be converted to usable energy by combustion, anaerobic digestion, hydrolysis, and pyrolysis.

In recent years, wood has been used as a major fuel in only the more primitive, low-energy-consuming regions, with the possible exception of India. In these regions nearly 40% of the energy is derived from wood and an additional 20% from animal wastes. This practice has resulted in deforestation in large land masses of Asia and Africa.

In peat-rich regions the burning of this organic matter is another major source of energy. Ireland draws upon peat for nearly 10% of its electrical power and the USSR uses significant quantities of peat. Sizable peat reserves are also found in Canada and the United States.

As energy conservation becomes more prevalent, the use of organic wastes directly for heat production and for the production of industrial alcohols may become more important. Much of this energy is so dispersed that it may not be practical to collect and transport it to a usable facility. A number of cities (St. Louis, Missouri, for example) are already substantially increasing their energy supplies by recovering the energy from garbage. On the average, developed countries discard about 60% of usable energy (e.g., paper, cardboard, and foodstuffs) in normal activities. Animal wastes in large cattle feed lots are a substantial potential source of energy as well as a disposal problem (eutrophication). It has been estimated that the combined urban (15%) and argicultural (85%) organic wastes of the United States could furnish 30×10^{12} ft^3 methane annually, an amount in excess of the current consumption of natural gas.

In our highly trained, engineering-oriented society, it is a paradox that instead of utilizing wastes we have turned them into pollution problems (including thermal pollution). Alternatively, crops could be grown specifically to be used by microorganisms to produce ethanol or methane; the potential of this energy source seems substantial. Brazil's goal is to meet 20% of its transportation needs with ethanol produced from organic matter. Following microbial conversion to ethanol, the remaining wastes can be enriched with methane-producing microorganisms and the final waste product (which has retained initial amounts of nitrogen and phosphorus) can be used for fertilizer.

5.3.2.b. Geothermal Power

A recent in-depth study of the pollution problems resulting from the operation of a geothermal power plant in New Zealand found that small amounts of 25 chemicals (including arsenic, mercury, and H_2S) are discharged in air and water in addition to a substantial thermal return. Minor ecological effects were noted. Some geothermal sources are more pollution free, depending on the outflow of the steam.

World-wide geothermal energy is estimated to be about 1000 MW, the capacity of one small nuclear plant. In those areas where it abounds, it is a technologically feasible, relatively inexpensive source of energy that is particularly amenable to the construction of small plants, but it is not viewed as a long-term solution to the energy problem, even in those areas. Major reserves are found in the United States, New Zealand, Iceland, Japan, Chile, and other parts of Latin America, and the optimistic estimates are that they could contribute no more than 1% of world energy needs. If geothermal hot water and heat from hot rocks were included in this estimate, the amount of energy would be doubled.

5.3.2.c. Wind

Wind is a clean source of energy, and predictions have not suggested adverse environmental effects, even where large sources are tapped. The effects of this technology would not be aesthetically pleasing, and there have been few studies of the possible adverse effects of diverting such an energy source. A main drawback is that output varies as the cube of the wind velocity; thus, a drop in wind velocity could make a power unit worthless.

This inexhaustible source of energy (actually derived from solar energy) is one of the most controversial among energy experts. The power potential of the winds over the continental United States and its seashores exceeds by 10-fold or more the electrical energy needs for the immediate future, and winds are reasonably repeatable and predictable in some regions. Nonetheless, wind power is essentially dismissed as a potentially important contribution by most authorities; however, a minority suggests it could be used for the generation of at least 20% of the electrical power in the United States by the year 2000. Denmark has built facilities of 100 kW capacity, and substantial advances have been made since then for lightweight aeroturbines. Enthusiasts have recommended mass land use of wind mills, as well as the use of rafts in the ocean for the turbines that would produce electricity to convert seawater into hydrogen (electrolysis) to be piped to the mainland. This source of energy is amenable for use by small power facilities (100–500 kW), where wind use is feasible, and would require a relatively low input of capital and technology.

5.3.2.d. Ocean Sources

Sources of energy from the ocean are derived from the gravitational pull of the earth and sun, solar energy, or salinity differences in bodies of water. All are purported to be clean, inexhaustible energy sources, but large-scale use has received limited environmental study.

Thermal and salinity gradients. These are two major energy sources, but the use of salinity gradients has thus far received little attention. In areas with a substantial temperature differential between surface and ocean depths (at least 30°F), a technologically feasible solution to energy problems has been investigated, and supply has been estimated at up to 10% of world requirements. As the result of two early projects that had partial success, the United States is contemplating operation of a 25-MW unit utilizing huge floating units, a large portion of which is underwater, by the early 1980s. Warm water will cause vaporization of a low boiling point liquid, which will drive a turbine engine. The vapor will subsequently be cooled by cold water brought from the ocean depths. Tremendous quantities of water will be required, and the electricity generated might be used directly or for electrolysis with hydrogen as the ultimate source of energy.

Tides. This has been a somewhat misunderstood potential source of energy. The requirements of an adequate head of water for generation during incoming tide and adequate storage of water to permit generation during outgoing tide can be fulfilled in only a few areas in the world. The more optimistic estimates suggest a contribution of no more than 1% of world energy needs. The most successful operation is a 240-MW unit in France where there is a tide rise of 27 ft and a natural reservoir extending many miles.

Waves. This constant source of energy is attractive from the standpoint of the staggering amount of energy released. However, utilization appears to be confined to regions where generating equipment can be protected, and the potential world supply is estimated to be approximately that of potential tide energy. The United Kingdom and Japan have made recent contributions in this area, and experiments in these countries are directed toward the use of gigantic rafts in partially protected inlets. In this system, as thousands of units bob up and down in the waves, half cylinders are rotated to provide mechanical energy for a turbine.

5.3.2.e. Solar Energy

This tremendous source of clean, renewable energy is gaining more popularity among scientists and world leadership because it offers much greater versatility, as well as safety, than any other alternative energy source. Furthermore, when compared with fossil and nuclear energy, it has the advantage of not adding to the thermal pollution problem, for solar energy enters the total heat balance whether converted to other forms or not. It has the additional advantage of being adaptable to very small and very large units, and thus can be used in a variety of situations. In Central Africa, which lacks technology, capital, and resources for either fossil or nuclear fuels, solar energy has already been utilized with considerable promise.

If but a tiny fraction of the 47% of solar energy absorbed within the earth's atmosphere could be collected, the demand for energy could easily be met. Predictions at present estimate that the contribution from solar energy will be 5–10% of the world energy supply by the year 2000. A recent joint NSF–NASA energy panel was even more optimistic, predicting that by 2020 the sun could provide 20% of the nation's heating and cooling needs, 30% of its gaseous fuel, 10% of its liquid fuel, and 20% of its electricity.

The major difficulty in efficiently harnessing solar energy is that it is an inconsistent and diffuse source. Thus, it must be concentrated and collected, and some mechanism for storage is required.

Although there are many variations, solar energy collection may be visualized simply in two ways:

1. *Absorption of heat that is transferred to other substrates:* This may be accomplished by a variety of means, from sophisticated mirror-focusing devices that can attain temperatures of approximately 1500°F, to simple blackened sheets of metal in glass-covered boxes through which water is circulated. In any case, the heat is collected by a medium that eventually is able to translate it into usable energy for the production of heat, electricity, or perhaps a transportable medium (Figure 5.1A).

2. *Direct conversion of solar energy:* As a result of the NASA program, silica in cadmium solar cells has been utilized to convert solar energy photovoltaically into electricity. This is a necessary system in most spacecraft, but technology must increase efficiency by a factor of 100 to compete with present economical sources of electricity. In contrast to the thermodynamic considerations of concern with the use of other fuels, with photovoltaic conversion there are no moving parts, no circulating fluid, and no consumption of materials (Figure 5.1B).

The use of solar energy for heating homes and domestic and commercial water heating is already economically competitive in many situations and may become a major industry in the United States in the immediate future. Its use is not restricted to warmer climates; for example, a public building has been erected in Boston that obtains over 50% of its energy from the sun. The use of solar energy for heating water and homes is not an uncommon practice in Japan. Because nearly 20% of total energy use in the United States is for heating, and solar heat techology has reached the point of being able to meet this need, a decided reduction in the consumption of fossil fuels could result from the use of solar forms of energy in the not too distant future.

France recently completed a 64-kW solar generating plant, and a 10-MW plant is destined for completion in Barstow, California, by 1981. Saudi Arabia has signed a contract with a French company to build a 25-MW solar generating unit in that oil-rich region. In order to circumvent the day–night cycle, one study suggests solar collectors in space, which would collect 10 times the solar energy they would on the earth's surface and beam the electricity to earth.

Many in the scientific and engineering communities are convinced that the solution to the energy problem lies in the use of hydrogen. They point out that both solar and nuclear sources (located at considerable distances from populated areas) could be used to convert water hydrolytically to hydrogen. This rather versatile and clean-burning gas could be used as the main source of energy, and its ease of transport, storage, etc. is equal to that of fossil fuels.

5.4. Conservation of Energy

The energy growth in the United States during the period 1950–1979 has varied from 4 to 8%/year. Electricity has been the fastest growing segment, at 7%/year. Assuming that petroleum reserves will decline dramatically in the immediate

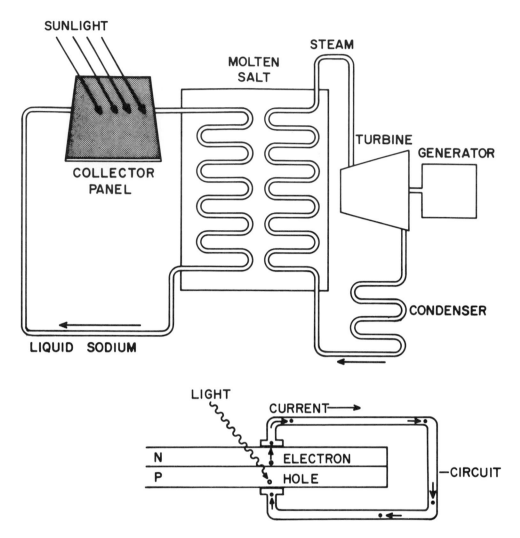

Figure 5.1 Solar energy devices proposed for conversion of solar energy to electricity. *A (top):* Sunlight falls on collectors and raises the temperature of the collection medium; the heat energy is transformed to steam, which drives a turbine engine. *B (bottom):* Solar cell contains a semiconductor made up of negative *(N)* and positive *(P)* layers that attract electrons. An electron from the P layer is dislodged by a photon of light and migrates to the N layer, creating a positively charged "hole" in the crystal. Because electrons and holes are oppositely charged, they attract. When the N electrons attempt to enter the hole they left at the P layer, a circuit is created. (From Energy and Power by C.M. Summers. Copyright © 1971 by Scientific American, Inc. All rights reserved.)

future, a preferred objective now would be to reduce yearly growth rates appreciably in order to buy time and avoid an economic crash. An electrical energy economy is forecast by the mid 2000s with coal, nuclear, and it is hoped, solar sources providing the necessary energy. This prediction is for energy with power-generating technologies already in existence. A decrease from 8% growth to 4% growth would be an extremely difficult goal to attain, and even this would mean that in the year 2000 oil and gas demand would be 80% greater than in 1970, total energy output 143%, and coal and electric power 270% larger. Obviously, realization of such projections will require more initiative from all sectors (government, business, and the public) than has been evident for the past several decades.

Some decided measures have been taken to conserve energy, not as a result of a desire to save fuel, but because the Arab embargo increased the price of fuel and there was a mandated incentive to save. Attempts to conserve have been made in the industrial (decreased heat loss via air and water cooling methods), transportation (smaller cars, more efficient engines, car pooling), and residential–commercial (lowered thermostats, insulation, energy-efficient appliances) sectors. Without delineating each specific energy-saving point, it seems reasonable to assume that the United States could reduce energy use by 25% without a serious change in life style. Energy consciousness and the desire to conserve are the main elements necessary to achieve such a goal, and the necessity for a long-term commitment seems obvious.

It is difficult to discuss conservation in the United States without appearing to be patronizing, for this nation has a more wasteful economy than any other in the world. The curtailment of waste is one of the most significant measures that can be taken to cut energy consumption sharply in the future. The average citizen can easily see the direct ways to conserve energy—use cars less, turn down the thermostat, turn off the lights, etc. A small segment of the population has made a conscious effort to conserve, but wonders why when Las Vegas is ablaze 365 nights a year. Few persons, however, comprehend the importance of conserving other resources that are habitually wasted. Each resource used has been developed at an expenditure of energy, and when usable resources are discarded, that energy expenditure is also lost. If our leaders could gain the cooperation of society in conserving *total energy* (take greater advantage of the Second Law of Thermodynamics and utilize resources to the optimum), the reduction in energy consumption would be tremendous.

5.5. Future Energy Policy

Our present rates of growth in energy production, raw material consumption, population, and pollution cannot be sustained. Thoughtful people have appreciated this for some time. Will it be possible for the rest of the world—often dedicated to immediate profit only—to understand and take action?

The main problem may not be that of maintaining a supply of energy; it is more apt to be that of maintaining a supply of energy that is safe, available to all technologies, and inexhaustable.

One must only take note of the problem-solving difficulty in the United States—an enlightened, democratic country that has no formal energy policy and as of this writing appears to be in no hurry to formulate one—to appreciate the reluctance for change. At this writing, Congress is in the final stages of enacting a highly modified version of President Carter's energy bill. Since the late 1930s Congress has been adequately informed of the pending energy crisis. Despite appreciable recent problems, no sense of urgency to solve one of the most crucial problems of this century is evident. Recent experience suggests that the educational background on which Congress bases decisions may be too narrow and the influence of vested interests (via well-placed congressmen) too broad for the solution of problems of this magnitude in this phase of our nation's history.

Suggested Reading

Doolittle, J.S. Energy: A Crisis, a Dilemma, or Just Another Problem. Champaign, Ill.: Matrix, 1977.

Energy and Power, Readings from Scientific American. San Francisco: Freeman, 1971.

Executive Office of the President. The National Energy Plan. Washington D.C.: Superintendent of Documents, 1977.

Ford Foundation. A Time to Choose: America's Energy Future. Cambridge, Mass.: Ballinger, 1974.

Goen, R.L., White, R.K. Comparison of energy consumption between West Germany and the United States. Prepared for Federal Energy Administration, June 1975. Contract 14-01-001-1885. Final Report, Research Institute, Henlo Park, California.

Institute for Contemporary Studies. Options for U.S. Energy Policy. San Francisco, 1977.

Lenihan, J., Fletcher, W. W. Energy Resources and the Environment, Vol. 1, Environment and Man. New York: Academic Press, 1976.

Power from the sun and world energy supplies. UNESCO Courier, Jan. 1974.

Special Issue on Energy Matters. Nature 249, June 1974.

Tuve, G.L. Energy, Environment, Populations, and Food. New York: Wiley, 1976.

David H. Martin

6

Nuclear Power

6.1. Introduction

Nuclear power had its beginning as an industry about 1960, when early estimates indicated that economy of scale (use of large reactors) would produce low-cost electricity. Since that time, the introduction of radiation from nuclear power into the biosphere has been small compared with other man-made radiation, such as that from bomb tests or medical X-rays. This situation, however, leaves no room for complacency, as nuclear power is unique in its potential for future pollution. Unfortunately, early workers did not foresee or did not consider seriously the possible mechanisms for environmental disasters before considerable development was underway. For example, the problem of containment of large power reactors under meltdown conditions was not brought out until the mid 1960s; terrorism as a real threat became evident in the early 1970s; and the as yet unresolved problem of final storage of nuclear wastes only recently became an intensely debated issue.

Whether or not these or similar problems, left unsolved, will result in unacceptably large increases in environmental radioactivity is actually not known, but, because of the potential harm, it is generally assumed that satisfactory solutions must be found. Nuclear power currently contributes about 12% of electricity in the United States and only about 3% of total energy. Planned construction, with the growth of other forms of energy, might increase the latter figure to approximately 5% by the year 2000. Thus, abandonment or phase-out of nuclear power in the United States remains a possibility if its problems become (or are perceived of as) insoluble.

In discussing nuclear power–produced radiation in the environment, we should note some differences from other types of pollution. First, although plant and animal life may be important in concentrating or dispersing radioisotopes, the effects of principal concern are felt directly by humans. Furthermore, the more serious health effects of low-level radiation are generally long delayed.

Nevertheless, they may be treated statistically. Thus, a given increase in radiation, if spread over a large population, might be small or even undetectable as an increase above background; nevertheless, real health effects will occur, based on the radiation increase. In such a treatment, a "linear hypothesis" is assumed—twice the dose produces twice the health effects—in contrast to nonlinear relationships for other types of pollution.

In this chapter, the steps in the uranium fuel cycle and the operation of nuclear reactors are discussed, with emphasis on possible radioactivity release mechanisms and the probabilities of their occurrence.

6.2. Mining and Processing of Uranium

6.2.1. Mining

About one-half of the uranium ore reserves in the United States are above and about one-half below a depth of 400 ft. As this depth is the approximate economic limit for strip mining, it is not surprising that the mines in our country divide about equally between open-pit and underground mines. Although both types of mines handle large quantities of uranium ore, the physical situation that determines radioactive releases is obviously different for each. The principle concern here is with the release and subsequent effects of ^{238}U and its daughter products, particularly radium and radon. In the case of open-pit or strip mining, gaseous products (i.e., radon) are released directly into the atmosphere and contribute to a diffuse, widespread background. Wind-borne radioactive dust particles may also present at least a minor problem.

Underground mining, on the other hand, tends to concentrate the gaseous alpha emitter, radon. Since radon is a noble gas, it tends to be expelled by the lungs and is much less dangerous than its daughter, ^{218}Po, which is mostly retained. If good ventilation can be maintained in underground mines, then the 3.8-day radon can be swept out before build-up of the 3-min ^{218}Po, and the large lung doses received by miners in the past can be avoided.

Both under- and aboveground mining present the problem of radioisotopes leached out in large quantities of mine drainage water.

6.2.2. Milling

After extraction from a mine, uranium ore is taken to a mill, usually close by, where the ore is crushed and the uranium removed by a chemical process. The final product, ammonium diuranate, is called "yellowcake." During the chemical processing, radium remains with the original ore, which passes to a tailings pond for permanent storage. Eventually the water from the tailings pond will evaporate, leaving a dry residue. During this process there is, of course, the chance of loss of radioactive solution by leakage, seepage, or other means. After dehydration, the tailings may become wind borne. However, the most significant release is that of radon gas, which will add to background radiation away from the site.

The tailings will produce radon for on the order of 100,000 years, and there are some 26 million tons of abandoned tailings in the western United States, in addition to more recent output. This source is currently considered by the

Nuclear Regulatory Commission (NRC) to be the major contributor to radiation exposure from the nuclear fuel cycle.

6.2.3. Conversion/Separation

The yellowcake produced from milling is next converted, by one of two chemical processes, to uranium hexaflouride (UF_6), which is needed to feed the gaseous diffusion separation process. As U_3O_8–UF_6 conversion and ^{235}U–^{238}U separation are both contained processes with small external losses, they are discussed together. Since we are still dealing with natural uranium, the materials processed are not highly radioactive and are easily handled. The gaseous diffusion process depends on the difference in diffusion rates of different masses, i.e., that of $^{235}UF_6$ and $^{238}UF_6$. In passing through a porous medium, the two isotopes are slowly separated, and thus a large number of stages, and large amounts of electrical energy, are required (approximately 98% of that consumed in the entire fuel cycle).

Development of a centrifuge and a laser-actuated method of separation is under way, and future separation plants may be of one of these types.

In the case of UF_6 conversion, wastes containing uranium are either buried or returned to a uranium mill for recycling. In separation, an enrichment of 2–4% ^{235}U is obtained; the depleted uranium (about 0.2% ^{235}U) is stored as UF_6.

6.2.4. Fuel Fabrication

Enriched uranium in the form of UF_6 from the separation plant is converted, at the fuel fabrication plant, to uranium dioxide (UO_2), which is then pelletized, sintered, and loaded into Zircaloy tubing to form fuel rods. Losses inherent in these operations are small, as they are in the isotope separation process. In both cases, because enriched uranium is handled, there is a possibility of a critical accident. However, the enrichment is too low to cause a bomb-type explosion (about 90% is needed for bomb production; thus conventional reactors also cannot explode as a bomb); in addition, a critical accident would most likely not last long enough to build up enough radioactivity to cause serious off-site contamination.

6.3. Nuclear Reactors

The basis for nuclear power is the neutron chain reaction, which operates as follows: The reactor core consists of slightly enriched uranium rods with water flowing between them. To start the reaction a neutron is necessary, perhaps from a special neutron source or from the natural background. If the neutron is relatively slow (close to a "thermal" velocity) there is a high probability (a high cross section) that it will interact with a ^{235}U nucleus so as to produce fission.

A fission reaction results in fission fragments (fission products, some of which are radioactive), alpha, beta, and gamma rays, about 200 MeV (3.2×10^{-11} J) energy, and an average of more than two neutrons. These neutrons are fast (energetic) and must be slowed down before they will have a high probability of causing further fission needed to sustain the chain reaction. Collisions of the fast neutrons with the hydrogen in the water mentioned above results in their slowing down to a desirable speed. Some of the neutrons find their way out of the reactor, or are lost to competing reactions; but to continue the chain reaction, at least one neutron from each fission must find and induce fission in another ^{235}U nucleus.

Nuclear reactors are built to sustain and control many chain reactions simultaneously, while removing the heat produced and using it to generate electricity in a more or less conventional manner. The heart of the reactor, the core, is composed of many thousands of fuel rods, set in a lattice array that is housed in a cylindrical, thick-walled (about 8-in thick), stainless steel pressure vessel (Figure 6.1). This vessel, which is mounted vertically, may be 16 ft in diameter and 40–50 ft long. Two types of reactors, the pressurized water reactor

Figure 6.1 Typical pressurized water reactor containment. (From Nuclear Regulatory Commission. Reactor Safety Study. WASH 1400, 1975.)

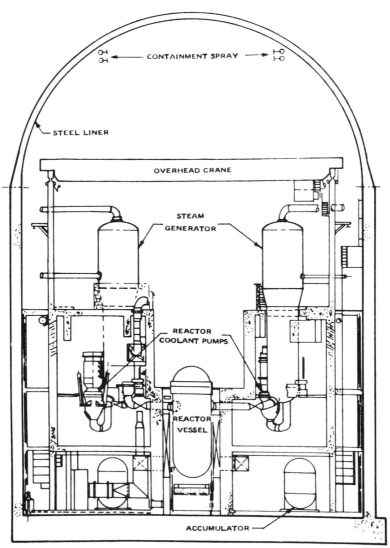

(PWR) and the boiling water reactor (BWR), are in use in the United States. Various design features, including the pressure vessel, are somewhat different for each type, but the basic operation is the same.

Control and shutdown of the reactor are accomplished by neutron-absorbing (boron) rods, which are moved in or out of the core to cause either a decrease or increase of power, respectively.

Water at a high pressure (about 2200 psi for the pressurized water reactor) is pumped at a high velocity through the core, where it picks up the heat produced by the fission reaction and rises to a temperature of about 600°F. This high-pressure fluid is used either directly (BWR) or via a heat exchanger and a secondary loop (PWR) to drive a turbine and an electrical generator (Figure 6.2). To reduce the pressure in the system, cooling is provided by direct evaporation either from a cooling lake or from cooling towers. Since the generating system that we are describing is basically that of a heat engine, Carnot's efficiency applies, and close to 70% of the nuclear-produced heat must be disposed of, mostly by evaporation of water. Because the operating temperature of nuclear-fired plants is lower than that of coal-fired plants (for safety reasons), the amount of heat released into the environment (thermal pollution) and water evaporated by nuclear plants is usually much larger than that released by coal-fired plants of the same rated output. Consumptive water losses for a 1000-MW$_e$ (megawatts of electrical output) plant might be of the order of 15 million gallons per day.

If cooling towers are used, a fraction of the water lost to the atmosphere is in the form of droplets (drift) that are blown out of the tower plume. These droplets carry certain chemicals and also some radioisotopes that enter the cooling system from reactor operation.

Some of the pathways that radioisotopes follow in escaping from a nuclear plant are as follows: Most directly, the fission products, which are formed in

Figure 6.2 Pressurized water reactor power system components. (From Report to the APS by the study group on light-water safety. Rev. Mod. Phys. 47, Suppl 1: 5–16, 1975. Used with permission.)

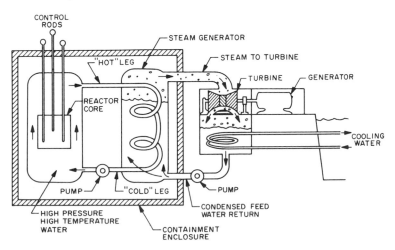

great abundance in the uranium fuel, leak out through pinholes and fissures in the fuel cladding (tritium will, to some extent diffuse through the cladding) and appear in the primary coolant water. In the PWR, borated water is used in the primary loop for control purposes, and the boron, when bombarded by neutrons, forms an additional source of tritium. Other radioisotopes are produced in the coolant water from neutron reactions with corrosion products, and from both neutron and proton interactions with oxygen. All of these radioisotopes may find leakage routes from the coolant loops, or they may be purposely released, with or without holdup for decay, from a gas-handling system.

In addition to the release of radioisotopes, a certain amount of direct radiation and "skyshine" (gamma radiation reflected or scattered from the atmosphere) will reach the boundaries of the plant. This problem is more severe in the BWR, where ^{16}N spreads into the steam turbine, the condenser, and the remainder of the steam system, forming an extended source of 6.28-MeV gamma rays.

6.4. Transportation

Transportation of radioactive materials may be necessary at various points in the uranium fuel cycle. However, since we are interested in the potentially more significant environmental releases, it is probably most appropriate to discuss the subject of transportation occurring immediately after reactor irradiation; with the present limited fuel cycle used in the United States (no reprocessing), spent fuel provides the greatest potential for radioisotope release to the environment. The current generation of light water reactors each contains about 100 tons uranium. It has been calculated that after 1 year of operation, a 1000-MW$_e$ reactor will have a fission product inventory equivalent to well over 1000 Hiroshima-sized bombs. This analogy has limited value—for example, the half-lives of remaining radioisotopes will be quite different in the two cases—but the comparison is useful to show the reason for so much concern over the possibility of the escape of even a small fraction of the fission product inventory.

About one-third of the reactor fuel is replaced each year and deposited in a storage pool at the reactor site. This spent fuel, after a "cooling-off" period of at least 150 days, will be shipped to a government interim storage facility, and then (after some years) to terminal storage, when such a site is available. Shipment will be either by truck or rail. The truck shipping containers, or casks, will each hold about 0.5 t (about 0.5% of a reactor core load), and the rail casks about 3.2 t (about 3.2% of a core load). The casks will be heavily constructed and heavily shielded, and we may assume that radioisotope releases to the environment would probably be related to accidents rather than routine use.

Normal operation of a reactor, besides creating spent fuel, also generates a considerable amount of low-level waste, which is shipped to burial grounds for disposal. Release to the environment would be through accidents, and the potential contamination would be small for any given shipment.

It should be mentioned here that a 1000-MW$_e$ reactor creates 200–300 kg ^{239}Pu per year. The ^{239}Pu is produced from neutron bombardment of ^{238}U, and thus is not a fission product. If separated from spent fuel and shipped as plutonium oxide, a potential for large environmental contamination exists, as plutonium oxide is a fine powder and is spread by the wind.

6.5. Reprocessing

A proposed procedure is to ship the spent fuel from a power reactor to a reprocessing plant, where the cladding would be removed mechanically, and uranium, plutonium, and the fission products would be separated by some variation of the (chemical) Purex process. Under this system, the slightly depleted uranium would be reenriched and recycled as reactor fuel; the plutonium would be stored, mixed with uranium for fuel, or used in a breeder reactor. The fission products (high-level wastes) would be removed for interim and/or final storage.

In the past, during reprocessing essentially all of the ^{85}Kr and most of the tritium present in the fuel were released to the environment. It is uncertain whether this would be the case in the future. For other radioisotopes, reprocessing represents a sensitive stage of handling; because large quantities of fission products are handled, only minute fractions may be allowed to escape. Accidents or sabotage could cause large releases at this point.

No commerical reprocessing plants are operating in the United States at the present time. Government policy is to forego reprocessing for the near future in order to reduce nuclear proliferation (diversion of plutonium for bomb use); however, the recent experience of private industries that have attempted to start or to continue commercial reprocessing has indicated that it is probably not economical at present.

6.6. Storage

Whether or not reprocessing becomes a link in the fuel cycle, radioactive waste is fast building up—spent fuel storage pools at reactor sites have in a few cases already filled—and some provisions for storage must be made soon. The history of the waste storage program has included a number of changes in policy, particularly with regard to emphasis on aboveground versus underground disposal. The present proposal is to maintain wastes (in the form of spent fuel, since reprocessing is not available) for an indefinite period in interim, aboveground storage, after which they are to be placed underground, probably in an irretrievable arrangement. (An obvious possible conflict exists here, since the nuclear industry would prefer to retain spent fuel to be used in the breeder reactor, if it should reach commercial development). The waste material may be coated with glass (glassified) and stored at depths on the order of 2000 ft. Geological formations of current interest for storage sites are salt beds, granite, and sedimentary clays.

No terminal storage program including choice of suitable site has been demonstrated as yet for either military or civilian high-level wastes (military and civilian wastes are currently about equal in radioactivity, although the military wastes are much greater in volume). Although geological formations of interest are widespread in the United States, attempts at fixing one or more sites have so far failed, due to either technical difficulties with the site itself or opposition within the state to the site location.

For interim storage, the same concerns regarding radioisotope releases apply as for reprocessing: The greatest releases would come from accidents, natural disruptions, and sabotage. Because a large fission product inventory is handled, percent releases must be very small. In the case of terminal storage, accidents, disruptions, and sabotage are of much less concern. Major problems would probably come from migration of wastes by leaching or through fissures created, perhaps, by earth motion, or by heat from the fission products.

Some of the more significant fission products present in spent reactor fuel are listed in Table 6.1. To these must be added activation products and, in particular, the actinides neptunium, plutonium, americium, and curium.

6.7. Normal Releases from the Fuel Cycle

It is customary to categorize radioisotope releases as being either normal or accidental. This distinction is rather arbitrary, since certain types of "accidents" occur on a routine basis. We will, however, stay with convention in listing normal, or planned releases, at the same time acknowledging that these values may not always be conservative or necessarily realistic.

Table 6.1 Representative Quantities of Potentially Significant Fission Products in Spent Reactor Fuels

Isotope	Half-life (years)	Quantity Ci/t	Quantity g/t	Release state
^{3}H	12.3	800	0.083	Gas
^{85}Kr	10.7	10,500	27	Gas
^{99}Tc	2.13×10^5	15	880	Semivolatile
^{103}Ru	0.11	180,000	5.7	Semivolatile
^{106}Ru	1.01	820,000	240	Semivolatile
^{125m}Te	0.16	6,500	0.36	Semivolatile
^{127m}Te	0.30	25,000	2.7	Semivolatile
^{129m}Te	0.09	13,000	0.42	Semivolatile
^{129}I	17×10^6	0.04	250	Volatile
^{131}I	0.02	2.0	<0.01	Volatile
^{134}Cs	2.05	100,000	77	Semivolatile
^{135}Cs	3×10^6	1.2	1400	Semivolatile
^{137}Cs	30.2	106,000	1200	Semivolatile
^{89}Sr	0.14	100,000	3.5	Solid
^{90}Sr	28.9	60,000	430	Solid
^{91}Y	0.16	190,000	7.8	Solid
^{93}Zr	0.95×10^6	2	490	Solid
^{95}Zr	0.18	400,000	19	Solid
^{95}Nb	0.10	800,000	21	Solid
^{125}Sb	2.73	13,000	12	Solid
^{141}Ce	0.09	80,000	2.8	Solid
^{144}Ce	0.78	800,000	250	Solid
^{147}Pm	2.62	200,000	220	Solid
^{155}Eu	5.0	40,000	87	Solid

Burnup is 33 GWd (thermal)/t; cooling time is 150 days.

Source: Environmental Protection Agency. Environmental Radiation Dose Commitment: An Application to the Nuclear Power Industry. EPA 520/4-73-002, 1974.

Table 6.2 lists the more significant expected yearly radioisotope releases from the fuel cycle associated with a 1000-MW$_e$ power plant. Overall releases for the industry may be obtained by multiplying by the current number of operating reactors in the United States (approximately 69), or by a projection (say, 100–300) for the year 2000. Direct radiation is not included, because it is mostly restricted to the environment of the nuclear worker; however, recent studies of long-term health effects of irradiated Hanford, Washington, workers indicate the possibility of such radiation having a much larger impact than previously thought.

Table 6.2 omits releases in mining, largely relating to radon gas, which, though they have significant effects on the miners, are small contributors to the exterior environment.

The inventory of spent fuel fission products removed from a 1000-MW$_e$ reactor is about 5.17×10^9 Ci/year. (Total inventory of the reactor is about three times this number.) After a cooling period of 150 days before shipping, the spent fuel activity drops to about 1.35×10^8 Ci. This number decreases only slightly during the period when the fuel is in a reprocessing plant. In addition, almost 300 kg plutonium are removed from the reactor per year.

In 1974, the EPA estimated the fractional releases due to handling of the actinides (^{238}Pu, ^{239}Pu, ^{240}Pu, ^{241}Pu, ^{241}Am, ^{242}Cm, ^{244}Cm) produced by the nuclear industry. The fraction of the total actinides handled assumed to reach the environment was 1 part in 10^6. Estimates for solid fission products were not made.

Unfortunately, routine industrial releases, producing a cumulative "dose commitment" over future years, will be known with accuracy only through experience.

Table 6.2   Expected Annual Radioisotope Releases from the Uranium Fuel Cycle in a 1000-MW$_e$ Reactor

Stage	Release state	Isotope	Amount (Ci)	
Milling	Gas	^{222}Rn	56.7	
	Liquid	U	1.9	
		^{230}Th	3.2	
	Solid (86,200t tailings)	^{230}Th	53.5	
		^{226}Ra	56.6	
			BWR	PWR
Reactor	Gas	^{3}H	10	50
		^{131}I	0.3	0.8
		Kr + Xe	50,000	7,000
	Liquid	^{3}H	90	450
		other	5	5
Reprocessing	Gas	^{85}Kr	3.73×10^5	
		^{3}H	20,580	
		^{129}I, ^{131}I	0.06	
		Other	0.918	
	Liquid	^{3}H	3,340	
		^{106}Ru	3.67	

Source: Pigford, T. H. Environmental aspects of nuclear energy production. Reproduced, with permission, from the *Annual Review of Nuclear Science*, Volume 24. © 1974 by Annual Reviews Inc.

Some difficulties inherent in interpreting radioisotope releases in terms of effects on humans might be mentioned at this point. First, the radioisotope may have radioactive "daughter" decay products that are different in half-life, emissions, and other properties from the parent. Furthermore, the radioisotope may be concentrated by biological or other means, so that it reaches humans as a much more intense source than when released. This situation is of particular concern when a food chain is involved. A classic example is the concentration of radioiodine in the food chain: if deposited in a disperse manner on grass that is eaten by a cow, it is concentrated in this process, and again by the cow's production of milk; the radioiodine is again concentrated in the human who drinks the milk, since iodine is selectively directed to the thyroid gland.

Bioaccumulation factors have been measured for various elements that are accumulated by different forms of aquatic life. These factors, which are given in units such as pCi/kg per pCi/liter, may range in magnitude from less than 1 (uranium in algae) to 500,000 (phosphorus in algae).

It is important to consider the relationship of released radioisotopes to natural background radiation. The yearly background dose to man is typically on the order of 100 mrems, and is due to the following:

Cosmic radiation	40 mrems
Environmental radioactivity	40 mrems
Radioactivity in the body	20 mrems

Because artificially created radioisotopes that are released into the environment produce radiation sources at different locations than natural sources, are sometimes concentrated, have varying half-lives, etc., a meaningful comparison with natural background is probably best made by comparing population doses in the two cases. Particularly misleading is an earlier rationalization, occasionally still used, that if the release of a radioisotope caused little or no measurable increase in background level, then its effect was negligible. This approach may lead to gross underestimation of health hazards, as, for example, was the case with the earlier treatment of uranium mill tailings. It was recently realized that the overall long-term dose to the population from mine tailings would eventually produce significant health effects. These effects are statistically calculable and must be given serious consideration even though they are not directly traceable to the source.

6.8. Accidental Releases

As mentioned above, the routine operation of the nuclear industry will lead to a more or less routine release of radioactivity. Some of this release will be due to minor accidents, spills, fires, etc., which are a part of every industry. Reliable data on these occurrences will be available only with time.

The subject of this section is those more serious accidents that could individually cause radioisotope releases of major concern. The subject of nuclear accidents is a controversial one and, of course, will not be settled by a brief discussion; our object here is to formulate the questions that should be asked and to point out the limitations of the present answers. The first unknown is the quantity of radioisotopes that might be released in case of an accident. The fission product inventory of a 1000-MW$_e$ power reactor, as noted above, is approximately 5.17×10^9 Ci/year. Approximately 20% of the fission products are volatile, so that a breech of all fuel containments would release a considerable amount of radioactive gas. Under direct exposure of the core to the atmosphere, high core temperatures, rapid oxidation, and gas explosions could combine to produce large amounts of fine radioactive particulate matter, much of which would be borne by the wind when released.

It is next appropriate to ask if there are mechanisms (i.e., physical processes) that could cause penetration or rupture of a 4–6 ft reinforced concrete dome, an 8-in. thick pressure vessel, and Zircaloy cladding of the fuel. Among the obvious external possibilities are earthquakes, plane crashes (large jets), and perhaps tornados and floods. Internal causes of greatest concern are meltdowns (due to loss of coolant) and pressure vessel failures.

About 1965, engineers at the Oak Ridge National Laboratory realized that a meltdown in a large reactor probably would not be contained by the reactor housing. Such an accident might begin by coolant pipe rupture, pump failure, or blockage of coolant passages with foreign matter (for example, a loose piece of metal caused a partial meltdown at the Enrico Fermi Reactor) or perhaps by warpage or distortion. Loss of coolant for slightly less than 1 min is sufficient to cause overheating of the fuel by the decaying fission products, which continue to release energy even though the chain reaction may already have stopped. At this point it is too late for the emergency core cooling system, designed to feed in fresh water, and it is assumed that the reactor core will melt and most of the 100 tons of uranium fuel will slump as a molten mass to the bottom of the pressure vessel. Because cooling is no longer possible, the molten core is expected to continue to heat, until it melts through the pressure vessel and the concrete pad beneath and starts moving downward through the earth "toward China"—the so-called China syndrome. Under these conditions, fissures or other passages in the earth might allow escape of fission products. If such openings are not present, violent metal–water reactions or hydrogen–oxygen explosions could occur to force a breech.

Pressure vessel failure is also a potential problem. This could originate from metal fatigue, radiation damage, or overpressurization caused by power transients in the reactor core. Pressure vessel failure could lead to a meltdown similar to loss of coolant accidents. On the other hand, a great deal of energy is stored in the core coolant, which is at a pressure of about 2200 psi and a temperature of 600°F, and it is possible that the pressure vessel end cap, or some other object, could form a missile to penetrate the reactor housing.

The next consideration is the circumstances immediately following a major release of radioisotopes. A cloud of mixed gases and small particles leaving an accident site will tend to diffuse, with particulate matter slowly descending to earth, forming a more or less elliptical fallout pattern. In the case of large releases, individuals downwind of the site could receive direct radiation doses that could be lethal at distances up to 100 miles, and significant contamination could occur at distances up to several hundred miles and over thousands of square miles of area (Figure 6.3). These are, of course, the "worst" results from a selected range of variation of parameters such as weather conditions and particle size (they are not necessarily the worst possible results). Worst conditions must, of course, be considered for public health considerations.

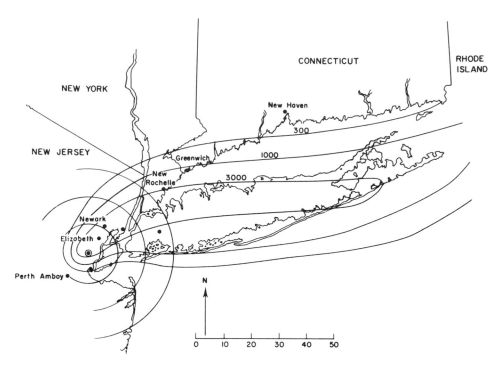

Figure 6.3 Bikini bomb test fallout pattern overlaid on the New York City area. Isodoses are in roentgens. This bomb had a fallout capability similar to that of a modern 1000-MW$_e$ reactor operated for 1 year. Serious reactor accidents could yield fallout patterns of this type. (From Mark, J.C. Global consequences of nuclear weaponry. Reproduced, with permission, from the Annual Review of Nuclear Science, Volume 26. © 1976 by Annual Reviews Inc.)

Finally, the most controversial issue is the probability of the occurrence of accidents involving large radioisotope releases. Early Atomic Energy Commission (AEC) accident studies (in 1957 and 1965) did not address this problem; rather, a given fraction of the reactor fission product inventory was assumed to be released, and the results were estimated. More recently an attempt to evaluate probabilities was made in the 1975 AEC Rasmussen Report (WASH 1400), in which estimates of the likelihood of various reactor events were combined to calculate the overall probability of an accident.

The findings of this study are, in part, that there is a negligible risk of pressure vessel failure (in sharp contrast to results of British studies and 1973 AEC results) and that overall meltdown probability is 1:20,000 per reactor-year—an unacceptably high value if we consider the number of reactor-years planned. Other portions of the Rasmussen Report, however, treat the releases from various meltdown conditions and it is concluded that the overall probability of significant off-site damage is extremely small.

Reactions to this report have included both approval and considerable criticism, perhaps the most significant being that of an American Physical Society review, which concluded in 1975 that a statistical study of this type is useful in comparing two different reactor systems but is not valid in calculating absolute numbers for overall probabilities. A group commissioned by the NRC (the Lewis Committee) published similar results in 1978, and the NRC has since withdrawn its support from quoted safety probabilities based on the Rasmussen Report. The Rasmussen Report was concerned with probabilities of equipment failure. An accident at the Three Mile Island plant near Harrisburg, Pennsylvania, in 1979, which received wide publicity, has cast doubt on the ability of nuclear engineers to predict the course of accidents and on the ability of plant personnel to maintain the exacting level of performance necessary for safe plant operation. Thus, at the present time, nuclear power cannot be stated to be safe, and, from the standpoint of public safety, should probably be considered unsafe.

6.9. Sabotage: Planned Accidents

True accidents are difficult to predict; predictions of intentional "accidents" (sabotage) are highly speculative. Controversy has arisen over both the likelihood and the outcome of such activities; however, it is clear that knowledgeable saboteurs could induce the type of accidents that we have mentioned. With sufficient explosives, it is also clear that such individuals could disperse the contents of a reactor, a spent fuel storage pool, a shipping cask, or a portion of the inventory of a reprocessing plant.

The General Accounting Office has indicated in a 1976 report that a small group of armed individuals could, under security measures prevailing at the time, take over a nuclear plant. Probabilities of the occurrence of this or similar actions have not been published; however, it is clear that the threat of massive environmental contamination as a result of terrorist activities may be as great or greater than that likely to occur by other means.

6.10. Future Sources of Radiation

Continued use of nuclear power beyond the next 30–50 years would, because of diminishing natural uranium supplies, necessitate the development and use of the breeder reactor. This reactor differs from the conventional thermal light water reactor in that it is designed to accentuate the reaction of neutrons with ^{238}U, which leads, after a short decay, to ^{239}Pu. Thus, while burning ^{235}U, new plutonium fuel is prepared from the more plentiful ^{238}U. The breeder of current interest uses liquid sodium as a coolant (moderation is not required, and the heat removal properties of a liquid metal are desirable owing to the high energy density of the core).

The breeder is believed by many to have more safety problems than light water reactors; an obvious additional potential for environmental contamination stems from the large quantities of plutonium that would be handled if breeders were used extensively. Estimates of the annual amount of plutonium reprocessed in a "plutonium economy" by the year 2000 have been on the order of 100 tons.

Development of the breeder has proceeded abroad, and to a less extent in the United States. Its use here is, however, dependent on implementation of reprocessing.

A final possible future source of man-made environmental radiopollution is the fusion reactor, which would operate on the energy produced when certain light nuclei combine (as opposed to fission). The principal radioisotope released is tritium, which is one of the fusing nuclei in the schemes of greatest interest. Unfortunately, tritium, like hydrogen, tends to diffuse through metals and losses on the order of curies per day might be expected from a reactor.

In addition, high-energy neutrons would result from the fusion reactions and would cause radioactivity in the reactor and adjoining materials. In comparison with the breeder, however, it has been estimated that the amount of long-lived waste would be 10^2–10^5 lower, and volatile radioactivity would be 10^4–10^6 lower.

Suggested Reading

Environmental Protection Agency. Environmental Radiation Dose Commitment: An Application to the Nuclear Power Industry. EPA-520/4-73-002. Washington, D.C., Feb. 1974.

Inglis, D.R. Nuclear Energy: Its Physics and Its Social Challenge. Reading, Mass.: Addison-Wesley, 1973.

Nuclear Power Costs, Twenty-Third Report by the Committee on Government Operations. 95th Congress, 2nd Session. House Report No. 95-1090, April 1978.

Pigford, T.H. Environmental aspects of nuclear energy production. Annu. Rev. Nucl. Sci. 24: 515–559, 1974.

Report to the American Physical Society by the study group on light-water reactor safety. Rev. Mod. Phys. 47 [Suppl. 1], 1975.

Report to the American Physical Society by the study group on nuclear fuel cycles and waste management. Rev. Mod. Phys. 50, No. 1, Part II, 1978.

Union of Concerned Scientists. The Nuclear Fuel Cycle, a Survey of the Public Health, Environmental and National Security Effects of Nuclear Power. MIT Branch Sta., Cambridge, Mass., Oct. 1973. (Other reports on nuclear safety have been released by this organization.)

U.S. Atomic Energy Commission. Environmental Survey of the Uranium Fuel Cycle. WASH-1248. Apr. 1974.

U.S. General Accounting Office. Reports EMD-77-32 and EMD-77-46, April 1977 and June 1977 on Nuclear Security and Nuclear Waste Storage.

U.S. Nuclear Regulatory Commission. Reactor Safety Study, An Assessment of Accident Risks in U.S. Commercial Nuclear Power Plants. WASH-1400 (NUREG-75/014). Oct. 1975 (known as the Rasmussen Report).

Frank E. Guthrie

7

Human Populations

7.1. Introduction

Problems of environmental pollution are primarily related to the activities of humans, for this species, especially in the so-called developed countries, has the capacity to alter the environment and indeed has done so dramatically. In view of the problems created by this minority of the world population, and the fact that the majority of the world population is desperately striving to improve its economic conditions by utilization of rapidly decreasing world resources, increased population growth is an important issue; furthermore, each increment adds both human and chemical wastes and increases the possibility of greater disease problems. If man cannot control human population in his finite world, evolution will obviously do it for him—and some think in the not too distant future.

The ominous threat of overpopulation was first expressed in Malthus' now famous "Essay on Growth" in 1798. Simply stated, he suggested that the human population was growing geometrically while the supply of necessary resources to accommodate the population was growing arithmetically. Technology, especially improved agricultural productivity, temporarily deferred the realization of Malthus' prediction; however, recent studies indicate that, barring a technological miracle, the population will outgrow our resources (and our humanistic values) within the next few decades unless growth is drastically reduced. Even in the event of such a miracle, mankind must ultimately accept the fact that the world is finite, the logic of which seems to elude most business and political leaders. Figure 7.1, depicting recent world population estimates, dramatically illustrates the critical trend toward overpopulation.

Those countries that are able and willing to control their own populations will be unable to construct barriers, real or imagined, that will prevent a drastic confrontation with those nations that are unable or unwilling to control their populations. Perhaps the best example of an approaching crisis is that between

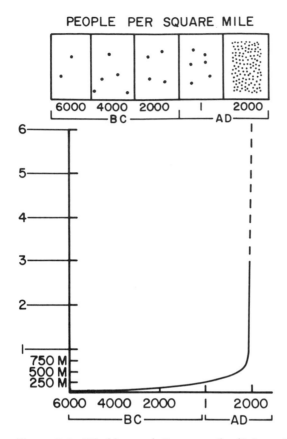

Figure 7.1 World population growth. (Adapted from United Nations, Vital Statistics Report: Populations, 1962.)

the United States and Mexico. Mexico, an already overpopulated country, will double its present population in the 21st century. No major geographical barrier separates this resource-limited country from one of the most affluent nations in the world, a stark contrast that exists nowhere else on this planet.

The commitment to over 100×10^6 babies born each year initially requires relatively few resources. However, during the next 50 years, a very large commitment in resources—food, housing, clothing, education, jobs, transportation—is made. For a child born in the United States, this resource burden includes 56×10^6 gal water, 21,000 gal gasoline, 10,000 lb meat, 28,000 lb milk and cream, more than 10 automobiles, 4500 ft³ wood, etc.

7.2. Population Estimates

Estimates of projected world population by the year 2000 vary from approximately 4.5 billion to nearly 7×10^9. A recent study of major areas since 1965, and projected to 1985, was conducted by the United Nations (Table 7.1). The contrast between the "developed and developing" countries of the world is dramatic. A similar UN estimate made in 1963 predicated a population of 187×10^6 less

Table 7.1 Population Estimates for Major Areas of the World

Area	Estimated population ($\times 10^6$)			Increase 1965–1985 (%)	Annual growth rate (%)
	1965	1976	1985		
World	3289	4022	4933	50	2.1
Developed countries	1037	1147	1275	23	1.1
Developing countries	2252	2874	3658	62	2.4
East Asia	852	1011	1182	39	1.8
South Asia	981	1296	1693	72	2.7
Europe	445	479	515	16	0.7
USSR	231	256	287	24	1.1
Africa	303	395	530	74	2.4
Northern America	214	243	280	26	1.2
Latin America	246	327	435	76	2.9
Oceania	18	22	27	50	2.1

Source: Adapted from New findings on population trends. Population Newsletter 7:1969.

people than is now estimated for 1985. One must recognize that population projections are occasionally, and quickly, reversed. The United States population trend, which had been toward rapid growth, changed from an average of nearly four children per family in the mid 1950s to two children per family in 1972 without any directed program toward this decrease (Figure 7.2). The reported decrease in population growth rate in the most heavily populated country in the world (the People's Republic of China) was not projected by any population estimates of the mid-1950s. This must be contrasted to growth rates in Zaire 3.9%, Mexico 3.2%, and Thailand 3.1%), as examples of three large countries without noticeable restrictions. The rate of natural increase is determined by subtracting deaths from births. If the world birth rate is 34/1000 and the death rate is 14/1000, the population growth rate is 20/1000, or 2%. A 2% growth rate doubles the population in 35 years because 2 persons per year are added to each 100 and those added also reproduce.

7.2.1. Population Doubling

The doubling times of the world population were 102 years between the first and second billion persons (1825–1927) and 48 years between the second and fourth billion; at the present rate of growth, the doubling time to 8×10^9 would be but 33 years. It seems safe to predict that children born today are uncomfortably close to realizing a ceiling of population expansion. Even if it were possible for the world to approach a zero rate of population increase, the lag time would be such that nearly 1 billion additional people would be born before populations were stabilized. The contrast between developed and underdeveloped countries is striking, for within 1 century (assuming present growth rates) the developed countries will have a population of less than 2×10^9 while the population of the underdeveloped countries will approach 40 billion.

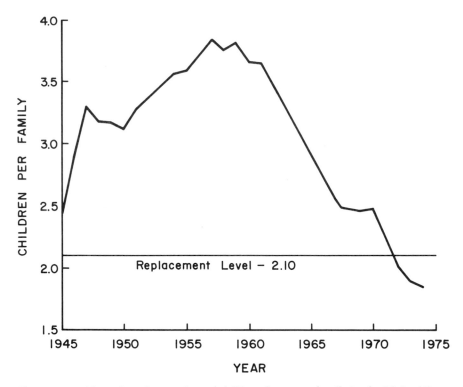

Figure 7.2 Alterations in number of children born per family in the United States during three decades (total fertility rate). The growth rate in three selected years was 0.71 (1945), 1.83 (1956), and 0.71 (1977). (Adapted from Turk, A., et al. Environmental Science. Philadelphia: W.B. Saunders, 1974.)

7.2.2. Age Structure Relative to Growth Rate

The age structure of the population is a very important component of growth. Due to the post–World War II population explosion—which resulted from the control of malaria and similar population-controlling diseases and a concomitant high birth rate—in the less developed countries, the number of people in the younger age groups greatly increased while the number in the older age groups remained stable. In the developed countries, such a trend was not apparent to any significant extent. Figure 7.3 depicts the age distribution in three contrasting situations and shows that the increased child-bearing population will cause a critical problem for several decades, especially in developing countries. The age pyramid for India (typical of the first curve) is an excellent example of the consequences of unrelenting population growth. Each year the number of people reaching reproductive age greatly exceeds the number of those outgrowing the reproductive years or dying. This trend will persist for several generations until the progeny of the former gradually diminish in numbers proportional to the latter in the simple case of illustration. Even if growth decreases to the replacement level (2%) by 1985, the 1971 population of 570×10^6 would still grow to over 1×10^9 before it stabilized in the middle of the next century.

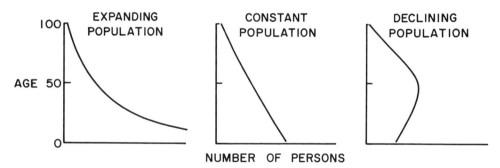

Figure 7.3 Population age distribution scheme illustrating the effect that the number of people in the child-bearing age might have on population growth.

7.2.3. Urban Growth

A problem of growth closely related to that of total population is the movement of a large number of people to cities. In many underdeveloped countries the increase in large city populations has exceeded 200%, and it has been estimated that by 1990 over 80% of the world's population will live in heavily populated areas. The slums of Calcutta, Lima, and Mexico City, which are horrendous today, will become indescribable within a decade. The reason for this movement has defied explanation, for the migrants are usually worse off in cities than in the areas from which they migrated. The elusive promises of jobs or of government care, which instigated the heavy migration, have not been fulfilled by the governments involved, in part because this major, unusually rapid sociological change was unanticipated.

Every city's problems—municipal wastes, air pollution, water pollution, housing, schools, etc.—have become magnified beyond the city's ability to cope. The possible long-term effects of human crowding were examined in simulated laboratory conditions by overcrowding mice in an otherwise Utopian situation. Although the animals had food, water, and space in apparent abundance, when their unrestricted population growth reached approximately two-thirds the capacity of the environment, catastrophe occurred. With no apparent disease problem, populations fell drastically, and adverse behavior patterns developed. Perhaps extrapolation to the human situation is far fetched, but it must at least be considered. Humans have lived for very long periods in extremely crowded conditions, and in places such as Singapore the basic needs of the population have been provided surprisingly well. However, the "old" cities have attained these populations slowly. It is estimated that by the 1980s the population of 150 cities will have increased to 1×10^6 (and there will be 2000 such cities by the year 2000); these cities will lack the experience gained through 100 or more years of growth, and problems may develop more rapidly than governments can cope with them.

7.3. Causes of Overpopulation

The overpopulation problem that has rapidly developed is largely due to the gap between progress in health and progress in other areas of society. The death rate has been drastically reduced by all the miracles of modern medicine. The statistical increase in longevity is largely due to decreased infant mortality; if one excludes the figures on infant mortality, individuals in developed countries do not actually live significantly longer than their grandparents did. The ability to care for the large population resulting from adequate health care has temporarily kept pace with the rate of increase. A major malthusian check to population growth, necessary food, has been circumvented, largely by the import of food to areas unable to support their populations; thus hundreds of millions more people will reach child-bearing age.

The birth rate per se has not undergone a major change. People are no more amorous than they were 1000 years ago, when the birth rate was 40/1000, about that of many populations today. The developed countries experienced a slower rate of birth over a period of a few hundred years, so that their birth rate is now approximately 25/1000. However, health technology became available in the underdeveloped world over a comparatively short period, and only the death rate has been affected to any extent; a concomitant decline in birth rate is yet to be realized.

Extremists argue that the more developed countries should have placed severe restrictions on population growth in the less affluent countries: An increment of population control should have been a requirement for an increment of technology or food in the opinion of many.

7.4. Carrying Capacity of Earth

Some leaders do not believe that unrestricted population growth is a problem. The United Nations and other concerned bodies have made estimates of the human population the earth has the capacity to carry. It would be almost impossible to prevent a world growth to at least 10×10^9 persons as we will have a population of 6.5×10^9 by the year 2000, regardless of what is done. Given present resources, one must project the sort of sustenance that would be acceptable to that population. With every conceivable advantage in weather and technology, and a population willing to accept a minimum of food and shelter, the most extreme estimates have suggested that the world might even accommodate 40 billion. Whether or not such a world would still be called "civilized" is debatable.

7.5. Controversy of Population Stabilization

Both developed and underdeveloped countries have expressed alarm whenever population growth has been drastically curtailed or such curtailment has been suggested. Politics and racial discrimination are often elements of concern in stabilization programs. Adverse economic effects and problems associated with an aging population recently caused both Japan and Rumania to reverse growth declines.

The poorer the nation or ethnic group, the more there is to be gained by population stabilization. This seems irrefutable, but spokespersons for these countries and groups claim that such population limitations are favored by more powerful groups for the purpose of maintaining dominance.

Scholars and leaders of third world countries have expressed the suspicion that colonial and imperialistic countries are limiting population growth for nonaltruistic reasons. They believe that economic redistribution and reform will solve the problem over time, and lower growth rates will occur as a consequence, not a precondition, of economic development. The developed countries, however, started with favorable conditions for economic growth: for example, lower initial populations, ample natural resources, large-scale immigration, and ample time. As these conditions do not prevail in the less-developed countries, it may be unwise to expect economic development to occur there in a manner similar to the former situation.

7.6. Meeting the Population Crisis

The two primary ways to meet the population crisis appear to be an increased effort toward reducing growth (primarily a reduction in the birth rate) and adequate adjustments to produce the needed food.

7.6.1. Controlling Population Growth

Methods to control population seem to be available, for large segments of the population have been able to utilize them effectively. The dramatic changes made in urban China over the past two decades are ample proof that a decrease in population growth can be attained even in a relatively underdeveloped country. Few democratic nations would condone the methods necessary for this rapid change, for a disciplined population coupled with a highly autocratic government seems to be necessary. The governmental structure required to effect change is unlikely to be benevolent.

The primary methods of reducing population growth involve contraception, sterilization, and abortion. There are ethical concerns, however, that must be considered in the development of programs designed to control population growth. If people do not voluntarily choose not to have children, what is the next move? What administrative unit in a democratic society will decide which persons are permitted to be parents? Are coupons to be given each person at puberty entitling the holder to children? If so, can they be traded for other values? No person, government, or religion can answer these questions, and yet unchecked population growth may lead to this ethical dilemma.

Although it is perhaps too simplistic an explanation, the problems encountered in population control are due to custom (regarding social security), religion, and lack of education and minimal affluence. The first two factors are often closely interrelated.

7.6.1.a. Custom

For many hundreds of years large segments of populations, particularly in Asia, have survived in a social system in which the children ultimately care for the parents. Thus, production of children, especially males, has been encouraged as a positive mechanism for old age security. Prior to recent developments, an "extra" child was encouraged to ensure at least one living male. As death rates have lowered, the necessity for excess children has declined. This desirable change has not been in evidence for a sufficiently long period to be "trusted" by the producing populations, and the numbers of children being conceived have not decreased in accord with diminished necessity. Even the better educated members of these cultures seem committed to three children as a desired minimum. Without an adequate governmental social welfare system, it seems likely that continuance of "extra" births for "insurance" will be manifest for many years. In addition to the custom of high birth rate for the sake of security, in many areas of the world it is a sign of male virility. A man "must" have large families or lose esteem among his peers. Especially where adequate care cannot be provided, this is surely chauvinism in its most ludicrous form.

7.6.1.b. Religion

Although populations that have religious beliefs opposing direct birth control methods have been able to effect a low growth rate among highly educated groups (in Italy, for example), this is not the case in countries with poorly educated populations. The effect is most easily seen in South America, with its predominantly one-religion, anti-birth-control system. Many federal governments seem as unconcerned as the church in some instances. During the past 10 years the official policy of the Mexican government has been encouragement of births. Many other religions are just as opposed to reduction of the birth rate by direct methods as is the Roman Catholic Church.

7.6.1.c. Education

In addition to the closely related problems discussed above, which are perhaps related to inadequate education, the obvious lack of instruction of impoverished groups is a major cause of difficulty in population control. To aggravate the problem, in many heavily populated regions it is literally impossible to travel more than a few miles per day. Therefore, "carrying the word" to these people, even when they are receptive, is a major problem. It requires an extremely dedicated government and a critical mass of educated persons whose energies are solely directed to this important sociological problem, as in the People's Republic of China, where the growth rate is reported to have decreased from 2.3% to 1.8%, at least in urban areas, in less than two decades.

7.6.1.d. Minimal Affluence

Many knowledgeable experts are of the opinion that the ultimate solution to the population problem can only be achieved through an appropriate rise in the standard of living of the afflicted populations and improved health care. This viewpoint would appear to involve a self-contradiction, but recent experience has shown that birth rates do not decline until the food supply is assured, infant mortality is reduced, minimal literacy is attained, and at least rudimentary health services are available to make population growth predictable. Only then has there been any movement toward stabilization of population. Several factors complicate this well-advised approach, the primary one being time. It will take at least one decade for any underdeveloped country to reach a minimal state of affluence even under optimal availability of resources, education, and leadership. During this period populations will increase dramatically, making the realization of such goals even more difficult.

The only large populations able to lower growth rates rapidly in the past were Japan and the People's Republic of China, both of whom had characteristics of leadership, mass discipline, and education quite atypical of other societies.

Other countries that have managed desirable population changes have built the base for such changes over many decades. One UN report suggests that for a total cost of 6×10^9/year, significant world progress could be made in establishing the base needed for population control. Several countries spend this amount each month for defense.

7.6.2. Increased Food Production

It has been the hope of developing countries, and many well-placed persons in developed countries, that the carrying capacity of the earth is perhaps 5–10 times that of the present population. Examination of the rationale for this belief seems appropriate at this time, especially regarding the production of food. Increased pressure on global food supply will continue if substantial economic and social progress is not made. The two most practical ways to increase world food production are through expansion of agricultural lands and increased productivity (technology).

7.6.2.a. Expansion of Available Land

Until approximately the middle of the present century, expansion of cultivable land was the major way to attain increased food production. However, during the period 1950–1970, about one-fifth of the food increase was due to the addition of new land to production and four-fifths to new agricultural technology.

The two major areas of the world that have large land masses not in agricultural production are Africa and South America. For the most part these are heavily forested, tropical areas that have thus far defied attempts at large-scale agricultural use, although they can be used to sustain small populations of primitive people. When such areas are placed in cultivation, the topsoil becomes rapidly unproductive after a period of 2–3 years, and serious erosion can result if the land is poorly managed.

One must also recall that growing urban populations and technology per se have removed a significant amount of land, often the most productive land, from agricultural use. Perhaps the best example of such a loss in potential production is the southern California area, where millions of acres of fertile croplands have succumbed to urban sprawl.

Almost all agricultural experts agree that any discovery of additional land to be placed into agricultural production could make only a relatively insignificant contribution to production (barring scientific developments allowing the utilization of tropical and semitropical land masses).

7.6.2.b. Increased Productivity

The average yields from underdeveloped countries are considerably below those from developed countries (Figure 7.4). Good land in Japan may produce, on the average, six times as much as good land in India, in large part due to energy input. Obviously, world technology must make gigantic strides to adjust productivity on a more equitable basis. It required two decades of experience for agricultural technology experts from developed countries to realize that the substitution of methods from developed to underdeveloped countries is not a

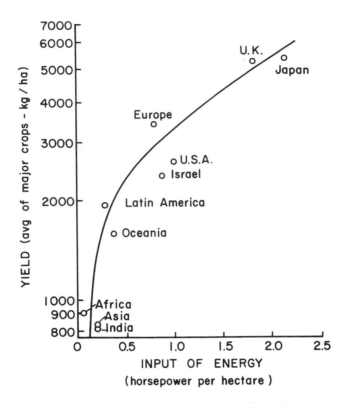

Figure 7.4   Relationship between crop yields and energy input. (Adapted from Turk, A., et al. Environmental Science. Philadelphia: W.B. Saunders, 1974.)

simple solution to complex problems. Only when these experts recognized that the methodology and culture of the developing countries had to be adapted to the new technology was progress made.

The "Green Revolution" that resulted in a large number of those previously production-poor areas showed that substantial progress can be made. New strains were developed that matured more rapidly and were less sensitive to day length, permitting two or more plantings per year in some situations. Yields were 25–100% higher in many areas than they had been in past decades, and India became self-sufficient in grain for the first time since World War II. Although some new problems have arisen (rich become richer, labor-saving devices cause unemployment, newer varieties are more prone to disease, fertilizer responses require capital, etc.), the new technology has at least kept pace with the rising population up to the present time. However, it must be noted that despite these examples, nonmodern, underdeveloped, land-short, and food-short countries are least capable of incorporating technology in agriculture, and grain yields in these countries are usually one-third those in more developed areas.

The Green Revolution has resulted in a dramatic increase in carbohydrate production, but a similar increase in high-protein crops has not been realized. Although there has been a dramatic world-wide increase in soybean production (a protein-rich grain, low only in methionine), the increment has often been due to substitution for other crops or the use of land removed from reserves. Soybean yields have increased only slightly, perhaps because soybean is a legume and not likely to respond to fertilization as dramatically as nonlegumes.

One must note, however, that as populations double within the next 30 or so years, certain realities of food production problems will be encountered.

Plateau of crop yields. Although initial gains from new varieties and other agricultural advances have been large for relatively small increments in technology, a plateau will eventually be reached (Figure 7.5).

Plateau of technological improvement. The cost of increased production rapidly reaches a point at which additional financial investment does not produce a corresponding increase in production.

Limitation of water. The water supply is rapidly becoming critically short. Population demands are in direct confrontation with a finite supply of water, particularly in certain areas of the world where water has always been in short supply.

Loss of cropland. In developing countries cropland has not yet been lost due to urbanization, but the recent losses in more affluent countries would appear to indicate such a loss will take place.

Energy shortage. The energy supply required for agricultural technology is becoming critically short. This is particularly true of petroleum, and the less developed countries with the larger populations will be the first to suffer from energy declines.

Figure 7.5 Relationship between technology and crop yield, illustrating diminishing gains.

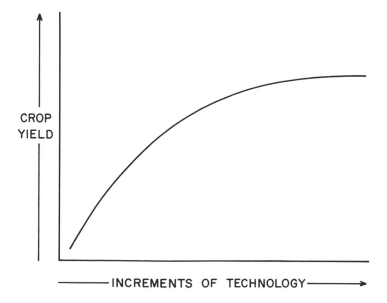

Fertilizer shortage. The shortage of fertilizer is partially associated with the pending shortage of energy (used to produce fertilizers), but also apparent is simply a shortage of resources. The new crop varieties require fertilizer if maximum yields are to be realized. If underdeveloped countries initiate fertilizer use at rates equal to those of developed countries, demand will exceed supply in the near future.

Ocean sources. The ocean has been considered to be a likely source of increased protein-rich food production. Thus far, a breakthrough in fish production has seemed unlikely. The harvest of ocean fish has actually been decreasing in recent years, and some countries that rely heavily on this source of food are expressing concern. Part of the problem concerns fish quality. If the less desirable fish were utilized, a sizable increase (perhaps 20%) in fish production could be immediately realized. Relatively little attention has been given to raising total fish production, and research to date in sizeable, controlled areas has not suggested that fish management would be more lucrative than other means of food production.

7.6.2.c. New Sources of Food and Food Fortification

The utilization of protein concentrates was tried with limited success during World War II. Although concentrates might be acceptable to persons living at marginal levels, they have little chance of acceptance by more affluent societies.

A number of other means of increasing essential food chemicals, both synthetic and natural, have been suggested. Utilization of wastes by microorganisms, or even directly by feeding wastes to animals, has been shown to be feasible. Although some increased production could be realized, the increment would be relatively minor, and some of the products would have questionable acceptance.

There are measures that could effect measurable changes in nutrition at the present time with better application of existing information. Where diets are adequate except for one or two essential ingredients (amino acids or vitamins), mass fortification of foods could be more judiciously practiced. This does not appear to be an insurmountable task, and the necessary educational and governmental programs could be realized with comparative ease in most countries.

Quantities of unused protein are wasted by many protein-poor populations. Many countries extract peanuts, coconuts, cotton seeds, etc. and discard a high-protein source of meal simply because their cultures are not adapted to this food source. Modifications here could appreciably affect short-term problems of nutrition.

Most populations can attain the necessary subsistence level for carbohydrates (approximately 2000 cal/day). On the other hand, the required level of protein (assuming appropriate essential amino acids) is 35 gr/day, and a large segment of the world population receives less than 20 g/day. In those countries (an estimated 1×10^9 persons), a high percentage of deaths of children under 5 years of age are directly traceable to malnutrition. A more subtle way of examining the problem is by comparing grain consumption in affluent and nonaffluent countries. People in affluent countries consume about one-fourth of their grain directly, and the remainder is used for indirect consumption through the production of animals and animal products. The food energy loss is, of course, tremendous, but the luxury of a more palatable diet is possible for the affluent. Less fortunate countries consume nearly the same amount of grain directly, but there is little to spare for conversion to animal feed.

It is cearly shown in Figure 7.6 that population increase rather than decreased food production is responsible for the pending nutrition problems. Although total food production has increased in both developed and underdeveloped countries, no substantial gains in food production per person have been seen where population growth has been high. On the other hand, in areas with low population growth greater total food production has allowed substantial improvements in individual diets.

Figure 7.6 Total (*solid line*) and per capita (*broken line*) food production as a reflection of population size. *Top:* Although total world food production has increased, per capita production has been less rapid. *Middle:* Economically developed countries with slow population increases show substantial gains in food per person. *Bottom:* In underdeveloped countries, where population growth rates are high, the availability of food per person has improved only slightly. (Adapted from Murdoch, W.W. (Ed.). Environment, second edition. Sunderland, Mass.: Sinauer Associates, p. 79, 1975.)

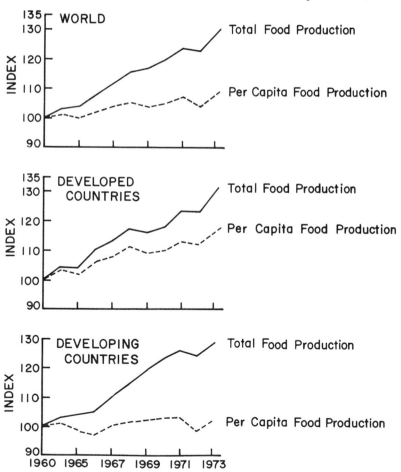

At the present time, the primary problem in providing food is the imbalance of food resources. There is presently no shortage of food, but the populations needing the food simply lack the monetary resources for purchase. It is a fact—sad, but true—that the majority of persons in developed countries are concerned about problems of obesity while some 1×10^9 persons in the world show signs of hunger or malnutrition.

7.6.3. Food Reserves

One alarming fact about food production that may be of importance, even for the present population, concerns reserves. Over the past decade the underdeveloped nations have barely been able to keep pace with food problems by increased agricultural technology. North America (and Australia and New Zealand to a less extent) has been able to back up grain production by maintaining a comfortable grain reserve (Table 7.2). However, the amount of land out of production (land bank) has steadily increased so that this valuable reserve has nearly disappeared (100 days reserve in 1960, 25 days in 1975). In the event of crop disasters in those countries with reserves (as might be expected to occur once or twice each century), the world food reserves would be lost within a year.

In addition to the concern for the food supply for the immediate decade (which we appear to be maintaining minimally at best), it is necessary to consider steps to prevent a disaster for the additional 2.5×10^9 persons expected by the early 21st century. Agricultural and industrial technologies have hidden costs that are usually overlooked in projections beyond the immediate future. Supplying large amounts of food to an uncontrolled population has both pollution and resource-depletion effects that may lead to environmental and economic disaster if limits are not defined. All aspects of agricultural technology (fertilizers, pesticides, petroleum, etc.) are inevitably related to toxic effects in the environment. The shipment of tremendous quantities of food from one continent to another will cause a measurable depletion of productivity due to loss of elements in time. Futhermore, the phenomenal success of American agriculture is based in part upon a huge input of fossil fuel. The energy required

Table 7.2 Pattern of World Grain Trade (t $\times$ 10⁶) 1930–1973

Region	1934–1938	1948–1952	1960	1973
North America	+ 5	+ 23	+ 39	+ 91
Latin America	+ 9	+ 1	0	− 3
Western Europe	− 24	− 22	− 25	− 19
Eastern Europe and USSR	+ 5	−	0	− 27
Africa	+ 1	0	− 2	− 5
Asia	+ 2	− 6	− 17	− 43
Australia and New Zealand	+ 3	+ 3	+ 6	+ 6

Source: Adapted from Murdoch, W.W. (Ed.). Environment, second edition. Sunderland, Mass.: Sinauer Associates, p. 88, 1975.

Symbols: +, net export; −, net import.

to produce some foods already appears to be greater than the energy derived therefrom.

7.6.4. Changing Pattern of Consumption

Populations in poor counties are sustained on 400 lb grain/year, whereas wealthier populations utilize nearly five times that amount, most of it indirectly through consumption of meat, eggs, and milk. A change in the consumption pattern of the latter population could make a sizable contribution to food conservation. The substitution of vegetable for animal fats and proteins holds much promise. Soya protein has been effectively substituted in many instances without a great outcry. High-protein vegetables could conceivably become an important source of protein with adequate education directed to effecting this needed change in consumption habits.

7.7. Summary

Many world leaders have not grasped the magnitude of the population problem. If the underdeveloped countries are not able to control populations within a few decades, an unimaginable degree of world-wide hunger may be commonplace. The great difficulty here lies in a struggle between time and the sharply rising population curve. One can perhaps envision the population doubling once, but a second population doubling seems untenable for persons accustomed to the standard of living enjoyed in Europe and North America; however, this seems quite likely to occur by the year 2050. If basic ecological concepts of population stability are as applicable to *Homo sapiens* as to other organisms, the steeply rising population curve will eventually become sigmoid. This leveling off, it is hoped, will be a reflection of man's superior intellect, not of such restraints as famine, disease, competition,and pollution.

In presenting this complex subject within a few pages, it is recognized that the viewpoint expressed may be both simplistic and pessimistic. For a more optimistic viewpoint, the reader is directed to the book by Bahr and colleagues.

Suggested Reading

Bahr, H. M., Chadwick, B. A., Thomas, D.L. Population, Resources, and the Future. Provo, Utah: Brigham Young University Press, 1974.

Calhoun, J. B. Population density and social pathology. Sci. Am. 206:139, 1962.

Davis, W. H. (Ed.). Readings in Human Population Ecology. Englewood Cliffs, N.J.: Prentice-Hall, 1971.

Food: A series of articles devoted to economics, nutrition, agricultural research and basic biology as they concern the world food problem. Science 188: 503, 1975.

Malthus, T. R. An Essay on the Principle of Population (1798). Middlesex, England: Penguin Books, 1970.

Murdoch, W. W. (Ed.). Environment, second edition. Sunderland, Mass.: Sinauer Associates, 1975.

Recheigl, M., Jr. (Ed.). Man, Food and Nutrition. Cleveland: CRC Press. 1973.

Treshow, M. The Human Environment. New York: McGraw-Hill, 1976.

Turk, A., Turk, J., Wittes, J. T., et al. Environmental Science. Philadelphia: Saunders, 1974.

Tuve, G. L. Energy, Environment, Population and Food. New York: Wiley, 1976.

George T. Barthalmus

8

Terrestrial Organisms

8.1. Introduction

Survival in terrestrial environments is a challenge. Seasonal changes, catastrophies such as flood, drought, fire, and earthquake, and disease, parasitism, famine, predation, and struggles for habitat and mates all probe the gene pool of populations for traits that will improve fitness and reproductive success. Pollutants are not unlike the above selection pressures in their impact on the gene pool. However, many chemicals synthesized via modern technology are new to all organisms, and species as well as ecosystems are challenged with pressures for which their long histories of evolution have no behavioral, physiological, or biochemical solutions. Excessive exposure to naturally occurring chemicals, frequent by-products of technology, is also an obvious threat to survival. When the above factors, plus loss of habitat, exert their impact on terrestrial species, it is surprising that extinction is not more commonplace. Terrestrial ecosystems are hardy—to a point.

Difficulties exist in determining the resilience of a species or ecosystem. Ecologists find it difficult to characterize the healthy ecosystem adequately (sometimes where healthy ecosystems do not exist). The monitoring of food webs and nutrient cycles, which is dependent upon effective sampling techniques, poses real and theoretical problems. Without confidence in these measurements, as well as adequate techniques for determining the presence and fate of contaminants, it is difficult to condemn any single chemical for declines in numbers of species and/or numbers within a given species. One merely has to witness courtroom proceedings centered on environmental impact statements to understand how emotions and inappropriate scientific investigations weaken the laws pertaining to environmental quality. When real estate, waterways, urbanization, and capital growth are weighed against wildlife habitat, scientific studies that characterize environmental impact cannot be conducted too carefully.

In this chapter some difficulties toxicologists encounter in formulating (and interpreting) data from field and laboratory studies are identified. The impact of pollutants on the components of terrestrial ecosystems are then examined. Finally, some of the effects of toxins on major taxonomic groups of vertebrates are discussed. Most of the studies discussed are centered on the effects of pesticides on terrestrial animal populations. However, hundreds of new chemicals, many of which are not pesticides, are introduced to a growing market each year. In addition, associated with new technologies are new by-products, some of which may be dangerous to wildlife. In preparing this chapter, it became clear that studies on nonagricultural chemicals have been neglected. In fact, field studies on the action of pesticides on animals are few and lack scope and methodological design. Research efforts to screen potentially dangerous compounds before their introduction into the environment are only now being developed.

8.2. Sampling Problems

Sampling vegetation is easier than sampling animal populations. Before sampling procedures and techniques are devised and employed to determine population size and the occurrence of agents in the tissues and other effects, one should be keenly familiar with the biology, ecology, and movements of the organisms to be sampled. The validity and interpretation of the sample data are dependent upon many factors in addition to the proverbial random sample. Are the animals migratory species, year-round residents, or nomadic? Do they have circadian feeding/activity rhythms? Are the bioenergetics of the species significantly variable by season and/or within a day? Was the usual food of the species scarce or abundant during the year of sampling and preceding years? Have there been harsh climatic conditions over the years in the sampling areas? Are the sampling techniques biased toward the capture of predominantly weaker or stronger individuals? If weaker animals dominate the sample one could easily overstate the toxicity of a chemical and/or one might find unusually high values of residues in the tissues. Capturing stronger individuals would tend to understate the toxicological problem. If a determination of the population size is the only datum desired as an index of good health, precautions must be taken not to conclude that live captures imply that exposure had no effect. Likewise, mere exposure of an animal to a pollutant does not guarantee an effect.

The point is that population fluctuations are expected even in healthy, uncontaminated habitats. The toxicologist should question whether fluctuations are the result of natural or unnatural causes. How else can one condemn a toxin for causing declines in population numbers and/or good health?

Many animals, particularly small mammals and birds, rely upon complexes of interacting biological and environmental factors to regulate their population size. For example, phytoestrogens are synthesized in the leaves of stunted desert annuals during a dry year. When eaten by California quail, the phytoestrogens apparently inhibit reproduction and prevent the production of young when adequate food would not be available. In a wet year, these plants grow vigorously, and very little of the estrogenic substances is produced. Quail then breed prolifically, and the abundant seed crop carries the enlarged population through winter. Ignorance of this interaction could lead a toxicologist to erroneous conclusions: that is, if a pesticide was sprayed on desert annuals at the onset of a dry season (when phytoestrogens are heavily synthesized), one might erroneously conclude, following population sampling, that the decline in numbers was caused by the pesticide. Detectable quantities of pesticide residues in the tissues might further incriminate the toxic agent.

Other sources of error and misinterpretation of data arise when residues in trapped and/or dead specimens are being measured. Some studies report tissue residue values on a wet weight (fresh weight) basis, while others are based upon dry weights. The inconsistency in units of measurement reported makes it difficult to compare and/or pool data, since usually greater than 70% of the water is removed for dry weight determinations. Therefore, dry weight samples contain three to four times more toxin. Furthermore, the tissues analyzed often vary between studies, making certain comparisons very difficult; for example, when organochlorine content is determined, the ratio of body fat to total body weight is important, since fat is a preferred site of organochlorine deposition. Similarly, when specimens are found dead in the field and are brought to the laboratory for residue analyses, the extent of dehydration is a major factor contributing to inflated levels of toxin found. Therefore, it is essential to compare these data with those obtained from fresh samples taken in the original habitat where the carcasses were found. The carcass may not always show inflated values; in fact, these values may be lower or negligible when compared with data on freshly killed animals. One reason is that a given pollutant may be metabolized after death, often to the point of leaving no residues. Therefore, we need to look at the activity of the enzymes these toxins affect.

Often, only one or a few carcasses are found, thus restricting adequate statistical analyses. Even residue data from animals exposed under controlled laboratory conditions have been questionable, since too few replicate determinations were made for each tissue. There are often notable variations between laboratories in the amounts of residues reported. Reasons can be traced to the experience of the residue specialist, the equipment and reagent quality used, and the number of replicate determinations made.

8.3. The Ecosystem

In 1971, approximately 1×10^9 lb of pesticides were applied to control some 2000 pest species. Unfortunately, less than 1.0% contacted the target organisms. In fact, frequently as little as 25–50% of the pesticide descends onto the crop area when applied by aircraft. The hazard to nontarget species is obvious, since 65% of all agroinsecticides are applied by aircraft. If chemicals were directed solely at the target pests, with no secondary intoxication, there would be less of a pollution problem with pesticides.

An analysis of how pollutants affect ecosystems is dependent upon a thorough understanding of the healthy, evolving ecosystem. Moreover, although not all pollutants are toxic, important effects may be noted. For example, ecosystems may change drastically when excessive nutrients (eutrophication) are available to producer organisms. The contaminants may exert an effect on consumer organisms only indirectly by altering the species diversity and numbers of the autotrophs. The species composition and density of producers largely determines species diversity and the number of consumer organisms by influencing the level of organic nutrients available, soil composition and chemistry, nutrient cycling, leaching, erosion, and physical habitat. Consequently, slight alterations in plant community structure can significantly affect all aspects of an ecosystem.

When the source of pollution is removed, ecosystems usually cleanse themselves. However, when contamination is chronic, or severe over a short period, one can expect two general effects on an ecosystem: (a) The loss of species tend to simplify the community by reducing the number of niches and trophic levels, and by reducing the ecological efficiency by which energy moves through the food chain. Community stability is undermined, and the abiotic components of the ecosystem exert greater control over the biotic components; consequently, one sees a loss of maturity and what might be considered a reversal of the community's succession toward the climax stage. (b) The ratio of photosynthesis to respiration is often reduced as the larger plants tend to lose their foliage, taking away primary photosynthetic sources and leaving the respiratory tissues of the stems, trunks, and bark intact. In general, smaller plants survive best in these situations, and the community changes are reflected in the variety and number of animals in the area and in the characteristics of the soil. Industrial chemical fallout in the form of sulphur dioxide or sodium sulfate has produced gradients of the above-mentioned effects.

8.3.1. Opportunism

Species that are intense exploiters of disturbed polluted areas are frequently hardy, broadly adapted species with great reproductive potential. Such animals (house sparrows, starlings, herring gulls, rats, and mice) usually have varied diets, while plants are easily classified as (or are similar to) weed species. Undesirable herbivorous animals frequently increase their numbers to outbreak levels after a toxin disappears from the affected ecosystems. Plants may adapt quickly to the effects of pollutants. Their adaptive responses to lead contamination along roadsides and around ore mining sites and smelters provide an excellent example of evolution in action. For example, the fact that lead tolerance develops along roadsides, but not in areas distant from roads, suggests that lead levels were sufficiently high to impose selection pressure for the evolution of tolerance in sensitive plant species. Consequently, what may appear to be a normal unaffected population of *Plantago lancelata* L. (ribwort plantain) growing on and off roadsides could really be two strains of this species, one tolerant and one intolerant.

8.3.2. Terrestrial Food Chains

The biomagnification of persistent, fat-soluble toxins is a particularly hazardous trait of food chains. This process has been misunderstood in the aquatic environment, where movement up the food chain is correlated with increasing levels of toxin. Here, bioaccumulation is not always a food chain effect; rather, the amount entering an animal may be a function of the volume of water passing over the highly vascularized gas exchange organs. The quantities stored are related directly to the lipid content, which frequently increases with the age and size of the animal. Although the large concentration factors between trophic levels may not be caused by predation of one organism by another, the fact that the toxins are in high concentration when the organism is eaten aggravates the toxic effect.

Bioaccumulation of toxins in terrestrial ecosystems is also well documented as a food chain effect. In this setting, carnivorous birds and mammals are affected more than herbivores. Mortality, population declines, and residue analyses support this supposition. Although carnivores are more heavily exposed through the food chain, it is not the higher concentrations alone that produce this effect. Herbivores exposed to doses of toxin that are lethal to carnivores are often unaffected. Chronic exposure of raccoons to 2 ppm dieldrin causes reproductive failure and may cause death, yet deer fed 25 ppm show only marginal effects. Doses of DDT and DDE (an impurity of Technical DDT) that have little affect on pheasants may kill kestrels. These differences in effect probably reflect physiological differences. Intestinal symbionts may assist herbivores in metabolizing toxins. The greater rate of pollutant loss in herbivores compared with carnivores, and the fact that eggshell thinning in herbivorous birds is rare compared with that in carnivores, suggests distinct differences in physiological tolerance and detoxification mechanisms. Even predaceous soil invertebrates are more readily killed by pesticides than are herbivores. Naturally, when the number of predators is reduced, one can expect outbreaks of herbivorous pests that attack crops. The problems encountered when pesticides are not used in maximal harmony with the agroecosystem are discussed in Chapter 22.

Numerous reports indicate that a major threat to raptorial birds, mammals, and invertebrates often arises shortly after pesticide application. Struggling target and nontarget worms, grubs, and insects attract predators that gorge themselves at a time when the prey is maximally toxic. Often, granivorous birds join the feeding frenzy.

Earthworms, with insecticide residues that often average nine times those of the soil, serve as a major route by which birds are killed. In DDT-treated areas earthworms contained 33–164 ppm DDT and 14–59 ppm DDE (dry weight). A 9-year study suggested that DDT residues pass from forest soil to earthworms and then to robins, a relationship that may persist for as long as 30 years. The older pesticides have had little impact on earthworm populations; however, their substitutes, such as chlordane, phorate, and carbaryl, are particularly lethal to earthworms. The carbamate, carbofuran, and the organophosphate, fensulfothion, are also toxic and may persist for 4 or more weeks in the soil. Copper-based fungicides are often used specifically to kill earthworms on golf courses.

Soil organisms, both micro- and macroinvertebrates, as well as microflora are essential as reducers and decomposers of organic litter. These organisms are differentially sensitive to heavy metals and various persistent and nonpersistent pesticides. Although their numbers may be reduced drastically in the early weeks and months following application, most authorities conclude that there is little evidence that microflora, soil animals, and soil fertility have been adversely affected. However, the most serious problem is in natural ecosystems, where toxic agents may interfere with processes of decay and soil formation.

8.4. Vertebrates

Precensus and postcensus determinations of the effects pollutants have on the health and population dynamics of terrestrial vertebrates are few. Studies on amphibians and reptiles are essentially nonexistent; most data are based upon casual observations incidental to other investigations. Most studies center on birds and mammals; however, too much emphasis has been placed upon agrochemicals alone. Unfortunately, important data from the many environmental impact studies conducted by consulting companies are not easily obtained or are not reported in scientific journals. Such investigations are usually designed to demonstrate precisely what is lacking in the literature—pre- and postcensus population measurements.

8.4.1. Amphibians

Amphibians are highly susceptible to pollutants due to three important factors: (a) the toxicant is poorly diluted in shallow waters; (b) the diluents and solvents used to disperse toxicants (e.g., pesticides) are especially toxic as they penetrate the permeable and highly vascularized amphibian skin; and (c) oil-laden insects struggling on the surface may also be eaten. Therefore, toxicosis may result from both oral and dermal exposures. These problems are heightened when temporary ditches, pools, and ponds are exposed to toxins. As water evaporates, the contaminants are concentrated. Additional stress results as these waters heat and the biochemical oxygen demand increases. For these reasons, larval forms are particularly vulnerable.

The extensive fat bodies in amphibians, combined with their low to moderate sensitivity to pollutants, causes them to accumulate large residues of potentially toxic chemicals. Delayed mortality in tadpoles exposed to DDT may occur when they metabolize stored fat during metamorphosis. Small tadpoles are more susceptible to these effects than larger ones. Unfortunately, most of the observations of pesticide effects on amphibians are made casually in the course of other studies.

Some laboratory studies, although neither comparable nor applicable to the field, have been helpful. For example, tadpoles of the western chorus frog (*Pseudacris triseriata*) and Fowler's toad (*Bufo woodhousii fowleri*) showed greater susceptibility to dieldrin, endrin, methoxychlor, DDD, carbophenothion, and malathion than to DDT. Methoxychlor has been shown to be more toxic than heptachlor and aldrin for a 96-hr exposure of toad tadpoles; however, all cyclodiene insecticides are more toxic than methoxychlor for a 30-day exposure of adult leopard frogs (*Rana pipiens*) fed periodically on uncontaminated food. Cyclodienes induce hyperresponsiveness to stimuli, followed by convulsions in frogs. Fowler's toads and cricket frogs (*Acris crepitans*), exposed for 36-hr to filter paper impregnated with insecticide, were susceptible to organochlorines in the following descending order: endrin > dieldrin > aldrin > toxaphene > DDT. Tests of mosquito larvicides at a concentration of 0.4 lb/acre on tadpoles of the bullfrog (*Rana catesbeiana*) and western toad (*Bufo boreas*) showed that carbophenothion caused 100% mortality, while azinphosmethyl, parathion, naled, fenitrothion, ronnel, and trichloronat caused no deaths. Parathion at 1.0 lb/acre kills most mosquitofish but is harmless to juvenile bullfrogs. Frogs, toads, snakes, and salamanders were unaffected in a New York forest sprayed with carbaryl at 1.25 lb/acre.

Salamanders (*Ambystoma tigrinum*) collected from a Texas pond polluted with polycyclic hydrocarbons were found to have high levels of aryl hydrocarbon hydroxylase (AHH), a hepatic enzyme of the microsomal mixed-function oxygenase group. The high AHH levels were correlated with high rates of spontaneous cancer. In another study, *A. tigrinum* taken from a polluted pond also had high levels of AHH. In 1970, 1 salamander in a sample of 2430 contained obvious abnormal tissue growth; by 1971, approximately 25% had abnormalities. This number increased to 40% by 1974. The highly invasive and malignant melanoma occurred at a rate of 1.0%/year with at least 10% of the second year salamanders exhibiting the carcinoma.

8.4.2. Reptiles

There are fewer toxicological field studies on reptiles than on amphibians. Pesticide studies dominate the literature; however, observations of pesticide effects are casually made in the course of other investigations. Reptiles appear less sensitive to insecticides than amphibians. Presumably, the heavily keratinized integument, coupled with respiration entirely through the lungs, provides protection that is in sharp contrast to the thin, permeable, well-vascularized skin of amphibians.

DDT concentrations of 2 ppm or greater have killed turtles and water snakes. A deciduous forest sprayed with 1 lb/acre DDT killed few water snakes; box turtle populations were unaffected when sprayed with DDT at 2 lb/acre for 5 consecutive years. Amphibians and reptiles of northern deciduous forests sprayed with malathion at 2 lb/acre and carbaryl at 1.25 lb/acre were unaffected. Water snakes, cottonmouths, and copperheads were unaffected when Louisiana woodlands were sprayed with phosphamidon at 1 lb/acre or dicrotophos at 0.25 lb/acre. Residues in the fat bodies of water snakes, exposed to various pesticides applied to a Texas agricultural flood plain, revealed that the common water snake retained the highest residues (ppm) of DDE (590), DDD (3.3), and DDT (20.4). The ribbon snake contained the highest concentration of dieldrin (8.9). DDT residues in the brain did not exceed 1.5 ppm. Residues in terrestrial snakes were significantly lower than in aquatic snakes. Residues of heptachlor epoxide as high as 172 ppm have been found in turtles (*Pseudemys*). These and other data suggest that such residue concentrations pose a serious threat to the terrestrial food chain. Consequently, agricultural areas may suffer from outbreaks of rodent and insect pests normally controlled by snakes and carnivorous birds.

8.4.3. Birds

Birds appear to be somewhat tolerant to low ambient levels of pollutants, even with chronic exposure. Nevertheless, experts are concerned with the effects of pollutants, especially pesticides, for the following reasons: (a) High mortality continues to occur in conjunction with heavy pollution. Contaminated areas accumulate potentially lethal levels of residues of heavy metals, polychlorinated biphenyls (PCBs), and numerous other agro- and industrial chemicals. (b)

Carnivores accumulate high residue levels by biomagnification through food chains. Carnivorous species suffer from higher mortality and reproductive failure rates than herbivorous species. Many local, state, and continental populations are endangered. (c) In general, the loss of wildlife habitat greatly enhances the loss of species and numbers within species by reducing adequate reproductive ranges and by forcing birds and mammals to live closer to urban sources of contamination.

8.4.3.a. Eggshell Thinning

It is now accepted that DDE is the primary pollutant implicated in eggshell thinning in numerous bird species. The controversy that shell thinning caused the population declines of peregrine falcons, sparrow hawks, Cooper's hawk, ospreys, bald eagles, golden eagles, brown pelicans, and others is a classic example of how inappropriate experimentation, inadequate residue sampling, poor historic population records, and varying species sensitivity to pollutants can lead to premature, often emotional, claims of cause and effect. This brief discussion is not intended to promote the continued use and development of persistent pesticides such as DDT (nor to decriminate them); rather, the discussion should serve to alert the reader to the need for better methodologies and more detailed population surveys, since future banning of chemicals will require irrefutable evidence in courts of law.

Studies reported in 1967 and 1968 provided evidence that British and American raptors had been suffering population declines since 1947, shortly after DDT came into common use. Since 1967, shell thinning has been noted in at least 54 species of birds. The many early investigations were misleading, since shells of eggs from chickens, quail, grouse, finches, doves, and other granivorous species were studies that exhibited no thinning in the field and little or no thinning in the laboratory. Despite the risk of obtaining data that are inapplicable to the sensitive species, research continues on the herbivorous birds, largely because they are available.

Regional differences in shell thickness were reported. For example, eggs of eastern brown pelicans had a thicker, heavier shell when found on the Florida Gulf coast than on the Atlantic coast. No explanation of this difference has been reported. Furthermore, the shell of eggs of some birds vary in thickness with the kind of ground upon which they are laid. The early interpretations of the correlation of eggshell thickness with residue analyses proved difficult. Often, PCB content equalled DDE content; therefore, it became difficult to place the blame exclusively on DDE. Interpretation was difficult because many scientists who analyzed for DDE failed to report the concentrations of other pollutants in the egg. Some studies showed positive correlations of shell thickness with mercury content; others demonstrated negative correlations with residues of DDE, DDT, DDD, dieldrin, and PCBs. However, DDE was consistently associated with significant thinning. Many studies showing a positive correlation were criticized for lack of statistical treatment and the fact that some eggs tested were partly incubated (incubated eggs lose some shell thickness). Moreover, some data showing a negative correlation between DDE content and shell thickness were not reported; some accused scientists of withholding data so that DDT would be banned. Some laboratory studies may have shown positive correlations because the birds were calcium deprived. Those birds given extra calcium had no shell problems. Similar studies produced conflicting results. For example, in one study, lindane at 100 mg/kg in chickens had no effect, while in another study, 0.1 mg/kg did produce shell thinning.

Laboratory studies have shown that a variety of pesticides can cause shell thinning (some cause shell thickening); however, there are no data that clearly implicate these chemicals in natural populations. The correlations of DDT levels in museum specimens, obtained before and after 1945, with population estimates during the years of collection are not always incriminating. First, U.S. population records are poor, and some experts believe that only large-scale declines in numbers would be noticeable. Second, a number of the implicated species had shown population declines before 1945. The osprey showed strong declines for a century; the peregrine falcon, since about 1932. In one study, a stable population of peregrine falcons in Canada had twice the levels of chlorinated hydrocarbons than the declining populations of British peregrines. This is not easily explained. Moreover, British populations of peregrine falcons increased rapidly from 1945 for several years, yet thin eggshells were reported in 1946 and were maximally affected in 1948.

The data for eagle populations are also confusing, since reports in 1921 and 1943 draw attention to the possible extinction of bald eagles as evidenced by declining population numbers. Bounties in Alaska and several western states total 120,000 eagles over the past 40 years. Between 1960 and 1968, the Patuxent Wildlife Research Center (Maryland) examined 147 eagles found dead in the United States. Only 9 were suspected of having died as a result of pesticide poisoning.

Although pesticides are implicated, a truly clear picture of avian reproductive failure in nature as a direct result of any chemical is not at hand. When one considers the reproductive requirements and habits of most birds of prey, the widespread slaughter for "fun," sport, or bounty, and the encroachment on their prime nesting sites by growing human populations, it is easy to account for endangered bird populations without consideration of the influence of agrochemicals.

8.4.3.b. Heavy Metals

Many studies, some as early as 1874, have reported wild waterfowl mortality due to heavy metals, particularly lead poisoning. These investigations were concerned with poisoning from lead shotgun pellets either directly introduced into the flesh of birds or by ingestion in the form of spent lead shot picked up from the bottom of lakes and streams as feed or gizzard grit. Lead intoxication of wild birds is a very serious problem; in fact, lead toxicosis causes more deaths in whistling swans than avian tuberculosis, coccidiosis, idiopathic impaction of the proventriculus, botulism, aspergillosis, or filariasis. A study at the Bitter Lake National Wildlife Refuge, New Mexico, determined that 59% of 162 soil samples taken randomly contained 1–5 lead shots. A minimum lead shot incidence of 98,985 shots/hectare (40,075/acre) was calculated. A further indication of how hunting practices involving lead shot contributed to bird mortality was reported in Tennessee. Biologists collected 1949 gizzards from mourning doves harvested on fields managed for public hunting. One percent of the doves had ingested between 1 and 24 lead shots. Pre- and posthunt soil samples, collected from a field with an 8-year history of dove management revealed that the top 0.38 in. soil contained 10,890 shots/acre before hunting and 43,560 shots/acre after hunting.

Birds affected by lead include bobwhite quail, pheasant, mourning doves, scaled quail, Canada geese, mallard and pintail ducks, pigeons, and the Andean condor. Wildlife biologists have recommended that lead shot pellets be replaced by steel pellets; however, hunters have complained that steel shot lacks the killing power of the denser lead shot.

Although methylmercury is no longer used as a seed dressing in Sweden, the United States, and numerous other countries, its use in Sweden during the 1960s caused mortality among mammals and seed-eating birds. Very serious secondary poisoning was seen in predators. The more serious problem with mercury was later traced to industrial effluent. Laboratory studies with birds have shown that mercury (a) potentiates the toxicity and biochemical effects of parathion, (b) affects reproduction by increasing embryonic and juvenile mortality and by reducing egg laying, and (c) affects approach–avoidance behavior as well as operant behaviors (quail and pigeons).

There are no examples of terrestrial wildlife being harmed by industrial arsenic pollution. However, deer and livestock have been killed after licking sodium arsenite from vegetation. Apart from the effects arsenic may have on humans occupationally exposed, many arsenic compounds are of low toxicity; in fact, arsenic has many medicinal uses. The most persistent arsenicals have a half-life in the body of only 60 hr. Copper acetoarsenite (Paris green) is used extensively in mosquito control because it is a highly selective larvicide that affects almost no organisms other than mosquito larvae. Accumulation of arsenic and copper is negligible in birds exposed to doses of Paris green higher than those they would encounter in nature. Wildlife biologists are concerned that unfounded fears could deprive us of one of the safest chemicals for mosquito control.

8.4.3.c. Polychlorinated Biphenols

The widespread distribution of PCBs in the environment and their effect on animal populations are matters of growing concern. PCBs are readily taken up by animal tissue and, like DDT and other lipid-soluble chemicals, accumulate in adipose tissue. In dosed birds, the highest PCB level is found in adipose tissue, followed by kidney, liver, brain, muscle, and blood. The lethal dietary toxicity of most Aroclors (trade name for PCBs) to experimental birds generally is less than that of DDE, DDT, or dieldrin. The reproductive effects are apt to have the most serious impact on bird and mammal populations; however, these effects are difficult to evaluate. The major reproductive effects in chickens are reduced egg production and hatchability. Also seen are deformities in chicks and depressed growth rates of young. No eggshell thinning has been shown in chickens, bobwhite quail, ringdoves, and mallards after low dietary exposure to PCBs. Residues in wild birds frequently are at concentrations known to have caused reproductive failure in chickens. When ringdoves were exposed to 10 ppm Aroclor 1245 during two generations, the reproductive success of the first generation was normal, but reproduction of the second generation was greatly reduced. Caged European robins fed PCBs showed increased migratory activity.

Similar effects have been seen in redstarts. The embryonic mortality of ringdoves may have resulted from reduced parental attentiveness. The above effects are not caused by all PCBs, nor are all species of birds equally sensitive.

8.4.4. Mammals

The effects of pollutants on wild mammals are not well understood for several reasons: (a) many reports of dead mammals are not published; (b) perhaps the more toxic commonly used organophosphate and carbamate insecticides are too short lived in the field, and in tissues, to kill appreciable numbers of mammals; and (c) many dead mammals are overlooked because they are secretive, are scarce, and/or range widely. For animals that range widely, exposure to a small contaminated area would be minimal.

Mammals can be killed by heavy applications of dieldrin, endrin, toxaphene, heptachlor, and azodrin. Dieldrin applied at 3 lbs/acre in Illinois resulted in extensive, well-documented deaths of nontarget species in the vicinity of application. Farm cats, ground squirrels, muskrats, and rabbits were effectively eliminated, and major losses were encountered in populations of short-tailed shrews, fox squirrels, woodchucks, and meadow mice. The whitefooted mouse (*Peromyscus*) was more resistant to dieldrin. Sheep in a nearby area were killed when dieldrin drifted across a road. The affected wildlife population showed substantial recovery 1 year later. In other studies, many British foxes died of secondary dieldrin poisoning by eating dead wood pigeons and other animals that had consumed dressed seed wheat. Cottontail rabbits that survive dieldrin poisoning breed normally; however, this is not true of dogs and raccoons. Some species of antelope that store little fat have been killed by small quantities of dieldrin and photodieldrin.

The use of heptachlor for control of fire ants in the southern United States killed a variety of mammals including raccoons, skunks, armadillos, opossums, nutria, rabbits, cotton and rice rats, and some mice. However, repopulation was rapid in the early years after treatment.

Since small mammals such as mice of the genera *Peromyscus*, *Microtus*, and *Mus* are very common and easily collected, biologists suggested that they might be ideal indicators of pesticide effects. Unfortunately, studies have shown the reverse to be true. The ubiquitous and abundant populations of *Peromyscus* are surprisingly resistant to dieldrin, Diazinon, endrin, heptachlor, parathion, methylparathion, aldrin, and DDT. An explanation for the tolerance observed arose from studies in which rates of loss of DDT were determined for *Peromyscus*, wild *Mus*, and laboratory *Mus*. It was known earlier that thousands of ppm of dietary DDT is withstood by *Peromyscus*, while DDT tracking powder controls common house mice. Loss rates for DDT, expressed as mean half-times for males, were 3.7 days for *P. leucopus*, 3.0 days for *P. maniculatus*, 3.8 days for laboratory mice, and 5.5 days for wild *Mus*.

The sublethal effects on wild populations are difficult to determine and are not well understood. However, field studies conducted on *Microtus* and *Peromyscus* exposed to 0.5 endrin lb/acre revealed differential long-term toxicological effects on *Peromyscus* but not on *Microtus*. Immediate and significant postspray declines in *Microtus* numbers occurred on the experimental plot, but no long-term effects were noted. The *Microtus* population rapidly recovered and in 2 years exceeded the prespray number and the corresponding control number in all 3 years of the study. It was suggested that reduced numbers and the presumed decrease in intraspecific aggression disrupted the social structure such that normal regulation of numbers was not possible.

Bat populations have declined significantly in recent years, and much evidence supports the hypothesis that pesticides are responsible. The Mexican free-tailed bat (*Tadarida brasiliencsis*) is a migratory and colonial species that migrates north from wintering areas in Mexico to maternity roosts in the southwestern United States. In the late 1950s and early 1960s, about 150 million bats were living in 20 colonies. Before the southward migration in October, this population would eat more than 18,000 metric tons of insects; clearly, they are important in pest control. However, populations at Carlsbad Caverns, New Mexico, declined from an estimated 8.7×10^6 in 1936 to 200,000 in 1973; the population at Eagle Creed Cave, Arizona, fell from 25×10^6 in 1964 to 6×10^5 in 1970. Pesticide residues in these bats showed no cause-and-effect relationship. Later, research indicated that the organochlorine (DDE, DDD, DDT, and dieldrin) residues in the fat of young free-tailed bats reached the brain and caused symptoms of poisoning after fat mobilization that took place during simulated migratory flight. Starved and exercised younger bats, containing more fat, contained 43 times more DDE in the brain than a reference group of bats (3.7 ppm) trapped and killed before migration. Exercised older bats containing less fat had brain DDE levels 123 times that of the control reference group (1.3 ppm). Consequently, low concentrations of residue in fat is deceiving, since migratory stress increases the blood and brain level many times. Other studies with big brown bats (*Eptesicus fuscus*) fed the PCB Aroclor 1254 revealed that PCB increased in brains of starving bats as carcass fat was mobilized. However, during starvation, PCB-dosed bats lost weight significantly more slowly than controls. It was suggested that PCBs may slow metabolic rates.

Marine mammals off the shores of industrial nations frequently contain high residues of DDT, DDE, mercury, and PCBs. Seals (*Phoca vitulina*) from the Dutch coast contained PCBs in concentrations that ranged from 385 to 2530 ppm (wet weight) in blubber and from 13 to 89 ppm in the brain. Mercury levels in the liver (257–326 ppm) and the brain (9.6–30 ppm) were high. However, healthy seals had 40–218 ppm mercury in liver. In fact, organs of dolphins and porpoises from other areas have similar levels of mercury. Consequently, it is difficult to determine whether mercury or PCBs are responsible for deaths. Mercury may be responsible, since a sick seal (*Pusa hispida saimensis*) in Finland was found to be ataxic and contained 197 ppm mercury in muscle and 210 ppm in liver—levels that could cause ataxia.

Much attention was directed toward marine mammals in 1973 when sea lions were studied off southern California. Sea lions produced a small number of premature young, most of which died. Residue analyses identified several times more DDT and PCBs in the blubber and liver of affected females than of normal females. The brains of premature pups had more DDT and PCBs than those of normal pups. Of interest was the determination that the percentages of fat in livers of affected (1.7) and normal females (4.4), and in brains of pups (3.3 in affected, 4.8 normal) suggested that fat depletion may have been a more important factor than the residues present. A definite explanation of this situation is not yet at hand.

The importance of recognizing the differential sensitivity between species to pollutants is well illustrated by a problem that mink ranchers of the Great Lakes region faced in the middle 1960s. Ranchers claimed that Great Lakes fish fed to mink caused reduced reproduction. Researchers substituted Coho salmon from Lake Michigan as food for mink; the mortality of newborn mink (kit) increased dramatically. Rancidity, chlorinated hydrocarbons, and mercury poisoning were suspected. Other studies revealed that increasing the dietary percentage of Coho salmon to breeder mink resulted in increased embryonic death or kit mortality. Other Great Lakes fishes caused reproductive failure (but to a less extent). Rancidity and mercury contamination of various fish were discounted as causative factors; however, hydrocarbon pesticide contamination (total DDT isomers or dieldrin) of fish food was inversely related to the number of mink born per female. These curious results may have been related to the fat content of the fish. However, when diets containing excessive amounts of DDT and isomers or dieldrin failed to produce the effects seen when mink were fed salmon, the problem attracted much attention.

Because PCBs were known to contaminate Lake Michigan and its fishes, PCBs were studied. When adult female mink were fed a control diet containing 30% oceanic fish, the same diet but with 30% Coho salmon, or the control diet plus 30 ppm PCBs (10 ppm each of Aroclors 1242, 1248, and 1254), the latter two diets resulted in no births. In addition all females fed supplemental PCBs died by the end of the normal birthing (whelping) period. Those that survived showed no signs of whelping. No controls died. The PCB tissue residues in organs of mink that died were strikingly similar in the two diets. Brain contained nearly twice the levels of most other organs. Other experiments determined that 10 ppm Aroclor 1254, when fed continuously to growing mink, depressed growth rates. An extension of the same study revealed that raw or cooked Coho salmon and 15 ppm PCB totally inhibited reproduction, while 5 ppm PCB markedly reduced reproduction. With 1.0 ppm PCB, only a slight reduction in reproduction was seen. The addition of DDT and dieldrin to the 5 ppm PCB diet produced no synergistic effects.

The above studies focus on the acute effects of PCBs (reproductive failure, death, and ataxia). The possible impact of PCBs on humans, considering the knowledge that affected birds and mammals display signs of neurotoxicity, becomes alarming when complex behavioral disruptions are seen in the off-spring of female rhesus monkeys fed PCB (Aroclor 1248). Eight monkeys fed 2.5 ppm PCB in their daily diet conceived, delivered, and nursed five infants, three of which survived past weaning at 4 months of age. The exposure period terminated at the end of 3 months. Residues in the fat of infants at 8, 10.5, and 23 months of age declined linearly when plotted as log concentration versus time. These functions extrapolated to peak levels of 21, 114, and 123 μg/g fat at 4 months of age. Behavioral tests on these infants and controls revealed hyper-locomotor activity at 6 and 12 months of age. This behavior correlated with peak PCB body burdens. Higher PCB burdens also correlated with increased errors in five of 9 learning tasks conducted between 8 and 24 months of age. Even the monkey carrying only 21 ppm PCB at 4 months of age exhibited some behavior deficits that persisted through the final tests at 24 months of age.

About one-third of all Americans contain measurable residues of PCBs. Studies such as that of the rhesus monkeys exposed chronically to PCBs *in utero* and in mother's milk draw attention to a possible mode by which PCBs may affect human populations. Similar behavioral deficits in humans will be difficult to determine in infants and toddlers. By the time effects are noted, the damage may have been done to the young, developing nervous system.

8.5. Conclusions

Although environmental contamination has taken its toll on terrestrial wildlife, and it continues to do so today, some brighter considerations should be recognized and supported. First, the majority of species appear to be flourishing and multiplying where physical habitat is not limiting. Second, residue levels of persistent pesticides in the environment are on the decline. Third, public awareness has prompted the establishment of legal and regulatory government agencies that deal with environmental toxins in a positive and unprecedented manner. These points are encouraging, for they provide the incentive to seek answers to the difficult problems yet unsolved. Hopefully, the careful screening of new chemicals and the development of new industrial manufacturing procedures that pollute less will eliminate the majority of deleterious substances in the environment.

Suggested Reading

Antonovics, J., Bradshaw, A. D., Turner, R. G. Heavy metal tolerance in plants. Adv. Ecol. Res. 84:1–85, 1971.

Bowman, R. E., Heironomus, M. P., Allen, J. R. Correlation of PCB body burden with behavioral toxicology in monkeys. Pharmacol. Biochem. Behav. 9:49–56, 1978.

Brown, A. W. A. Ecology of Pesticides. New York: Wiley, 1978.

Cooke, A. S. Response of *Rana temporaria* tadpoles to chronic doses of p,p'-DDT. Copeia 4:647–652, 1973.

Cooke, A. S. Shell thinning in avian eggs by environmental pollutants. Environ. Pollut. 4:85–102, 1973.

DeLong, R. L., Gilmartin, W. G., Simpson, J. G. Premature births in California sea lions: Association with high organochlorine pollutant residue levels. Science 181:1168–1169, 1973.

Edwards, C. A., Thompson, A. R. Pesticides and the soil fauna. Residue Rev. 45:1–79, 1973.

Geluso, K. N., Altenbach, J. S. Bat mortality: Pesticide poisoning and migratory stress. Science 194:184–186, 1976.

Ringer, R. K., Aulerich, R. J., Zabik, M. Effect of dietary polychlorinated biphenyls on growth and reproduction of mink. Preprints of papers presented at the 164th National Meeting of the American Chemical Society, 1972.

Stickel, W. H. Some effects of pollutants in terrestrial ecosystems. In McIntyre, A. D. Mills, C. F. (Eds.). Ecological Research—Effects of Heavy Metals and Organohologen Compounds. New York: Plenum, pp. 25–74, 1975.

R. B. Leidy

9

Aquatic Organisms

9.1. Introduction

Prior to 1970, some 100 organic compounds had been identified in water. With the development of more efficient analytical techniques and sensitive detectors, more than 1500 organic compounds have been identified in all types of water, including ground water, industrial waste water, lakes, and rivers. Between 400 and 500 compounds have been identified in drinking water throughout the world. It has been postulated that if 5% of the 2 million organic compounds get into water, approximately 100,000 compounds might be identified in the world's waters.

The external and internal chemical environment of an organism determines whether that organism grows, survives, and perpetuates itself. The internal chemical balance is mediated by the organism's genetic make-up, the external chemical milieu in which it lives, and all other environmental factors. In aquatic environments, the chemical effect on living organisms is very important, as the organism is in intimate contact with chemicals in solution or suspension, and these pass through the body via the integument, membranes, gills, and mouth. As the number of chemicals entering the aquatic environment increases, two extreme types of aquatic contamination can occur: a highly enriched overproductive region resulting from detergents, fertilizers, and sewage, which add to the nutrient supply, or a body of water poisoned by chemicals.

In this chapter the properties of water and the factors affecting chemical toxicity in water are discussed. Food webs and food chains are related to residues of chemicals in aquatic animals and the effects of pollutants on the Great Lakes are briefly discussed.

9.2. **Properties of Water**

The concentration of water to the earth's surface area is 273 liters per square centimeter. However, 269 liters are sea water, and less than 1% of the remainder is distributed as fresh water in ground water, lakes, rivers, streams, and water vapor. There are many properties of this ubiquitous molecule that have allowed life to develop and thrive. At the same time, the same properties have caused severe problems in the environment.

9. 2.1. Chemical Bonding

Water is the universal solvent that can solubilize many molecules. In their solubilized form these molecules are able to enter an organism and perhaps cause undesirable effects. The water molecule is a dipolar molecule containing a "positive end" (two hydrogen atoms) and a "negative end" (one oxygen atom). These atoms are joined by covalent bonds (a covalent bond is one in which an electron pair is shared between two atoms) (Figure 9.1). Many chemicals have structures held together by ionic bonds (an exchange of electrons between atoms of the chemical), and when in contact with water, these atoms lose or gain electrons, and thus become ionized. The formation of sodium and chlorine ions from sodium chloride in contact with water is a typical example of ion formation. Other chemicals are soluble because the water molecule can form a hydrogen bond to certain groups attached to the chemical. A hydrogen bond results from the sharing of a hydrogen atom between two electron-donor atoms, one which is either the hydrogen or the oxygen of water and the other, the atom to which the hydrogen is bonded or the atom that is attracting a hydrogen atom of water. Although this is a weak bond, sufficient numbers give a large collective bond strength to compounds. Thus, many of the anomalous properties of water can be explained on the basis of hydrogen bonding.

9.2.2. Surface Tension

Within the interior of water, the molecules are hydrogen bonded to neighboring molecules on all sides by an average force, but molecules on the surface are unattached on one side. In order for molecules to move from the interior to the surface, both energy and an increase in surface area (due to the increased number of surface molecules) are required. Thus the water surface has a higher potential energy than the interior.

When aggregates of molecules come in contact with the water surface, those forces holding them together can be overcome by dispersal forces in the form of the kinetic motion of the water. The surface energy dissipates as a result of the separation of the aggregate into a film at the surface. The energy consumed per unit area increase at the surface is the surface tension (expressed in ergs/cm^2). Water has a high surface tension, which is very important to adsorption of pollutants to solids suspended in water. Those substances that lower the surface tension between the water and the particulate matter become positively adsorbed to the particulate. Local concentration of a material can be greatly affected by the interfacial tensions between the material and water.

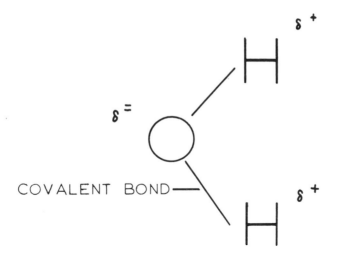

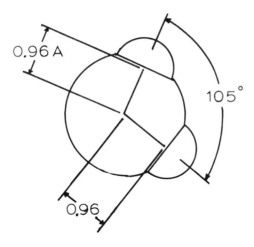

Figure 9.1 Chemical structure of water molecule. Top: Charge distribution. Bottom: Bond angle and O–H distance.

9.2.3. Thermal Properties

Large bodies of water do not fluctuate in temperature as do land masses, because water stores heat. Therefore, a large amount of heat must be applied to water to produce a given temperature rise. The specific heat of water is 1 cal. It takes 1 cal of heat to raise 1 g water 1°C at 15°C. In comparison, standard chemicals such as ethanol and sulfuric acid require 0.54 cal and 0.27 cal, respectively, to raise 1 g 1°C. A tremendous amount of heat (540 cal/g) is required to turn liquid water to a gaseous state (called the heat of vaporization), and 80 cal/g are required to change ice to liquid water (heat of fusion). The heats of vaporization for ethanol and sulfuric acid are 204 and 122 cal/g, respectively, and the heats of fusion are 25 and 24 cal/g, respectively. Because so much heat is required for these processes, a protective barrier is provided to aquatic species. The density of water is 10% greater than that of ice. When water freezes, it expands and will float on the water surface. This prevents large open bodies of water from freezing solid as the ice forms at the surface and freezes downward. Hydrogen bonding is responsible for these phenomena.

9.2.4. Inert Material

Another property of water is its inertness. The properties of water are not altered when most substances are dissolved in it, nor are the properties of the materials dissolved changed. These materials can be transported into a living cell in this state and, if harmful, can begin producing undesirable effects. Because water is an inert material, it is renewable in that contaminated water can evaporate, leaving the contaminant behind, and recondense to fall as unpolluted rain.

9.3. Factors Affecting Water Purity

Many factors influence water quality. Some of the factors occur naturally, whereas others have resulted from man-made events. Generally, the factors to be discussed include temperature, pH, dissolved carbon dioxide and oxygen, suspended solids, and turbidity. Other chapters in this book are concerned with agricultural, industrial, and urban pollutants, so little will be said concerning these.

9.3.1. Temperature

Large fresh-water lakes have three temperature zones called, from the surface to the bottom, the epilimnion, the thermocline, and the hypolimnion. Temperatures decrease as one passes through these zones; the thermocline is a transition zone in which temperature decreases rapidly. Therefore, the water becomes more dense at greater depths and dissolved gases and nutrients do not pass readily between the zones. There is a mixing of the layers, usually in the fall and spring when surface waters cool and become more dense than the hypolimnion, and this process redistributes the gases and nutrients throughout all zones. Conditions could arise in which the water temperature rises to a level of which animals and plants could not adapt and there would be a drastic alteration of their populations. This could be caused by such events as diversion of industrial cooling system water into rivers or lakes, removal of vegetation along shore lines, and increased erosion resulting from clearing of land.

Diatoms, used as a food source by higher forms, decrease in number above 20°C and are replaced by blue-green algae. At 35°C the diatoms disappear and the blue-green algae predominate. These organisms are a source of water blooms that kill the biota and make water unfit for human consumption. Every

10°C increase in temperature reduces the solubility of essential gases (e.g., oxygen decreases 17% as the temperature rises from 20° to 30°C), and, at the same time, the metabolic rate of aquatic species can double for a 10°C increase. These two conditions place an even greater stress on the aquatic species. Elevated temperatures cause an increased solubility of salts, which can become more concentrated as the evaporation rate of water increases. This, too, places a strain on an organism's metabolism, which could make adaption to environmental factors more difficult.

9.3.2. pH

The term "pH" is used to express the negative log of the hydrogen ion concentration and is a measure of alkalinity and acidity of a solution. pH is measured on a scale of 0 to 14; pH 7 is neutral. Below pH 7, a solution is considered acidic and above pH 7 it is alkaline. pH 6 is equivalent to 10^{-6} (0.000001) g hydrogen ions (H^+) per liter, and a drop of one pH unit to 5 (equivalent to 0.00001 g H^+/liter) increases the concentration ten-fold. Surface waters normally have a pH range of 6–9, which is regulated by the relationship of carbon dioxide (CO_2), bicarbonate ion (HCO_3^-), and carbonate ion (CO_3^{2-}) (Figure 9.2). These ions have an important influence upon the chemistry of water. Many minerals are deposited as salts of CO_3^{2-}. The equilibria established among atmospheric CO_2, aqueous CO_3^{2-}, aqueous HCO_3^-, and solid carbonate minerals have a strongly stabilizing effect on the pH of an aquatic environment by forming a buffer system. Buffers are subtances that have the ability to bind with or release H^+ in solution, thus maintaining the pH of the solution relatively constant even if considerable quantities of acid or alkali are added. Because the tolerance limit of most aquatic organisms is pH 5–9, serious problems can result if the buffering capacity of their habitat is disrupted.

9.3.2.a. Carbon Dioxide

Because the atmosphere contains such small concentrations of CO_2 (0.3 ml/liter), equilibrium experiments with pure water show concentrations of approximately 0.5 ml at 0°C (32°F) and 0.2 ml at 24°C (75°F). However, in aquatic environments much larger concentrations of CO_2 are present. These larger concentrations result from decomposition of organic material, respiration of aquatic animals and plants, and the production of calcium carbonate ($CaCo_3$) by aquatic plants, shell accumulation, or soil leaching. Based upon its form in water, CO_2 can be discussed in terms of free CO_2 (Co_2 and H_2CO_3) or combined CO_2 (HCO_3^- and CO_3^{2-}) (Figure 9.2). The pH of the water can be affected by the free and combined forms. For example, if sufficient quantities of a strong mineral acid (e.g., H_2SO_4) from mine drainage were to get into an aquatic environment, the combined forms would convert to the free form, thus decreasing the pH of the water. On the other hand, abundant aquatic plant life could reduce the concentration of free CO_2 through photosynthetic processes causing both a rise in pH and inhibition of further plant growth.

Not only aquatic plants are affected by CO_2 levels, but also aquatic animal species can be affected. Some metabolic processes increase with high CO_2 levels,

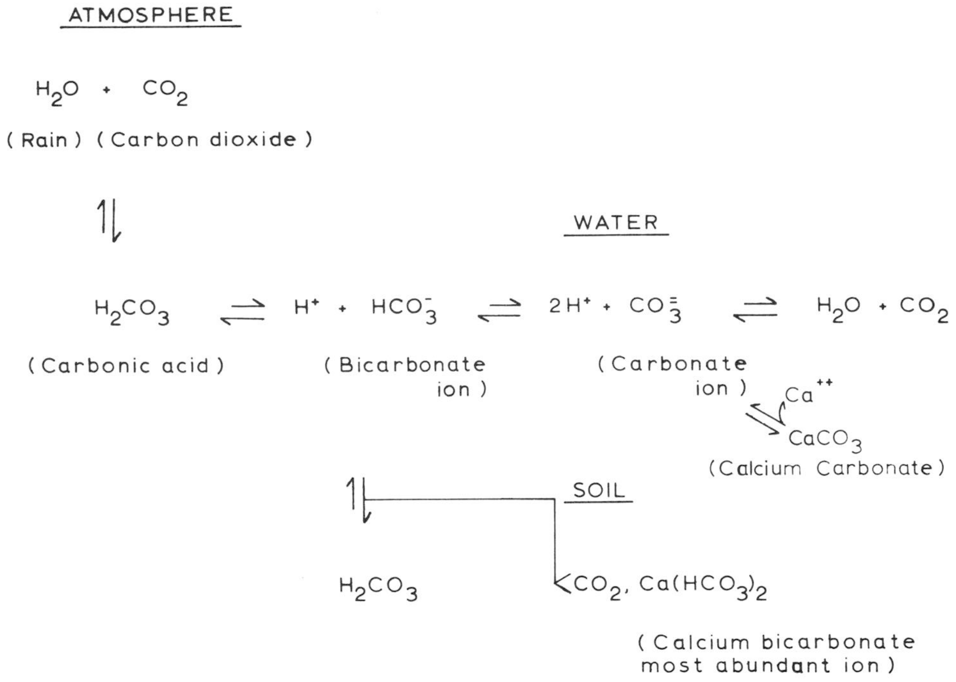

ATMOSPHERE

H_2O + CO_2

(Rain) (Carbon dioxide)

WATER

H_2CO_3 ⇌ H^+ + HCO_3^- ⇌ $2H^+$ + $CO_3^=$ ⇌ H_2O + CO_2

(Carbonic acid)   (Bicarbonate   (Carbonate
                         ion)   ion) Ca^{++}
                                                         $CaCO_3$
                                                         (Calcium Carbonate)

SOIL

H_2CO_3 CO_2, $Ca(HCO_3)_2$

(Calcium bicarbonate
most abundant ion)

Figure 9.2   Molecules involved in maintaining the buffering capacity of water. Contributions from air and soil are shown.

whereas other processes are inhibited at the same level. For example, the respiratory rate is increased in some arthropod and mollusk species and in vertebrates by increased CO_2 concentrations, whereas other species show no apparent effect. Increased CO_2 content affects its equilibrium concentration in the blood of aquatic animals. Excess CO_2 decreases the blood pH, since it forms carbonic acid (H_2CO_3). Excess CO_2 also decreases the oxygen-carrying capacity of the hemoglobin in red blood cells. Gases move from one point to another by diffusion against a pressure gradient (i.e., the gas diffuses from a point of high pressure to one of a lower pressure); thus, an increased CO_2 level will cause an increase in the CO_2 pressure in the blood, which decreases blood pH and allows more CO_2 to bind to hemoglobin. Both effects reduce the hemoglobin molecules' affinity for oxygen. Some pigments (e.g., hemocyanins) of invertebrate species are affected similarly. Thus, those species with blood types affected strongly by CO_2 levels would experience difficulty in obtaining sufficient quantities of oxygen.

9.3.2.b. Calcium Carbonate

Carbon dioxide influences the formation of calcium carbonate ($CaCO_3$) (Figure 9.2) and its dissolution to Ca^{2+} and CO_3^{2-}. The equilibrium of this reaction depends upon the CO_2 concentration. High levels of CO_2 favor the ion formation by lowering the pH and making H^+ available to react with CO_3^{2-}. Low levels (e.g., from photosynthesis) result in the formation of $CaCO_3$, which precipitates as a deposit within and on the tissues of aquatic plants. This effect is seen in those lakes and ponds containing large quantities of Ca^+ ions. In lakes with an acidic pH, both Ca^{2+} and CO_3^{2-} tend to stay in solution and their concentrations are much lower. This affects a number of invertebrate species (e.g., arthropods and mollusks); relatively few are found in lakes with low pH. These species require $CaCO_3$ for shell and exoskeleton formation, and the absence or low levels of $CaCO_3$ limit their habitats. Of course, Ca^{2+} affects membrane permeability and other physiological reactions in both aquatic plants and animals. Low concentrations of Ca^{2+} would have limiting effects on these species.

Various chemicals, depending on their physical and structural properties, react differently to pH changes. For example, a decreased pH increases the toxicity of the pesticide, pentachlorophenol, nickel cyanide, and sodium sulfide. Highly dissociated acids (e.g., H_2SO_4) and bases (e.g., NaOH) are relatively nontoxic between pH 5 and pH 9.

If pollutants can be prevented from entering streams and lakes, natural cleansing can occur and the pH balance may be restored. The buffering capacity of this ecosystem could return through biological processes, including photosynthesis and respiration, and by the addition of essential minerals from rocks and sediment.

9.3.3. Dissolved Oxygen

Many aquatic species obtain oxygen required for respiration from gaseous oxygen dissolved in the water. Dissolved oxygen (DO) is defined as a body of water maintaining certain minimal concentrations of oxygen. In southern regions of the United States, the aquatic species require a DO content of 5 mg/liter (equivalent to 5.0 ppm oxygen), whereas northern region species require 6.0 ppm. The amount of DO at any one time depends on the following factors: water temperature (the lower the temperature, the greater the DO content); altitude, which is related to the partial pressure of atmospheric oxygen in contact with water (e.g., at 25°C, the DO content at sea level is 8.3 ppm, and at 6000 ft it is 6.6 ppm); and natural sources such as photosynthetic processes of algae and higher aquatic plants.

As long as water remains relatively free of waste materials, the DO content will support aquatic life. However, pollutants, primarily organic compounds, cause a reduction in DO. These pollutants come primarily from untreated sewage, industrial wastes, food processing plants, and feed lots. By combining these materials with the DO, aquatic bacteria have an available food source. As more organic material becomes available for bacterial utilization their population increases, the demand for oxygen to break down the organic material increases, and a severe depletion of oxygen results. Unless the water can be reaerated rapidly, as by agitation, the oxygen content will become depleted to the point where higher aquatic species cannot survive. Other oxidations (e.g., of nitrogenous or sulfur-containing compounds) from chemical and or biological reactions further reduce the water's oxygen content. A standard test, the BOD, was developed to measure the amount of organic material in water samples. This test measures the quantity of oxygen utilized by aquatic microorganisms over a 5-day period. Thus, the degree of organic pollution can be determined.

A new method, called the chemical oxygen demand (COD), uses a strong oxidizing agent (dichromate ion in 50% sulfuric acid) to break down completely the organic material in a water sample. It is much faster than the BOD test but normally gives higher results because bacteria will not completely break down all organic materials and this method will. A third method, the total organic carbon (TOC) analysis, uses high temperatures to reduce organic materials to CO_2, which can be analyzed by infrared spectroscopy in a matter of minutes.

An aquatic environment can have a BOD of 5 mg/liter (5 ppm) and be polluted. However, severely polluted lakes can have BODs of 600 mg/liter and greater. Adverse physiological effects on fish resulting from the low DO content include reduced swimming speed, loss of weight and appetite, small and weak fry, and a reduced ability to convert food to energy. Aquatic plants require oxygen to support young plant growth as well as to support respiration. In its absence, metabolic reactions continue, but as carbohydrates are broken down, ethanol accumulates and poisons the cells and eventually kills the plant. If the BOD reaches the point where aerobic microorganisms (those requiring molecular oxygen for metabolic processes) cannot survive, anaerobic forms (those that grow in the absence of molecular oxygen) become predominant, producing materials that are unpleasant to smell such as hydrogen sulfide (H_2S) or methane gas (CH_4), thus decreasing water quality. Eventually bodies of water can be returned to a noncontaminated state if the sources of organic pollution can be eliminated.

9.3.4. Suspended Solids and Turbidity

In addition to the problems caused by organic molecules, many inorganic materials entering the aquatic environment cause serious problems. The primary source of these materials is surface runoff resulting from erosion. It has been calculated that erosion from roadsides and cultivated land contributes 5.1×10^{10} kg (56×10^6 tons) and 2.7×10^{12} kg (3×10^9 tons) respectively, of solid materials per year to aquatic environments in the United States.

These solid materials can be categorized as either solid sediment, such as rocks and sand, or colloids. Colloidal particles range in size from 0.001 to 1.0 μm and are significant from the standpoint of chemical interactions because they have a large surface area per unit weight. It is known that the interfaces between these particles and molecules are important regions that facilitate chemical reactions. Some algae, bacteria, many metals and minerals, organic pollutants, and proteinaceous material exist as colloids. Of these particles, clays are the most common materials found in natural waters. Clays have an important role in the transport of chemicals, gases, and organic wastes in the aquatic environment. In some respects, the adsorption of chemicals to the clay surface exerts a purifying effect as it prevents the chemical from producing an effect. Some of the bacterial chemical reactions, such as the degradation of organic matter, occur on the clay surface. Furthermore, heavy metals can become solubilized from otherwise insoluble metal compounds. This facilitates their entry into aquatic organisms, resulting in a number of detrimental effects. Many of the inorganic materials serve as nutrients for aquatic plant life. It should also be pointed out that many inorganic materials are products arising from the oxidation of organic compounds that can be used as nutrients for the subsequent growth of other organisms.

This process, called eutrophication, is a naturally occurring phenomenon in which nutrients are carried by rivers and streams to estuaries and lakes and are used by plant life. Most of the nutrients available to the plants are present in excess amounts, but the so-called limiting nutrients—carbon, nitrogen, and phosphorous (in the ratio of 106 parts carbon to 10 parts nitrogen to 1 part phosphorous)—are critical for plant growth. If only a limited amount of one of these is available, it determines how much of the other nutrients will be used. An overabundance of these elements, caused by erosion and runoff, accelerates the growth of plant life (including blue-green and green algae, diatoms, and larger plants) because there is no limiting nutrient. The rapid growth of these plants causes algal blooms, unsightly plant growth, and, as the algae and plants die and are broken down by bacteria, unpleasant odors and off-flavored water. These changes can cause the population to change as species leave to seek more favorable environments.

In addition to contributing to the eutrophication process, the suspended solids make water turbid or opaque. Naturally occurring suspended solids, including inorganic and organic detritus, plankton, and silt, produce some turbidity. The majority of these solids are added by erosion, mining, quarrying, and atmospheric dust, producing adverse effects on the aquatic biota. As water becomes more opaque, light penetration decreases. For example, 150 ppm particulate matter will reduce light penetration to 8 cm (3 in.) in water. Consequently, light absorption by aquatic plants is restricted and photosynthetic processes either are slowed or cease. Since plant life forms the basis of the food web (see Section 9.4.1), deviations in either population or productivity can alter the population of other species.

In areas where particulate material is coarse, abrasive effects and actual clogging have been observed on gill-breathing species, affecting metabolism and respiration. Much of the solid material settles out, affecting spawning sites and eradicating benthic organisms (bottom-feeding species). Once settled, the material can become a site for bacterial and fungal growth.

A third problem is the large amounts of inorganic salts that enter the aquatic environment, primarily from highway runoff during deicing operations in winter, acid–base neutralizations from industrial processes, and mine drainage. These inorganic salts damage aquatic life through osmotic processes. When the concentration of dissolved materials is greater in the surrounding water than in a living cell, water will flow from the cell until the concentration of material is equalized between the inside and the outside of the cell. This can lead to a fatally high concentration within the cell.

9.3.5. Metals

Natural water supplies contain trace amounts of metals from soil leaching and runoff, erosion, and breakdown of mineral deposits. However, the concentrations of naturally occurring and other metals have increased in the environment because industrial and mining processes allowed the metals to escape and enter water supplies. Many metals are toxic at low levels, while others are essential components of metabolic processes. It is difficult to determine the biological effects on aquatic organisms. The amount or form of metal absorbed by an organism is difficult to determine because many of these metals are adsorbed onto colloidal particles. The degree of adsorption determines the amount of metal entering the organism. In order to enter the organism, the metal must either be phagocytized (i.e., engulfed by specialized cells) or be in a solubilized form.

An important factor in absorption is the degree and type of complex the metal might be in with an organic molecule. The common term applied to this complex formation is chelation. Organic molecules involved in chelation processes with metal ions are called ligands. More properly, the ligand is that portion of the organic molecule involved in the binding process and includes atoms of nitrogen, oxygen, and sulfur (these atoms are electron donors). Cyclic structures that involve the formation of at least one covalent bond result when the chelate is formed. Other chemical factors are involved in chelation reactions, but they are beyond the scope of this chapter. Chelates perform a number of functions in biological systems: for example, they can alter reactions (e.g., activate or inhibit metal-activated enzymes), alter membrane permeability, and affect the reactivity of metal ion concentrations by regulating amounts available to change metabolic reaction rates.

The chemical and physical conditions of the water itself, including the pH, and the size and nature of the particles present, affect the toxicity of the metal. In addition, the organism itself would influence the rate of metal absorption, based on its age, health, metabolic rate, and species. Little is known about the effects produced by many of the metals now present in the aquatic environment. Others have been studied extensively.

9.3.5.a. Cadmium and Zinc

These two metals are related chemically and both are used in various aspects of the electroplating, metal, and plastics industries. Both are found in high concentrations in mine drainage. In 1969, the EPA reported that 2.5% of water samples taken in the United States contained cadmium and the mean value was 9.5 ppb. This survey also found that 76.5% of the samples had zinc, with a mean value of 64 ppb. Studies with cadmium have shown harmful effects on some fish at concentrations of 0.2 ppm. Zinc toxicities seem to depend upon its form (i.e., an ionic species or a fine precipitate), but it is not as toxic as cadmium.

Cadmium might replace zinc in some enzyme systems, changing the three-dimensional structure and altering the catalytic activity. Both metals inhibit reactions where phosphate and sulfhydryl groups are involved. Mitochondrial synthesis of adenosine triphosphate (ATP) is impaired by both metals. ATP is the carrier of chemical energy resulting from the oxidation of food to processes or reactions in a cell requiring a supply of chemical energy. In addition, zinc inhibits the mitochondrial electron transport system by affecting some cytochromes and alters the membrane permeability of mitochondria to potassium. Both zinc and cadmium are considered dangerous to aquatic environments.

9.3.5.b. Copper

This metal is present in natural water supplies as a result of the breakdown of rock containing this element. Industry and mining contribute high levels to some waters. Like zinc, copper is an essential trace metal and is a component of many enzymes. The mean concentration of copper found in the 1969 EPA survey was 15 ppb, however, concentrations as high as 280 ppb were found. The toxicity of copper is related strongly to the pH of the water. When the pH increases, the free copper in solution decreases and becomes a finely divided group of particles. This form appears to be more toxic than the copper in solution. Studies have shown that these particles adhere to the mucous coating and gills of fish and perhaps are absorbed at higher rates through the gill membrane at higher pH. Copper alters the permeability of plasma membranes, but other events appear to be necessary to produce toxic effects.

9.3.5.c. Lead

This metal normally enters the environment from lead-bearing limestone, but industrial waste, construction sites, lead-based paint deterioration, organic lead from gasoline combustion, and lead shot from spent shells have added large quantities to aquatic habitats. In 1969 lead was found in 19% of natural waters with a mean value of 23 ppb.

The physiological affects of lead are not clear in fish, aquatic invertebrates, or plant life under natural conditions. High lead concentrations affect plasma membranes, sulfhydryl groups in enzymes, and synthesis of hemoglobin and cytochromes. Since lead is an undesirable component of drinking water, a maximum limit of 0.05 ppb has been set by the Public Health Service.

9.3.5.d. Mercury

Because few natural sources of mercury exist, this metal was never considered an environmental hazard in the Unites States. However, in 1970 mercury was found in fish, and subsequent sampling found this metal widely distributed in the environment. Industrial processes (e.g., those employing alloys and catalysts), mining operations, and agricultural runoff of fungicides containing mercury have contributed to the contamination. Ionic forms of inorganic mercury are toxic to fish at relatively high concentrations (approximately 1.0 ppm); however, surveys of fish and fish-eating birds have shown much higher concentrations. Studies revealed that the high concentrations resulted from the conversion of the inorganic form to organic forms of mercury primarily by anaerobic bacteria inhabiting the sediment of lakes and streams.

Like other heavy metals, mercury binds to sulfhydryl groups of enzymes, altering their catalytic properties. Many studies have shown that mercury binds to cell membranes and alters the permeability to hydrogen and potassium ions, amino acids, and carbohydrates. Unfortunately, there is no practical method of eliminating mercury from aquatic environments, and this problem will continue for years.

9.3.5.e. Other Metals

Other metals have been implicated as having toxic effects on aquatic organisms but their mechanisms of action are obscure. For example, beryllium, chromium, and vanadium appear to be toxic, but current methodology limits meaningful conclusions. Difficulties in determining the absorbed dose and the inability to define both the chemical and physiological conditions under which the experiments are conducted have made the interpretation of data most difficult. These are the primary reasons that data on heavy metal toxicity to aquatic organisms are scarce.

9.3.6. Other Factors

Two broad categories of factors that affect water quality should be discussed briefly. There are natural environmental factors that directly or indirectly contribute to water quality changes. Air temperature and wind speed and direction have important roles in regulating the amount and degree of oxygen saturation. Wind is very effective in aerating the upper layers of lakes when water is able to circulate freely. Animal and plant detritus contribute a significant portion of nutrients to plankton and filter-feeding bivalve species. Since many pollutants are carried by air currents, precipitation could deposit undesirable quantities into aquatic habitats. Solids and rock substrates are dissolved slowly by water, and the minerals and metals released not only provide essential nutrients for inhabitants but also aid in the maintenance of the water's buffering capacity. As mentioned previously, these factors can produce an unfavorable environment, especially if pollutants resulting from man's indifference are present.

The other factor is the effects urbanization has had on water quality. Large areas of land are being cleared for shopping and residential areas and corporate farms. Flood plains have been replaced with asphalt, causing flooding, erosion, and increased sedimentation. This, in turn, can adversely affect both water flow in streams and the attractiveness of streams, since flooding erodes banks and destroys much of the plant life.

One must remember that all of these factors are interrelated, and no single entity will destroy the ecology of an aquatic environment. Too many well-meaning groups tend to single out one source as the reason the environment is deteriorating. They fail to look at other possible sources. It is easy to say that a nuclear power plant's cooling water or a city's sewage system is causing all of the problems without considering erosion, industrial sources, urbanization, and other factors, both natural and man-made, that are contributing to environmental degradation. Some of these contributions might be small, but when taken as a whole, the amounts and types of material entering the aquatic environment stagger the imagination.

Thus far, the factors contributing to aquatic pollution have been discussed with little mention made of the complexity of the aquatic ecosystem. In the next section, a typical ecosystem is discussed in general terms, with an emphasis on the changes made when the quality of water entering this system deteriorates.

9.4. Aquatic Ecosystem

As in any complex society, the inhabitants of the aquatic environment rely on one another for materials to aid in their growth and reproduction. Aquatic populations can be divided into producers, consumers, and transformers. The consumers and producers are organized into nutritional or trophic levels. Within each level, groups of organisms feed on similar food sources. Producer organisms are those utilizing photosynthetic processes for food production, while consumers feed upon both producers and consumers in different trophic levels. Transformers are those organisms that break down dead organic material into nutrients used by the producers. These organisms form the base of the food web.

9.4.1. Food Chains and Food Webs

Within trophic levels there are food chains that involve the transfer of food energy from plants through various animal species, with one being devoured by another. An interconnection of many food chains is called a food web (Figure 9.3). The lowest level of a food chain contains plant life that uses solar energy to produce food. These producers are eaten by herbivorous organisms at the second level. The herbivores are eaten by small carnivores, these are eaten by larger carnivores, etc. Generally, the farther removed from the lower levels a species is, the greater the probability that it will feed on more than one level.

The food web is in delicate balance and can be altered quite easily. It has been mentioned that some pollutants (e.g., mercury) are found in higher concentrations in certain animals than in the lower species they feed upon. This phenomenon is referred to as bioaccumulation or biomagnification. It is possible that one or more species in a trophic level could be killed as a result of the large concentrations of a pollutant ingested from lower level feeding. If this were to occur, those species at higher trophic levels would lose a food source, forcing them to leave the area in search of new sources. Ingestion of large quantities of a pollutant might not kill a species, yet detrimental effects such as reproductive failure or general debilitation would have adverse effects on the food web. These organisms could become easier prey for species that would normally not utilize them as a food source. The addition of materials other than toxic chemicals has produced significant alterations not only in the water quality and inhabitants of small lakes and streams, but in large bodies of water as well.

9.4.2. Pollution of Lake Erie

In the early 1900s, the Great Lakes region of the United States was both a haven for naturalists and a production site for commercial fishing. By the 1940s, commercial fish catches in Lake Erie were less than one-half of what they had been 20 years before. Some of the decline was attributed to overfishing and the introduction of the sea lamprey and predatory, nongame fish. Much of the decline, however, occurred because of the accumulation of materials from agriculture and industrial sources surrounding the lake. As a result, the natural aging process of Lake Erie was accelerated. Under normal circumstances lakes change from the oligotrophic (nutrient-poor) to the eutrophic (nutrient-rich) state, which results in an overproduction of plant species, primarily algae. Two of the materials that have caused the large algal blooms in Lake Erie in the past are nitrate (NO_3), as inorganic fertilizer applied to the 78×10^3 km² (30×10^3 miles²) of farmland and some 9×10^3 kg (20×10^3 lb) phosphate (PO_4) per day from detergents. When the algae died, the decay resulting from bacterial action produced an area 6700 km² (2600 miles²) devoid of oxygen 3 meters from the bottom and resulted in gross changes in the lake.

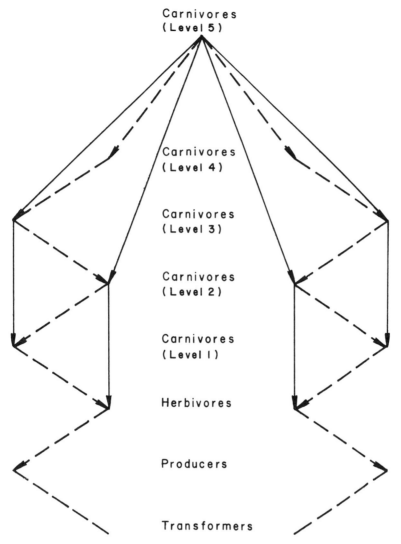

Figure 9.3 Food chain (*broken lines*) and food web (*solid lines*) involving various feeding levels.

In the early 1960s physical changes in the lake included a DO content in 70% of the hypolimnion of less than 3 ppm (10% saturation), a high specific conductance of 241.8 μmhos (a measure of electrical conductance of water showing high salinity), 180 ppm total dissolved solids (primarily calcium, chlorine, potassium, and sulfate), and a transparency of 4.5 m (14.8 ft). Fish populations declined due to reproductive failure. For example, 9.1×10^6 kg (10,000 tons) of lake herring were caught by commercial fishermen in 1925, compared to 3.2×10^3 kg (3.5 tons) in 1962; 6.8×10^6 kg (7500 tons) of blue pike were caught in 1957, compared to 4.5×10^2 kg (0.5 tons) in 1962. At the same time, the total catch has remained about the same, 22.7×10^6 kg (25,000 tons), because the game fish have been replaced by so-called "trash" fish including carp, sheepshead, smelt, and yellow perch.

With increased public awareness and federal and state regulations, many areas of the lake have been cleaned up and game fish are returning to this and the other Great Lakes. Many rivers, notably the Hudson and the Thames are showing signs of revival since extensive cleanup has been undertaken by industry. However, the fight against aquatic pollution is one that must be continued if we hope to preserve these areas for future generations. Chapters 17–20 are devoted to specific estuaries, lakes, and rivers, and the methods being used to return them to the beautiful and productive systems that they once were.

Suggested Reading

Brown, A.W.A. Ecology of Pesticides. New York: Wiley, 1978.

Dugan, P.R. Biochemical Ecology of Water Pollution. New York: Plenum Press, 1972.

McCaull, J., Crossland, J. Water Pollution. New York: Harcourt Brace Jovanovich, 1974.

Miller, S.S. (Ed.). Water Pollution. Washington, D.C.: American Chemical Society, 1974.

Stoher, H.S., Seager, S.L. Environmental Chemistry: Air and Water Pollution. Dallas, Tex.: Scott, Foresman, 1976.

Wilber, C.G. The Biological Aspects of Water Pollution. Springfield, Ill.: Thomas, 1969.

Walter W. Heck
Charles E. Anderson

10

Effects of Air Pollutants on Plants

10.1. Introduction

Historically, injury to vegetation has been one of the earliest manifestations of air pollution. Sulfur dioxide (SO_2) and fluoride gases were first investigated about the middle of the 19th century in Europe, primarily in Germany. The effects of SO_2 were often ignored by industry in the early part of this century, as evidenced by major pollution problems that occurred near Trail, British Columbia, Canada; Sudbury, Ontario, Canada; and Ducktown (Copper Hill), Tennessee. Copper sulfide at Ducktown was roasted in piles by huge bonfires until about 1900. The trees that were not cut for fuel were killed by the SO_2, and the land was denuded for several miles around the source.

Today, extensive injury to vegetation near sources of SO_2 rarely occurs because either there has been a reduction in emissions or tall stacks have been constructed. However, the SO_2 problem is of increasing concern because high-capacity power plants are being developed that use sulfur-containing fossil fuels. These plants, with their high stacks, will increase the area exposed to SO_2 pollution and will contribute to the acidity of precipitation.

Injury to vegetation by fluorides [primary hydrogen fluoride (HF)] from industrial sources was well described by the early 1900s, but fluoride did not become a serious threat to vegetation until industrial expansion began about 1940. By this time, characteristic fluoride symptoms were known and the concept of a spectrum of sensitivity among species was developed. Fluoride was shown to be an accumulative poison, and foliar analysis for fluoride content was an accepted diagnostic tool. The most important fluoride problem in agriculture, other than direct effects on plants, is the effects on grazing animals that have ingested forage containing elevated fluoride concentrations (>30 ppm).

Injury to vegetation was the earliest recognized biological effect of photochemical air pollution in the Los Angeles, California, area. This type of injury was recognized over a large segment of southern California and in the San Francisco

Bay area by 1950. Components of photochemical pollution have injured plants in most, if not all, of the major metropolitan areas throughout the world and in many rural areas. Three important phytotoxic oxidants have been identified in the photochemical complex: ozone (O_3), PAN, and nitrogen dioxide (NO_2).

Ethylene is a major product of automobile exhaust. It was first identified as a toxic component of illuminating gas in commercial greenhouses near the turn of the century. Later research suggested that ethylene is more than 50 times as phytotoxic as other hydrocarbon gases and that it contributes to the formation of photochemical oxidants. Concentrations in metropolitan areas, primarily from automobile exhaust, are sufficiently high to cause early senescence and possibly reductions in yield.

Other phytotoxic air pollutants include air-borne pesticides, chlorine, heavy metals, acid aerosols, ammonia, aldehydes, hydrogen chloride, hydrogen sulfide, and particulates such as cement dust. These pollutants are released primarily from industrial sources or as agricultural applications, but are either less widespread or less concentrated than the major pollutants. Thus they have been studied less and their effects are less well understood.

10.2. Air Pollution Effects

The effects of air pollutants on vegetation can be either visible or subtle. Visible effects are identifiable morphological, pigmented, chlorotic, or necrotic foliar patterns that result from major physiological disturbances in plant cells. Subtle effects are those that do not result in visible injury but are measurable as growth or physiological changes in the plant; they may affect yield and the reproductive or genetic systems of plants. The cumulative changes within plant systems subjected to air pollution stress may result in changes in plant populations and communities.

10.2.1. Visible Injury

Visible injury is classified as acute or chronic. Acute symptoms are associated with short exposures (measured in hours) to relatively high concentrations of a pollutant and usually appear within 24–48 hr after exposure. Chronic symptoms are normally associated with long-term or intermittent exposures (measured in days) to lower concentrations of a pollutant.

Acute injury from air pollutants results in the plasmolysis and death of some cells and subsequent collapse of the tissue. The injury may occur in one specific leaf tissue or in several tissues indiscriminately. In most cases, the first visible symptom on the intact leaf is a slightly water-soaked or bruised appearance. The affected areas generally dry out, producing the necrotic pattern characteristic of the toxicant.

Tissue injured by air pollutants often has a characteristic color; bleaching is associated with SO_2, yellowing with ammonia, and browning with fluoride. A dark band of color often marks the edge of necrotic tissues injured by fluoride. The pigmentation (stipple) of small areas of the palisade tissues seems to be characteristic of O_3 injury in some plants. A silvering or bronzing of the under surface of some leaves (spongy tissue) is associated with PAN injury. Chlorosis may appear in association with necrotic tissue after exposure to SO_2 or oxidants.

Chronic injury may be mild or severe but does not initially result in cell death. Initial disruption of normal cellular activity may be followed by chlorosis or other color or pigment changes that may eventually lead to cell death. A more subtle symptom may be early leaf senescence with or without leaf abscission. Chronic injury patterns are generally not characteristic for a given pollutant and are easily confused with symptoms caused by parasitic diseases, insects, nutritional factors, other environmental stresses, or normal leaf senescence.

Although air pollution can cause growth reduction, it has been well established that few distinctive alterations of growth can be attributed to air pollutants. Herbicides such as 2,4-D act as plant growth regulators. When these drift out of desired spray patterns, they produce marked abnormalities (twisting and/or elongation of leaves and stems) in the growth of sensitive species. Ethylene is a normal constituent of plant tissues and, as such, acts as a plant growth regulator. It induces epinasty and abscission of plant parts.

10.2.2. Injury Patterns from Specific Pollutants

Only the common symptoms caused by the major air pollutants will be summarized here. Several reviews describing injury to vegetation and atlases of colored plates have been published.

10.2.2.a. Ozone

Leaf injuries are divided into three categories by plant type:

1. Broadleaf: pigmented, red-brown spots (stipple) appear on the upper surface: areas bleached tan to white (fleck) occur; small irregular bifacial collapsed (necrotic) areas may coalesce to form irregular necrotic blotches; chlorosis, premature senescence, and leaf abscission may occur.
2. Grasses: scattered bifacial necrotic areas (fleck) appear; sometimes larger lesions or necrotic streaking occurs; interveinal chlorosis may occur.
3. Conifers: brown-tan necrotic needle tips appear that show no distinct separation between dead and healthy tissue; chlorotic mottling occurs, especially in sensitive pine.

Sensitive plants: oat, petunia, snap bean, potato, radish, soybean, sycamore, tobacco, tomato, white ash, white pine.

Tolerant plants: beet, geranium, gladiolus, maple, mint, pepper, rice.

10.2.2.b. Sulfur Dioxide

Leaf injuries are divided into three categories by plant type:

1. Broadleaf: irregular, bifacial, marginal, and interveinal necrotic areas are bleached white to tan or brown; chlorosis may be associated with necrotic areas, or a general chlorosis of older leaves may develop; diffuse to stippled colors ranging from white to reddish brown have been observed.
2. Grasses: irregular, bifacial, necrotic streaking bleached light tan to white is seen between larger veins; chlorosis may be pronounced but develops as strips between the veins.

3. Conifers: brown necrotic needle tips appear, often with a banded appearance; generally chlorosis of adjacent tissue is found; needles of the same age are uniformly affected; chlorosis and premature abscission are common.

Sensitive plants: alfalfa, apple, barley, cotton, giant ragweed, pine, squash, wheat.

Tolerant plants: cantaloupe, celery, corn, oak, rhododendron.

10.2.2.c. *Hydrogen Fluoride*

Leaf injuries are divided into three categories by plant type:

1. Broadleaf: necrotic tips and/or leaf margins occur with occasional interveinal blotches; area between dead and living tissue is sharp and usually accentuated by a narrow, darker, brown-red band; a narrow chlorotic band may be found adjacent to the necrotic area; in some species, the necrotic area may fall off, leaving a "chewed" edge on a seemingly healthy leaf; citrus, sweet cherry, and certain other plants show a mottled interveinal chlorosis.
2. Grasses: brown necrotic tip burn extends in irregular streaks down the leaf and there is a sharp demarcation between dead and healthy tissue; some plants develop a chlorotic mottle that may be diffuse between the veins.
3. Conifers: brown to red-brown necrotic needle tips appear; necrosis may affect entire leaf; all needles of the same age are not uniformly affected; needle chlorosis may develop.

Sensitive plants: Chinese apricot, gladiolus (light-colored varieties are more sensitive than darker ones), grape, Italian prune, pine.

Tolerant plants: alfalfa, cotton, elm, pear, tobacco, tomato.

10.2.2.d. *Peroxyacetyl Nitrate*

Leaf injuries are divided into three categories by plant type:

1. Broadleaf: spongy mesophyll collapses, giving a glazed, silvered, or bronzed appearance to the underside of the leaf; some leaves show a bifacial collapse, usually in a banded pattern; plants often show an early senescence with leaf abscission.
2. Grasses: irregular collapsed banding bleached yellow to tan occurs, sometimes appearing more as a chlorotic or bleached band than necrotic.
3. Conifers: injury is not specific; needle blight with some chlorosis or bleaching occurs.

Sensitive plants: annual bluegrass, petunia, pinto bean, romaine lettuce.

Tolerant plants: broccoli, chrysanthemum, corn, cotton, sorghum.

10.2.3. Growth and Yield Effects

The major air pollutants are known to reduce the biomass and yield of sensitive plant species and cultivars. Generally, growth and yield is not affected without visible injury to the plants, but exceptions have been reported. The effects of the three major pollutants are discussed in this section.

10.2.3.a. Oxidants (Primarily Ozone)

Enough data are not available to develop specific equations for growth and yield effects of O_3 or ambient oxidants on plants. Graphs similar to those produced by McCune for fluoride (Section 10.2.3.c., Figure 10.1), however, may be of help in estimating oxidant dose–response relationships over time (Section 10.4).

Studies using controlled pollutant additions permit accurate determination of total dose for long-term chronic studies. Although these studies are suggestive of "real world" effects, cumulative acute exposures are probably responsible for most of the effects reported in the field. A summary of some long-term studies with O_3 or ambient oxidants is presented in Table 10.1. Plants in the field studies were grown in the field and enclosed in field chambers to ensure controlled O_3 dosages. Plants in the ambient studies were grown in chambers where the air was filtered or not filtered.

10.2.3.b. Sulfur Dioxide

Early research indicated that SO_2 did not affect alfalfa growth until at least 5% of the foliage was visibly injured, and that yield reductions from acute SO_2 injury were roughly equivalent to those occurring when the same amount of leaf tissue was manually removed.

Table 10.1 Effects of Long-Term Exposures to Ozone or Ambient Oxidants on Plant Growth

Plant species	Exposure type	Concentration and duration of exposure	Effects (percent reduction from control)
Geranium	Greenhouse	0.07–0.01 ppm, 9.5 hr/day, 90 days	50% Flowering
Radish	Greenhouse	0.05 ppm, 8 hr/day 5 days/wk, 5 wk	54% Root fresh wt.; 20% Leaf fresh wt.
Soybean	Greenhouse	0.10 ppm, 8 hr/day, 5 days/wk, 3 wk	24% Root fresh wt.; 21% Top fresh wt.
Bean, pinto	Greenhouse	0.15 ppm, 2 hr/day, 63 days	33% Plant dry wt.; 46% Pod fresh wt.
Soybean	Field, closed top chamber	0.10 ppm, 6 hr/day, 133 days	55% Seed wt. 65% Plant fresh wt.
Corn, sweet	Field, closed top chamber	0.10 ppm, 6 hr/day, 64 days	45% Kernel dry wt.; 35% Other yield measures
Corn, field	Field, open top chamber	0.15 ppm, 7 hr/day, 85 days	38% Kernel dry wt.
Spinach	Field, open top chamber	0.10 ppm, 7 hr/day, 37 days	32% Leaf fresh wt.
		0.13 ppm, 7 hr/day, 37 days	72% Leaf fresh wt.
Orange	Ambient	>0.10 ppm, often (over several years)	54% Yield
Grape	Ambient	>0.25 ppm, often (May–Sept.)	12% Yield, year one 61% Yield, year two
Tobacco (Bel W$_3$)	Ambient	0.05–0.10 ppm, often (June–Sept.)	30% Leaf fresh wt.

For alfalfa the relationship between decreased yield and the percentage of leaf area destroyed is well expressed by a simple regression equation:

$$y = a + bx \tag{10.1}$$

where y is the yield expressed as percent of control, a is a constant of approximately 100%, b is the slope of the yield–leaf destruction curve, and x is the percentage of leaf area destroyed. The following regressions were found upon exposure of alfalfa to 1–5 ppm SO_2 for 1–2 hr one, two, or three times during the growing season:

Single exposure $y = 99.5 - 0.30x$ (10.2)

Double exposure $y = 95.5. - 0.49x$ (10.3)

Triple exposure $y = 96.6 - 0.75x.$ (10.4)

A similar equation was developed for alfalfa using 0.1–3 ppm SO_2 exposure for 1–600 hr:

$$y = 99 - 0.37x. \tag{10.5}$$

Results with barley, wheat, and cotton differ from those with alfalfa because yield is not always directly proportional to vegetative growth. With these types of plants, pollutants have a greater effect during the blossom and fruit development stages than at other growth stages. Examples for barley illustrate this difference:

Early vegetative stage $y = 98 - 0.06x$ (10.6)

Heading out (flowering) stage $y = 98 - 0.40x.$ (10.7)

Decreased growth attributable to SO_2 has been reported in numerous publications. There is some information to suggest that growth reductions may occur with little or no visible injury, as found in ryegrass and radishes exposed to low concentrations of SO_2.

10.2.3.c. Hydrogen Fluoride

Fluoride can decrease the growth and yield of many plant species. Figure 10.1 is a log–log graph of the mean concentrations of atmospheric fluoride versus duration of exposure. These are simple representations but are probably the best possible with the limited data available. The figure includes injury, growth, and yield data.

Growth effects reported include decreased radial growth of trees, decreased dry weights of many plants (including rose, alfalfa, grass, lettuce, and sorghum), loss of flower quality and gladiolus corm size, and reduction in the number of flowers or fruits of tomato, citrus, sorghum, and bean. Decreased root growth is also reported. Effects of fluoride on fruit quality and number have been reported for peach (soft suture), apricot, pear, cherry, and citrus.

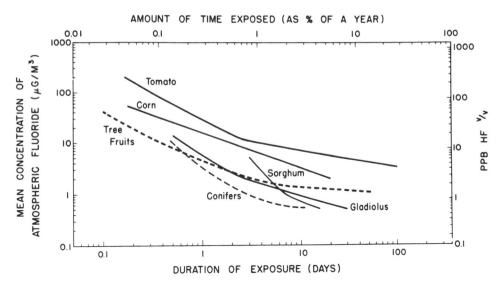

Figure 10.1 Possible response thresholds of different plant species for atmospheric fluoride (as HF). (From McCune, D.C. Air Quality Monograph 69-3. American Petroleum Institute, 1969.)

There is interest in relating the effects of fluoride to concentrations of fluoride in plant tissue. Linear regressions for orange and grapefruit yield against fluoride content of the leaves showed significant yield reductions at leaf fluoride concentrations below 50 ppm. Growth of pinto bean was decreased when the fluoride concentrations in the leaves exceeded 300 ppm; growth of alfalfa decreased at leaf concentrations above 200 ppm; and growth of citrus and Douglas fir may decrease at leaf concentrations near 100 ppm. Some highly sensitive plants may have a leaf concentration injury threshold of approximately 15–25 ppm and certainly under 150 ppm; resistant plants may tolerate tissue levels well above 200 ppm.

10.2.4. Physiological and Biochemical Effects

Physiological and biochemical effects are the underlying causes of measurable visible and growth effects. Early studies showed that SO_2 decreased net photosynthesis without visible injury but that plants recovered rapidly when exposure ended. Results have been similar for O_3, PAN, nitric oxide, and NO_2. This decrease in photosynthetic rate is associated with both stomatal regulation and rates of transpiration.

Stomata are the principal avenue of pollutant uptake by plant leaves. Stomatal closure will effectively protect plants from pollutant injury, except in the unusual case of NO_2 (dark exposures may produce more injury than light exposures). Thus, conditions that favor stomatal opening may result in increased gas entry and resultant injury. Stomatal closure in onion is related to a genetic factor; the stomata of the resistant onion plants close in response to O_3, whereas the stomata of sensitive plants do not close. Sulfur dioxide concentrations of 0.05–0.50 ppm stimulated stomatal opening in both bean and corn when relative humidity was 50–60%. The effect was noted in both well-watered and water-stressed plants.

In laboratory studies, isolated enzymes and enzyme systems have been affected by exposure to PAN, O_3, and fluoride (normally added as sodium fluoride): High pollutant concentrations were used in many of these studies but the concentrations at the reaction sites were unknown. However, it is recognized that strong oxidants may interfere with oxidation reactions within plant systems. Metabolic pools have been studied in terms of nitrogen (amino acids and proteins) and carbohydrate levels, and the sensitivity of plants to specific pollutants has been related to these pool concentrations. Sulfhydryl groups appear to be a key to understanding the mechanism of action of oxidant pollutants and perhaps of SO_2. Unsaturated lipid components of cell membranes are an early site of action for O_3 and possibly for PAN.

Any reasonable mechanistic explanation of acute dose–response symptoms and chronic growth–yield reductions must acknowledge that plant systems have repair capability. The acute response of plants to air pollutants must result from a massive dose that causes disruption of the cell membrane (in part through an attack on sulfhydryl linkages and/or unsaturated lipid linkages) and a loss of the differential permeability of the membrane. Cellular water and solutes may be lost and the cell may be plasmolyzed, which may cause cell death. However, if environmental conditions are not severe and if the exposure dose is minimal, some recovery may take place. The extent of recovery depends upon the severity of the external stresses and the ability of the cells to initiate repair. If we assume that a given tissue is growing under conditions that maximize its sensitivity to a particular pollutant, then the severity of the injury is a function of the inherent resistance of the plant. This inherent resistance is essentially the ability of the plant to "inactivate" the pollutant and to complete tissue repair.

Chronic injury and subtle effects result primarily from secondary reactions. Any membrane injury will induce secondary reactions that could disrupt cellular organelles or shift metabolic pathways, which in turn may induce additional adverse effects in cells. Sulfur dioxide is rapidly changed to sulfite, which may be used as a sulfur source, as a precursor in the production of hydrogen sulfide, or as a component in the initiation of other metabolic effects. Nitrogen dioxide can form nitrite in the cell, which can cause harmful secondary reactions. It can also be oxidized to nitrate or reduced to ammonia and be used as a nitrogen source. Ozone, PAN, and other oxidants can cause the formation of free radicals and/or other more stable oxidants (such as hydrogen peroxide), which in turn can cause secondary reactions. Any of these secondary reactions can, over time, cause senescence via the increased production of cellular ethylene.

10.2.5. Reproductive Effects

Ozone, ambient oxidants, and fluoride affect reproductive structures and may influence fruit set and yield in the absence of visible injury or any obvious effect on total biomass. Ethylene has long been known to stimulate floral abscission, although it is usually accompanied by either growth alterations and/or abscission of other plant parts.

Ozone can induce the formation of free radicals and may also cause genetic abnormalities. Ozone decreases tobacco pollen germination and pollen tube growth, and decreases flower production in carnations. Germination of petunia pollen is also lowered and is thought to be associated with a loss of organelles in the peripheral layer of cytoplasm.

An exposure of 0.3 ppm SO_2 for 1 hr inhibits pollen germination and growth of the pollen tube in pear. The size and development of Scots pine pollen was related to distance from industrial pollution where SO_2 was the major component.

Fluoride can affect reproductive structures and initiate genetic abnormalities. Exposure of sorghum to fluoride during tasseling and anthesis decreases the seed yield and top growth, while exposures before and after this relatively short developmental period have no effect on yield. Fluoride inhibits pollen germination and pollen tube length in tomato and sweet cherry, and decreases citrus yield when exposures occur during the bloom period. Fluoride also causes chromosomal aberrations in tomato, corn, and onion roots and phenotypic abnormalities in the second generation of tomato.

10.3. Factors Affecting Air Pollution Effects

Our understanding of the effect of any given factor on the sensitivity of a specific variety or species to an air pollutant cannot be predetermined by the response of related plants nor by the response to similar doses of different pollutants. Before we can predict how a plant variety will respond to a specific pollutant, we must understand many interrelated factors; some of the most relevant are discussed below.

10.3.1. Genetic and Age Factors

Knowledge of the influence of genetic variability on plant response to pollutants has been obtained from field observations and from chamber experiments with controlled additions of pollutants. Plant response varies between species of a given genus and between varieties within a given species. Such variation is a function of genetic variability as if affects plant morphological, physiological, and biochemical characteristics. Thus, pollutants may act as a selective pressure mechanism in native populations and in breeding experiments (whether planned or accidental).

The sensitivity of plants is also affected by leaf maturity. Cotton leaves are most sensitive to O_3 at about two-thirds full expansion, which is representative of studies with both O_3 and SO_2. Generally, studies show that young tissues are more sensitive to PAN and hydrogen sulfide, and maturing leaves are most sensitive to the other pollutants.

10.3.2. Environmental Factors

The effects of climatic, edaphic, and biological factors on the response of sensitive plants to air pollutants have been studied primarily under laboratory conditions. Most of the studies have dealt with individual factors and only one or two response measurements.

10.3.2.a. Climate

Environmental conditions before, during, and after the exposure of plants to air pollutants influence their response. Plants may change in sensitivity to a given pollutant after being grown under a different set of conditions for 1–5 days. Conditions after exposure are important, but probably less so than those before and during exposure.

Annual bluegrass, pinto bean, and certain tobacco varieties were much more sensitive to ambient oxidants or to O_3 when grown under an 8-hr photoperiod than under a 16-hr photoperiod. The response of annual bluegrass was independent of temperature variations during growth.

Light intensity during growth affects the sensitivity of pinto bean and tobacco to a subsequent O_3 exposure. Sensitivity increases with decreasing light intensities within the range of 4000–900 ft-c. However, the sensitivity of pinto bean of PAN increases with increasing light intensity. Buckwheat was more susceptible to SO_2 when grown at 3000 ft-c than at 7000 or 10,000 ft-c.

When pinto bean was exposed to O_3 at higher light intensities, sensitivity was increased at lower humidities (60%) but was not affected at higher humidities (>80%). At low light intensities, plant response is closely correlated with stomatal opening. However, since full stomatal opening frequently occurs at about 1000 ft-c, light intensity seems to have an effect on plant response in addition to its effect on stomatal opening.

Plants grown at temperatures below 5°C lose sensitivity to air pollutants. Generally, sensitivity to oxidants increases with increasing temperature up to about 30°C. Soybeans were more sensitive to O_3 when grown at 28°C than at 20°C.

The sensitivity of pinto bean and tobacco to O_3 decreased with increasing exposure temperature from about 17° to 30°C. Similar results were obtained for several other plants, but the reverse effect has been reported.

Field observations generally indicate that plants are more sensitive to air pollutants at higher humidities. However, field observations do not separate effects during growth from those during exposure. A 90% loss in sensitivity to SO_2 exposures was found when the relative humidity dropped from 100% to essentially zero. Sensitivity to O_3 in Virginia pine, pinto beans, snap bean, and tobacco increased with increasing relative humidity during exposure.

Plants are generally more sensitive in mid- to late morning and early afternoon. Under some conditions, depending on leaf maturity, there may be a midday loss of sensitivity. This time-of-day effect is related to the overall effects of the environment on plant physiological processes, including stomatal closure, which then directly affect the sensitivity of the plant to air pollutants.

10.3.2.b. Soil Conditions

Soil water and fertility affect the sensitivity of plants to air pollutants; however, edaphic effects are poorly understood. Ozone causes less injury as soil water stress (−0.4, −2.4, and −4.4 bars) is increased irrespective of O_3 dose. Soil water stress is the most significant edaphic factor affecting the response of plants to pollutants. Humidity and available soil water are the two primary factors that control overall water stress in plants. The relative importance of each of these two factors is difficult to distinguish under field conditions. Drought during growth causes physiological changes that increase the resistance of plants to pollution stress, and drought during exposure causes a decrease in stomatal opening, with a resultant reduction in the amount of pollutant in the leaves. Ozone may cause stomatal closure in some plants when they are under water stress.

There is a lack of understanding as to the effects of soil fertility on plant sensitivity to air pollutants, but ion availability must play a role. However, plants may be more sensitive when grown under low fertility. Nitrogen nutrition has received the most attention, but evidence on its effects is conflicting. An interaction between potassium and phosphorus has been reported in spinach exposed to O_3. Pinto bean and soybean were more sensitive to O_3 when the nutrient solution contained about one-sixth the normal potassium level. Tomato was more sensitive to O_3 with increased phosphorus. Plants are not as sensitive when grown in heavy-textured soils, possibly due to decreased soil oxygen tension or water availability. The effects of soil temperature, aeration, texture, compaction, and composition have not been studied.

10.3.2.c. Pollutant Interactions

Pollutants normally occur together in the atmosphere in various combinations and concentration ratios. Early research suggested that no interactions were present, or if present they were antagonistic. The first reported synergistic interaction was found when Bel W_3 tobacco was exposed to mixtures of O_3 and SO_2 at concentrations that were not independently injurious. These results have been substantiated for several species but antagonistic responses have been reported for other species. The relative concentration ratios are important in determining the degree of interaction. Mixtures of NO_2 and SO_2 injured six crop plants at concentrations that independently did not injure the plants.

10.3.2.d. Other Factors

The interactions between pollutants and various biological agents are receiving considerable attention, but the subject is still not well understood. Most pathogenic organisms induce protection from O_3 injury in the host plant. In general, pollution inhibits diseases caused by fungi but greatly increases the parasitism of Botrytis cinerea and Armillarea mellea on several plants. The systemic presence of three tobacco viruses enhances the sensitivity of tobacco to O_3 even when virus symptoms are not pronounced.

The problem of Ponderosa pine decline was related to oxidants and several species of bark beetles. There is general agreement that the beetles invade trees injured by oxidants and can increase the rate of pine decline. Pollution stress on sensitive tree species, such as sycamore, may result in increased feeding by insects such as lace bugs and mites, thereby promoting early leaf senescence and abscission.

10.4. Toxicological Considerations

Generally, toxicological data concern the dose of a given substance that enters a living system. In air pollution research, dose refers to the concentration of a substance in air over the duration of exposure (concentration × time). This definition of dose is used throughout this discussion. The dose that enters the organism is really the "effective" dose, but the effective dose is difficult to determine in air pollution studies.

An understanding of the effects of a given pollutant dose on plants is essential for the development of air quality standards and as a basis for understanding the effects of pollutants on the environment. The ideal criteria would be a set of standard equations that would relate response to concentration and duration of exposure (time), and would reflect the effects of all factors that control the response of a specific plant to a specific pollutant. Such a multivariate model would become so complex that it would be of little practical importance. If the model were to assess only the most critical resistance factors, if these factors could be easily measured, and if average values for these factors were to reflect a given number of plant susceptibility groupings, then such a model would be useful. Two types of models are required if we are to define "what is happening." These two models would not be mutually exclusive. One would explain the acute membrane response, and the second would explain the chronic and subtle responses (Section 10.2.4).

10.4.1. Acute Response

The first acute dose–response model attempted was an empirical relationship for SO_2 developed by O'Gara. This equation was developed from acute exposures of alfalfa to SO_2 when grown under conditions of maximum sensitivity. Visible injury was the response measure used. The equation was originally written in a form that emphasized the concept of a threshold concentration and dose:

$$t(c - a) = b \tag{10.8}$$

where t is the exposure time (hr), c is the concentration (ppm), a is a concentration threshold for a specific percentage of injury, and b is a constant reflecting the other components of the model, such as inherent plant resistance and the external factors affecting resistance. This equation is often written

$$c = a + b/t. \tag{10.9}$$

Other efforts have been made to express the relationship between the pollutant concentration and exposure duration and the plant response, but they all reflect the O'Gara approach.

None of these efforts adequately describes the variation in plant response as either time or concentration, or both, varies. However, an empirical model has been developed that gives a reasonable interpretation of dose–response data. This model, used to analyze data on the foliar response of 14 plant species to O_3, has two characteristics: a constant percentage of leaf surface is injured by an air pollutant concentration that is inversely proportional to exposure duration raised to an exponent (Figure 10.2); and, for a given exposure duration, the percentage leaf injury as a function of pollutant concentration fits a log-normal frequency distribution (Figure 10.3). The complete leaf injury equation combines the equations shown in Figures 10.2 and 10.3. This equation expresses pollutant concentration as a function of plant response (injury) and exposure duration:

$$c = m_{ghr}s_g{}^z t^p \tag{10.10}$$

where c is the concentration (ppm), m_{ghr} is the geometric mean concentration for a 1 = hr exposure, s_g is the standard geometric deviation, z is the number of standard deviations from the median (injury), t is time (hr), and p is the slope of the injury line as a logarithmic curve. From the data for pinto bean in Figures 10.2 and 10.3,

$$c = 0.31 \cdot 1.44^z \cdot t^{-0.57}. \tag{10.11}$$

Figure 10.2 Percentage leaf injury in pinto bean plants exposed to various ozone concentrations for various durations—concentration versus exposure duration. (From Larsen, R.I., Heck, W.W. J. Air Pollut. Control Assoc. 26:325–333, 1976. Used with permission.)

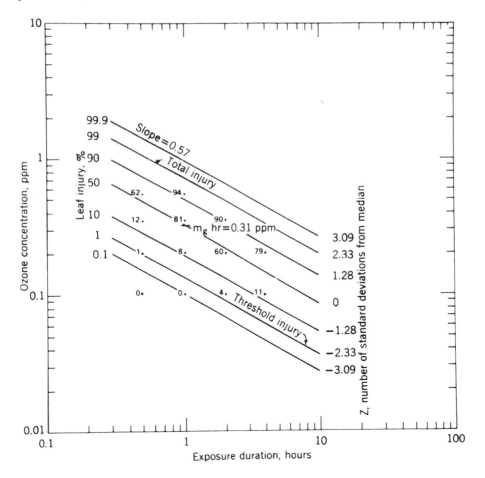

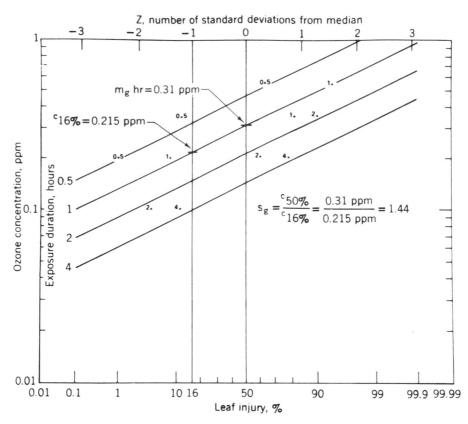

Figure 10.3 Percentage leaf injury in pinto bean plants exposed to various ozone concentrations for various durations—concentration versus percentage injury. (From Larsen, R.I., Heck, W.W. J. Air Pollut. Control Assoc. 26:325–333, 1976. Used with permission.)

Thus, a concentration of 0.104 ppm will injure 10% of the leaf surface in a 3-hr exposure. The O_3 concentrations required to cause 10% injury in a 3-hr exposure for tomato (cv. Roma), clover (cv. Pennscott Red), tobacco (cv. Bel W_3), and spinach (cv. Northland) are 0.095, 0.209, 0.088, and 0.395 ppm, respectively. From this analysis, it was suggested that average times of 1, 3, and 8 hr should be used in the development of oxidant standards for the protection of vegetation. This type of response data could be developed for SO_2 and for NO_2. Thus, this should be an effective approach to the development of criteria for use in establishing ambient air quality standards, whenever sufficient information is available.

Projected concentrations that would cause about 5% injury in three plant susceptibility groups for 1-, 3-, or 8-hr exposures are shown in Table 10.2 for O_3, SO_2, NO_2. These are subjective evaluations based on a review of available data. They can be used to predict effects in the field when ambient concentrations of the specific pollutant are known.

Table 10.2   Projected Pollutant Concentrations for Specific Exposure Durations That Will Produce About 5% Injury to Vegetation Grown Under Conditions of Varying Sensitivity

Pollutant	Time (hr)	Concentrations producing 5% injury		
		Sensitive	Intermediate	Resistant
Ozone	1.0	0.10–0.25	0.20–0.35	≥0.30
(ppm)	3.0	0.06–0.17	0.13–0.28	≥0.24
	8.0	0.03–0.12	0.10–0.22	≥0.20
Sulfur dioxide	1.0	0.50–2.5	2.0–7.5	≥7.0
(ppm)	3.0	0.22–1.6	1.2–4.0	≥3.5
	8.0	0.10–0.75	0.50–2.0	≥1.5
Nitrogen dioxide	1.0	3.0–10	9.0–20	≥18
(ppm)	3.0	2.2–6.5	6.0–13	≥11
	8.0	1.5–5.0	4.0–9.0	≥8.0
Hydrogen fluoride	8	1.6–4.8	4.0–24	≥20
(ppb)	24	0.8–3.2	2.4–16	≥12
	1 wk	0.60–1.6	1.2–6.4	≥5.6
	1 mo	0.40–0.8	0.8–4.0	≥2.4
	Growing season	0.24–0.56	0.40–1.6	≥0.8

10.4.2. Chronic Response

Although some efforts have been made to develop equations to predict long-term chronic responses, not enough data are available to test the equations adequately. However, a graphic presentation of available data was developed for fluoride (Figure 10.1) shown as HF. The available data for several plants or groups of plants were plotted. The data plots consist of a notation of responses (leaf symptoms, no symptoms yield effect, etc.) on a graph defined by the log of the mean atmospheric concentration (μg fluoride/m^3) and the log of exposure duration (da). From these plots, threshold curves were developed for various effects parameters for the plants listed. Although these are not calculated curves and may be subject to some error, they satisfy the concept of threshold values, below which no injury should occur. Figure 10.1 shows threshold curves for tomato, corn, sorghum, gladiolus, tree fruits, and conifers. The suggested threshold curves for the three most sensitive groups (gladiolus, sorghum, and conifers) terminate at 0.5 μg fluoride/m^3 over the exposure period used (2–4 weeks). The data for citrus (not shown in Figure 10.1) suggest 0.4 ppb HF or less as a long-term exposure limit (18 months). Projected concentration ranges of gaseous fluoride (as HF) that will injure three different susceptibility groups of plants on long-term exposure are shown in Table 10.2. This type of approach could be used for other pollutants when sufficient data are available.

10.5. Other Considerations

Our understanding of the relationship between air pollutants and vegetation would not be complete without a brief mention of several other aspects of this relationship. First, plants have long been used as indicators (monitors) of pollution stress. These studies have included both field and laboratory research. Second, pollution has had economic repercussions for many years; crop and forest losses to air pollutants have been well documented. Third, vegetation serves as both a passive (particulate and impaction) and active (gas sorption) removal mechanism for atmospheric contaminates. Finally, methods for the protection of crops against pollution insult have been studied and recommended.

10.5.1. Vegetation as a Biological Indicator (Monitor)

The use of plants to indicate air pollution problems has often permitted the early detection of these problems. Plants have also been used in field surveys to determine the accumulation of certain pollutants and in laboratory studies to determine the phytotoxicity of pollutants generated in chambers designed to study atmospheric reactions. Attempts to use plants as monitors of pollution concentration or of the phytotoxic potential of polluted atmosphere have not been very successful.

10.5.1.a. Field Surveys

Since plants are sensitive and may develop characteristic symptoms when exposed to certain air pollutants, they can serve as a useful indicator in field surveys. The field survey attempts to answer the question: Does this area have a significant air pollution problem?

If both the pollutant and its effects on vegetation are known, the area can be examined for a relatively few characteristic symptoms. The competent observer must then make a series of judgments concerning the tissue age, the site, the weather conditions, and the history of the monitoring plant. The observer should then be able to conclude whether an area has or has not been fumigated with a particular pollutant. However, the investigator can not deduce with a high degree of certainty the amount, duration, or number of exposures to an injurious pollutant. Three limitations to this approach are obvious. First, we can identify specific necrotic symptoms caused by only a relatively few pollutants—SO_2, fluoride, O_3, and PAN. Second, we are dependent upon the presence of susceptible varieties at a susceptible stage of growth when the exposures occur. Third, a knowledgeable observer must be present to observe the symptoms after they have developed but before they have become obscured by other changes.

The presence and abundance of lichen and moss species have been mapped for large urban or industrial areas for a number of years. Many of these investigations associated decreased abundance of these plants with increased air pollution, primarily SO_2. However, it is not possible to separate the various factors that influence the survival of lichen and moss communities. These communities probably respond to the general SO_2–dust–dirt–grime complex of an urban–industrial area. Therefore, lichens and mosses serve as general long-term indicators of the total environment and that may identify historical air pollution problems and other environmental imbalances, but they give little indication of current problems.

10.5.1.b. Pollutant Accumulation

In some cases (i.e., some salts, SO_2, and fluorides) accumulation of the pollutant in foliar tissue may indicate the cause of the observed symptoms. Salt injury along roads can often be confirmed by chloride analysis. In most situations involving occasional acute fumigations with SO_2, tissue analysis for sulfate will not satisfactorily confirm the causative agent because the normal sulfate content of leaf tissue varies over a wide range of values depending upon plant species, soil fertilizer practices, and other factors. However, in cases of chronic air pollution exposures or acute exposures imposed upon chronic exposures, sulfate levels in the leaf tissue may confirm SO_2 as the causative agent for the observed field symptoms. Fluoride accumulation in plant tissues has special significance, because even small amounts can indicate fluoride problems. Plants grown in areas free from fluoride air pollution problems rarely accumulate as much as 20 ppm fluoride on a dry weight basis. Measurements of fluoride accumulation have been used to help confirm the effects of fluoride injury in plants and levels of fluoride in forage that may harm grazing animals.

10.5.1.c. Bioassay as a Pollutant Indicator

Plants may be used as field indicators (monitors) after general field surveys have established the presence of specific pollutants or groups of pollutants. Some of the uncertainties of field surveys are reduced by exposing plants under controlled culture in field situations where surveys are conducted. Species or varieties are selected for pollutant specificity, sensitivity, and symptom characteristics. Plants may be cultured under controlled conditions, exposed to ambient air, and returned to a controlled environment for symptom development and evaluation. In other cases, plants are germinated and grown to a given stage under known cultural conditions, transplanted to the field, and "read" periodically in the field. Various modifications of these basic techniques have been used. These techniques improve the specificity and sensitivity of field indicators by exposing more uniform plant material over the entire growing season. Generally, our ability to quantitate the field problem is improved by use of these techniques.

10.5.1.d. Bioassay of Chemical Reaction Systems

The initial isolation and identification of phytotoxic components of the photochemical oxidant complex were complicated by the lack of adequate chemical techniques. Thus, several early chemical reaction chambers used plants to help elucidate the chemical nature of the phytotoxic components. Seven types of phytotoxicants were suggested from an analysis of the experimental results using the response of selected sensitive plant species. These results imply that additional phytotoxicants are present in the photochemical complex besides PAN and O_3.

10.5.2. Economic Considerations

A distinction can be made between "injury" and "damage." Injury is any identifiable and measurable response of a plant to air pollution. Damage is any identifiable and measurable adverse effect upon the desired or intended use or derived product of the plant. Leaf necrosis on soybean or lettuce is injury. In the case of lettuce, the economic value would be reduced (damage). However, in soybean, damage would depend upon whether a reduction in yield occurred. Metabolic changes that accompany low pollutant concentrations (injury) might not cause visible injury but may cause damage (economic loss).

It is difficult to assess the economic, ecological, or aesthetic costs of air pollution damage to vegetation. Estimates have ranged from a low of $135 million up to $500 million per year for economic losses of crop plants alone in the United States. None of the estimates includes possible growth and yield reductions in the absence of visible injury, effects on native ecosystems, decreased aesthetic value when ornamentals are injured, reduction in vigor, predisposition to invasion by pests, or other important considerations. If these diverse factors were included, the total annual cost estimate would probably exceed 1×10^9.

10.5.3. Vegetation as an Air Pollutant Sink

The value of vegetation in controlling air pollution has been discussed for years. The concept has received encouragement from the proponents of greenbelts as an aid in protecting urban areas from industrial pollution. Plant scientists favor the development of greenbelts for use as parks within large urban–industrial complexes, but have been skeptical of the greenbelt as a means of controlling pollution.

It has long been recognized that trees filter particulates. The larger the particulate and the more stable the atmospheric conditions, the better the tree screen will operate. With small particulates and increased turbulence, the effectiveness of the screen will decrease. To be effective, a screen must be several trees in depth.

The sink concept is of interest to atmospheric chemists and meteorologists who are developing air pollutant budgets. What are the ultimate sinks of air pollutants? Reports indicate that plants, soil, and soil organisms are effective sinks for gaseous air pollutants under certain conditions. Soil is apparently a minor sink per se, but the microbial constituents of the soil are effective via metabolic activity. Several attempts have been made to quantify pollutant uptake by plants; these data are then used to calculate the total uptake of each pollutant per acre of plants under given pollutant loads. This work suggests that vegetation is a significant pollutant sink.

It is one thing to find that plants are major pollutant sinks and another to extrapolate this information to support the development of greenbelts primarily for the purpose of decreasing pollutant concentration. Greenbelts will not serve as an effective barrier against gaseous pollutants, although they are of supplemental benefit since they are effective sinks. However, plants do not respond in a predictable way over time and are not active over the greater part of the year. Thus, they should not be expected to act as reliable pollutant filters and greenbelts should not be recommended as an air pollution control strategy.

10.5.4. Plant Protection from Air Pollutants

Studies show genetic variability in pollutant sensitivity within varieties of any given species. Thus there is a genetic basis for the sensitivity of plants to pollutants and it should be possible to breed resistant varieties. Some selection of resistant varieties has probably occurred, since plant breeders normally select plants with the highest yield and least injury regardless of cause. Natural selection pressures have, no doubt, increased the tolerance of populations of some native species located near urban–industrial areas.

An understanding of plant sensitivity to environmental effects enables the recommendation of certain practices that could be instituted during air pollution alerts. Recommendations have been made with regard to soil moisture for greenhouse- and irrigation-grown plants, since we know that infrequent watering during times of high air pollution potential will make sensitive crops more resistant. Some chemical sprays have been used experimentally to protect plants from air pollution. Lime sprays are recommended for protecting peaches against fluoride-induced soft suture. In general, chemical techniques are not presently recommended because of the frequency of application needed for continued resistance, the cost of chemicals, the possibility of undesirable residues, and the inability to predict accurately high pollution days.

Suggested Reading

Committee on Biologic Effects of Atmospheric Pollutants. Fluorides, Chap. 7 (1971); Chlorine and Hydrogen Chloride, Chap. 6 (1975); Nitrogen Oxides, Chap. 9 (1977); Photochemical Oxidants, Chaps. 11 and 12 (1977); Sulfur Oxides (1979). Washington, D.C.: National Academy of Sciences.

Dugger, W. M. (Ed.). Air Pollution Effects on Plant Growth. ACS Symposium Series 3. Washington, D. C.: American Chemical Society, 1974.

Heck, W. W., Taylor, O. C., Heggestad, H. E. Air pollution research needs: Herbaceous and ornamental plants and agriculturally generated pollutants. J. Air Pollut. Control Assoc. 23:257, 1973.

Heggestad, H. E., Heck, W.W. Nature, extent and variation of plant response to air pollutants. Adv. Agron. 23:111, 1971.

Jacobson, J. S., Hill, A. C. (Eds.). Recognition of Air Pollution Injury to Vegetation: A Pictorial Atlas. Pittsburgh: Air Pollution Control Association, 1970.

Lacasse, N. L., Treshow, M. (Eds.). Diagnosing vegetation injury caused by air pollution. Contract 68-02-1344. Research Triangle Park, N. C.: Environmental Protection Agency, 1976.

Mudd, J. B., Kozlowski, T.E. (Eds.). Response of Plants to Air Pollutants. New York: Academic Press, 1975.

Thomas, M. D. Gas damage to plants. Annu. Rev. Plant Physiol. 2:293, 1951.

van Haut, H., Stratmann, H. Farbtafelatlas uber Schwefeldixid-/Wirkungen an Pflanzen. Essen, Federal Republic of Germany: Girardet, 1970.

T. J. Sheets

11

Transport of Pollutants

11.1. Introduction

Many man-made pollutants are widely distributed in nature. Some can be found great distances from sites that are known to be points of discharge or release into the environment. Some, such as PCBs and DDT, are almost ubiquitous in nature, but the extensive distribution of these highly persistent, water-insoluble compounds was recognized only within the past two decades after ultrasensitive detection instruments were developed.

The movement of pollutants can be interpreted and understood through the laws of chemistry, physics, and biology. Movement occurs from the points of introduction into the environment, where the concentration is relatively high, to areas removed from the point of introduction, where concentrations are usually lower. In some situations, specific pollutants accumulate to levels exceeding the concentrations in surrounding media. Examples of such build-up, including biomagnification in top carnivores and high levels of food chains, are given in Chapter 9.

Transport of pollutants is promoted and sustained by wind and water movement and is influenced by temperature, the physical state and chemical properties of the pollutant, and other factors. Pollutants are moved to some extent regardless of their water solubility and physical and chemical properties. It is easy to visualize movement in water of pollutants that are water soluble (such as nitrate, sulfate, and chloride ions) or gases in air (such as sulfur dioxide and nitrous oxide) that are carried with air currents. On the other hand, it is more difficult for the layman to understand how compounds such as PCBs and DDT, which are extremely insoluble in water and exhibit very low vapor pressures, have been transported and deposited in areas remote from points of introduction into the environment. For most pollutants the ultimate sink or site of deposition is the depths of the oceans.

11.2. Movement in Air

The atmosphere is a dynamic system. Temperature and winds, in various compass directions and vertically in either direction, greatly influence the rate and volume of movement of dissolved or dispersed pollutants. Movement of pollutants can occur by diffusion and drift in air currents. Diffusion generally is slow and occurs over short distances. Drift of suspended particles can occur readily under windy conditions, and movement by drift will usually be for much greater distances within a specified time than that occurring by simple diffusion. Light gases that readily disperse in air are transported long distances in air currents.

A good example of local or short-distance movement through the air is the drift of pesticides from the point of application to adjacent areas. Such drift is in the direction of the flow of air, and the amount and distance of movement are related to the size of the particles (either dust or spray), the velocity of the wind, and the height above ground at which the pesticide is dispersed. Formulations of pesticides known as invert emulsions (water dispersed in oil instead of oil in water) have been developed that can be applied by aircraft with little or no drift. Such developments facilitate the application of such chemicals and minimize contamination of nontarget areas.

Manufacturing plants of various types are sometimes the source of air pollutants, and, as with the application of pesticides, drift and vapor movement can occur from these sites to other areas. Many years ago sulfur dioxide gas emitted from a copper smelting plant near Ducktown, Tennessee, killed vegetation over a large area around the smeltery. For several miles in all directions the hills were completely denuded. Extensive efforts to revegetate the area have met with limited success. In addition to being toxic to the vegetation, the sulfur dioxide, once deposited on the soil, increased the acidity to the extent that the soil would not support plant growth. Combined with the effect of denudation and acid soils, severe erosion resulted in the loss of all topsoil, exposing the highly acidic clay subsoils of very low fertility. Efforts are still being directed to revegetating the area, and much time will be required to restore the land to a productive state.

Salt sprays continuously affect coastal vegetation. Moreover, there are reports of salt carried from the ocean in air and deposited in rainwater on certain inland areas of the United States. Deposition over a long time may approach 100 kg/ha near the coast and 4–5 kg/ha several hundred kilometers inland. This is a natural phenomenon. It is not man's utilization of the environment alone that produces pollution; nature can do it also.

There are a few examples of long-distance movement of pollutants in winds. Smoke from factories has been carried from Ohio to the southeastern United States and from Germany to Scandinavia. In Arizona, DDT transport was reported for distances 80–100 km. The presence of DDT at sites downwind was determined by measuring residues deposited upon the soil surface over an extended period; as with many other examples of environmental pollution with DDT and related chlorinated hydrocarbons, it was possible to demonstrate the presence of these residues only with very sophisticated and sensitive instrumentation.

Other observations suggested that pesticides such as DDT were transported in the wind from the panhandle areas of Texas and Oklahoma to Cincinnati, Ohio. Similarly, transport in the wind over long distances from England (or Western Europe) to the western Atlantic is suspected for some pesticides. In such cases the amount transported is very small, and the results are often questioned because it is difficult to measure such small amounts as are purported to be present in air.

Movement of some pollutants is global. Radioactive elements from nuclear explosions are known to be widely distributed around the globe. Radioactive particles form nuclei for snowflakes and raindrops that fall to earth. Fallout, therefore, is generally greater in humid areas. The northwestern coast of the United States, adjacent areas of Canada, and the eastern half of the United States generally receive greater despositions of radioactive fallout than other areas of the two countries from nuclear explosions in the western Pacific area and Asia, and more fallout has occurred in the northern hemisphere than in the southern hemisphere.

Somewhat reminiscent of the fallout from nuclear explosions is the deposition of mercury after fossil fuels are burned. The mercury is widely distributed in low concentrations and fallout is generally accentuated by rainfall.

The presence of DDT and PCBs in Antarctica, in all likelihood, is due mainly to aerial transport and deposition there, but movement in ocean currents and migratory animals surely contribute to some extent.

11.3. Transport in Surface Water

Pollutants are transported in water as dissolved ions and molecules or on suspended particulate matter. Soluble forms of nitrates, sulfates, phosphates, and other salts are moved relatively freely by water. Similarly, some pesticides that are soluble in water and are not strongly adsorbed to particulate matter can be transported freely. In nature, some pesticides such as 2,4-D, though soluble or slightly soluble in water in some forms, are decomposed so rapidly and are applied in such a way that significant pollution is unlikely. A few, picloram for example, would be readily transported if they were discharged into water. Detergents, a major source of phosphate pollutants, and sulfuric acid, an undesirable by-product of coal mining, are highly soluble and are readily carried wherever the water goes.

The concentration of a contaminant in water usually decreases with time if the discharge does not recur. Water-soluble pollutants that move freely are diluted as uncontaminated water mixes with contaminated water. Concentrations of soluble pollutants, therefore, decrease as distance from the source of pollution increases in proportion to the volume of uncontaminated water entering a polluted stream.

Chemical and biological degradation reduces the concentration of contaminants, and most water-soluble organic compounds are biologically degraded within a few days or weeks. Adsorption to clay or organic colloids reduces the availability of pollutants and, hence, reduces their toxicity to biota.

The insoluble pollutants and those that are adsorbed to or associated with clay or organic colloids are moved as suspended particles. Transport of the suspended particles is usually much slower than transport of soluble forms; the pattern of movement is different and exposure of animals and plants is sometimes greater. Over a long time, total movement can be extensive and long distance, if the contaminant is persistent. Suspended particles settle out along a water course as velocity of flow recedes. The heavier the suspended particle, the sooner it settles. The smallest particles remain suspended longest and are therefore transported farthest.

Turbulent flow of water from storm runoff redistributes sediment deposits. As flow increases, deposits from previous flow are resuspended and moved farther downstream. With a series of such storms over extended periods, pollutants will be transported to estuaries and ultimately to the oceans. As with water-soluble forms, dilution occurs as insoluble and adsorbed pollutants are carried farther from the source and become mixed with uncontaminated sediment. Some dilution may also occur as, by mass action, adsorbed molecules are slowly desorbed and carried away as solutes in very dilute form.

Chemicals that persist in the environment for long periods can be deposited in sediment along streams and in other bodies of water and accumulate there. Ecologically sensitive sites where accumulation has occurred include farm ponds, lakes, estuaries, sounds, and shallow seas. Measurement of DDT levels in the water and sediment of the Tar River in North Carolina in 1967 and 1968 showed sediments containing concentrations of "apparent DDT"[1] 10–10,000 times greater than water flowing above the deposits. Similar differences have been observed for the lower Mississippi River and other delta regions. The ultimate sink is the ocean floor; but, in spite of its vastness, the ocean is not an unlimited sink into which we can forever deposit nondegradable toxic wastes.

According to estimates in a report of the National Academy of Sciences in 1971, 0.1% of the DDT produced annually reached the oceans by surface runoff and transport down rivers. The estimates placed the total amount at about 100 tons DDT/year. Similarly, PCB transport to oceans through North American rivers was estimated to be about 200 tons/year.

Other calculations show that if all of the nitrogen used as fertilizer in North Carolina were dissolved in all of the precipitation (in excess of that lost to the atmosphere by evapotranspiration), the average nitrate concentration would be 3 ppm. Uptake of nitrogen by plants and microorganisms was not considered in this calculation; on the other hand, some nitrate is deposited on the soil from the atmosphere. The hypothetical 3 ppm nitrate alone is insufficient to support eutrophication (see Chapter 14), but nitrogen from fertilization contributes to the nitrate load in streams and other bodies of water. Furthermore, nitrate from fertilizer, though a nonpoint source, is not evenly distributed in water from rainfall.

11.4. Movement in Soil

Several transfer processes act upon pollutants in soils and give rise to spatial displacement. Pollutant molecules may be absorbed by plants, adsorbed to soil particles, displaced downward into the soil profile, transported in surface runoff, or lost to the atmosphere by vaporization.

---

[1]The term "apparent DDT" refers to the value calculated from the total response on a gas chromatograph at the retention times of DDT and its isomers.

Molecules absorbed into plant roots may subsequently be transported within the plant. If plant parts containing pollutants such as lead, ^{40}K, or ^{226}Ra are harvested and removed, the chemical present within or on the plant tissue is also moved. In most cases, such movement accounts for very small (usually insignificant) amounts of pollutants, including pesticides. However, under some conditions sufficient contamination occurs to create a hazard to animals or people consuming plants grown on contaminated soil. For example, relatively high levels of lead, a by-product of combustion of leaded gasoline, have been found on vegetation near heavily traveled highways. In the recent past, potatoes and a few other food and feed commodities have been contaminated with residues of certain chlorinated hydrocarbon insecticides to levels exceeding official tolerance levels, forcing removal of such commodities from commerce.

Some pollutants are strongly bound to clays and organic matter in soils; others are adsorbed little or not at all. The amount and strength of binding depends on several factors: molecular structure, polarity, and basicity of the chemical pollutants and the type and amount of clay, amount of organic matter, and moisture content of the soil. Adsorption to soil particles retards or restricts leaching, vaporization, and other processes. It also reduces availability to plants and animals and consequently reduces or even eliminates toxicity. Paraquat, a widely used herbicide, is almost totally adsorbed to soil, and its toxic effect to plants is thereby eliminated when the chemical comes in contact with soil.

A few substances can be readily leached downward into the soil profile by percolating water. Water-soluble compounds and ions that are not adsorbed to soil particles are moved wherever water moves. The nitrate ion is a very mobile soil constituent and with heavy rainfall may be leached so deeply into the soil profile, especially sandy soils, that the beneficial effects of nitrate fertilization are reduced or eliminated.

Some pollutants, certain pesticides for example, are transported from cultivated land in surface flow during and after rainstorms. Contrary to common belief, insoluble chemicals are usually moved in greater amounts in surface runoff than soluble ones. Water-soluble compounds are readily leached and hence are displaced from the soil surface into the soil early during rainstorms, whereas insoluble chemicals remain on or near the surface and are eroded away by the impact of rain and by the force of surface flow. They become suspended in and are carried away by the surface runoff.

Total movement of an organic pollutant in surface runoff is also related to its persistence. Rapidly decomposing compounds do not remain long enough to be carried in significant amounts, except when erosive rains fall soon after application. Experiments have shown that only a very small portion of applied pesticides is displaced in surface runoff. Percentages based on the amounts applied are often less than 1% and usually are less than 5%.

Many pollutants, including some pesticides, are volatile. Highly volatile pesticides must be injected into the soil or incorporated by disking soon after application to maintain concentrations in the soil sufficient to control pests. Loss from soil surfaces is a function of vapor pressure of the chemical and is influenced by air and soil temperature, soil moisture, and adsorption of the pollutant molecules to soil particles.

The importance of the several transport processes varies widely with type of pollutant and environmental conditions. Relatively few pollutants are transported in significant amounts by all of the processes. Nitrate is a fertilizer constituent that can, under appropriate conditions, be moved by all of the transport processes discussed above. Phosphorous, on the other hand, doesn't leach readily; low solubility in water and binding usually restrict movement of phosphorous in soils. Arsenic, lead, and several other heavy metals do not leach appreciably. A few pesticides are moved relatively freely with percolating water (for example 2,4,5-T, picloram, fenac, and TCA), but most remain near the soil surface.

Water-soluble pollutants with a low affinity for clay and organic colloids in soils (nitrate ion, for example) may occasionally be leached to the water table. A favorable combination of factors must exist for such movement to occur. Conditions favoring movement to the water table include a shallow water table, coarse sandy soil, and high rainfall continuing for an extended period. Water must percolate downward in a sufficient quantity to reach the water table since the pollutant can be leached no farther than the water moves, and several centimeters of water are required to reach the water table in most soils.

11.5. Movement in Ground Water

Dissolved ions and molecules that reach the surface of the water table become mixed very little with the mass of water below. Water moves very slowly along the surface of the water table in the direction of a stream or other depression where the water table reaches the soil surface, and the slow moving water carries with it any substances in solution.

Contamination of ground water has been a point of concern with pollutants such as pesticides, nitrate, and certain others. Most contamination problems caused by pesticides have arisen from improper use, improper disposal, careless practices when filling spray tanks, and improper drainage around wells. In a few instances, pollutants from discarded wastes have moved along an aquifer as far as 3 km to contaminate water sources. Although such instances have been rare, the problem may become more acute with the increasing deposits of wastes from ever-expanding industrialization, and we must maintain an adequate surveillance system to avoid problems in the future.

11.6. Transport in Animals

Small but significant amounts of some pollutants are transported by animals. Fat-soluble molecules that are persistent in the environment (such as DDT and PCBs) are stored in animal fat (see Chapter 8). When animals containing pollutant molecules (PCBs, for example) migrate, the contaminants are transported and subsequently are excreted, or upon death are released into the environment. Volume of transport in migratory animals is relatively small, but significant effects occur when contaminated animals produce offspring or are consumed by other animals that are more sensitive to the toxicant. Excreted substances are usually diluted to the extent that biologically active amounts are not absorbed or consumed by other organisms. However, such sources contribute to the body burden of toxic compounds in animals and become a part of persistent toxicants that move through food chains.

11.7. Transfer from One Medium to Another

Transfer from one medium to another, e.g., from air to soil or water, soil to air or water, or water to soil or air, usually involves a change in the physical state of the ions and molecules being transferred. Volatilization, precipitation, absorption, adsorption, solubilization, sublimation, and codistillation are processes by which pollutants are exchanged between physical states and between media. The involvement of specific pollutants in some of these processes has been intensively studied. Volatilization is an important process by which a number of pesticides are lost from the soil surface. Adsorption effectively inactivates many pollutant molecules that might otherwise harm plants or animals. Oil slicks on the surfaces of oceans are diminished largely by evaporation of the lightest components; solubilization may contribute in a small way to dilution of oil spills.

Scientists are presently studying several of the transfer processes in oceans, with specific attention being given to the exchange of ions and molecules at interfaces: oil–water, oil–air, water–air, and sediment–water. The processes are influenced by environmental and weather factors such as temperature, wind, and precipitation and by properties and characteristics of pollutants such as vapor pressure, solubility, affinity for sediments, polarity, and charge. Increased knowledge of the transfer processes and the influence of various factors on specific pollutants will help to alleviate and avoid long-term pollutant problems.

Suggested Reading

Holt, R.F., Timmons, D.R., Latterell, J.J. Accumulation of phosphates in water. J. Agric. Food Chem. 18:781–784, 1970.

Kurtz, L.T. The fate of applied nutrients in soils. J. Agric. Food Chem. 18:773–780, 1970.

Letey, J., Farmer, W.J. Movement of pesticides in soil. In Guenzi, W.D. (Ed.). Pesticides in Soil and Water, Madison, Wisc.: Soil Science Society of America, 1974, pp. 67–97.

McClure, V.E. Transport of heavy chlorinated hydrocarbons in the atmosphere. Environ. Sci. Technol. 10:1223–1229, 1976.

Merkle, M.G., Bovey, R.W. Movement of pesticides in surface water. In Guenzi, W.D. (Ed.). Pesticides in Soil and Water. Madison, Wisc.: Soil Science Society of America, 1974, pp. 99–106.

U.S. Department of the Interior. Mercury in the Environment. Geological Survey Professional Paper 713. Washington, D.C., 1970.

Windom, H.L., Duce, R.A. Marine Pollutant Transfer. Lexington, Mass.: Heath, 1976.

George T. Barthalmus
Gary M. Rand

12

Behavioral Toxicology

12.1. Introduction

Neurobehavioral toxicology, a subdiscipline of neurotoxicology, has been re-emerging over the past 10 years. Our understanding of the neurochemical correlates of behavior, coupled with the development of new behavioral techniques and equipment, may provide sensitive indices of the toxic effects of a wide variety of environmental contaminants and specific information regarding the site of action of neurotoxins.

It is important to recognize at the onset that humans are unique in the quantity and complexity of their nervous system and the array of behaviors they display, and that these unique qualities are not due to any remarkable differences in their biochemistry or physiology, or in the structure of their cells, tissues, organs, and organ systems. Undermining of human behavior results in destruction of their uniqueness, as well as their capacity to survive in a dynamic environment. The last statement applies to all animals since behavior is the final integrated expression at the interface between animals and their total environment.

To date, toxicology has relied mostly on biochemical, cytological, and morphological criteria as indices of effects resulting from subchronic and chronic exposure to toxic agents. Frequently, the exposure levels are unrealistic and are not encountered in the environment. Neuropathologists and neurochemists have seen very subtle changes in nervous system structure and function. Often these changes precede detectable biochemical change, and this is perhaps the prime rationale for behavioral toxicology. Behavioral change may occur on a dose–response curve of toxic effects sooner than neurochemical or neurophysiological toxin-related changes.

Implicit in behavioral toxicological studies is the need to evaluate the intact organism, the behaviors that reflect its total internal biological state, and the concomitant responses it makes to its environment. To study behavior the scientist must discard the idea that survival following exposure implies no effect, a notion that has hindered the development of realistic environmental quality standards. Certainly, concentrations not causing death may disrupt or alter a myriad of genetically programmed behaviors, such as reflexes or phototaxes, that have survival importance and are essential to daily performance and adaptability within the environment. Behavioral toxicology studies should employ a level of toxin that produces no gross sign of intoxication. The expression of much of an animal's behavior is dependent on locomotor activity, and it is essential to employ toxicants at concentrations that do not at first impair locomotor activity. For example, if a fish cannot swim well, it obviously cannot be expected to avoid shocks in an aquatic shuttle apparatus.

An urgent priority in behavioral toxicological research is the development of simple, inexpensive, and sensitive batteries of behavioral screening tests for use by government agencies, industry, and private institutions. Such procedures will facilitate the evaluation of the hundreds of new compounds that are manufactured each year.

Incomplete knowledge of the parameters involved in normal behavior slows the rate of progress in neurobehavioral toxicology. In order to understand the etiological mechanisms of toxin-induced behavioral dysfunction we must first understand the normal and intact organism, its functioning nervous system, and the way the complete organism adjusts to a dynamic environment.

Early experimentation with poisons has contributed to our knowledge of the mode of action of neurotoxins such as nicotine and curare and the neurotoxicological consequences of exposure, and enhanced our understanding of the structure and function of the nervous system. Behavioral toxicology may therefore contribute to our understanding of nervous systems and the neurochemical correlates of normal and abnormal behavior.

12.2. Methodology

Since the underlying premise in behavioral toxicology is that animal behavior represents the expressed summation of sensory and motor functions of the nervous system, it is not surprising to find studies that report measurable behavioral dysfunctions from levels of exposure that produce no histopathological or morphological alterations in tissues. Experimentation in the Soviet Union has pioneered those behavioral measures that establish chronic toxicity standards for both the natural environment and the working environment of industrial workers. A comparison of recommended limits for 100 common contaminants showed Soviet maximum allowable concentrations (MAC) to be lower than American recommendations in 78 cases (Table 12.1). One factor contributing to this difference has been the use by Soviet toxicologists of behavioral and neurophysiological methods. This has prompted the development of behavioral toxicological research in the United States and the reduction of permissible levels of some agents (e.g., trichloroethylene).

We must recognize that any method employed to study behavioral phenomena involves difficulties. Paradoxically, preconceived ideas based largely on our awareness of the behavior of humans and animals can interfere with the objectivity so necessary in behavioral research. Additionally, behavior is dynamic, as it reflects changes in the interactions between the individual and the environment. These changes may be obvious or so subtle that elaborate techniques must be employed to measure them. A third difficulty is the loose definition of pollution (too much of anything), in that sufficient exposure to virtually anything can have behavioral consequences. The quantitative effect of an agent will usually depend upon the dose administered. In the past 35 years, experimental psychologists and behavioral pharmacologists have developed objective and quantitative techniques that are appropriate to pharmacological studies on behavior.

Many difficult questions concerning methodology remain: (a) Which procedures are most sensitive for a given test animal, dosage, and duration? (b) Does a change in behavior following exposure constitute an undesirable effect? (c) Can animal behavioral models apply to our understanding of toxicoses in humans? Despite their knowledge of the ways behavior is affected by drugs, behavioral pharmacologists are frequently confronted with these questions in the application of their techniques to behavioral toxicology.

Table 12.1 Ratios of U.S. to Soviet Maximum Allowable Concentrations (mg/m^3) for the Substances with the Highest Ratios

Substance	U.S. MAC	Soviet MAC	Ratio U.S./Soviet
Propylene oxide	240	1	240
Aniline	19	0.1	190
Ethyl bromide	890	5	178
Morpholine	70	0.5	140
Mesityl oxide	100	1	100
α-Methylstyrene	480	5.0	96
Methylchloroform	1900	20	95
Ethylene oxide	90	1	90
Methyl bromide	80	1	80
Acetaldehyde	360	5	72
p-Nitroaniline	6	1	60
Ethyl chloride	2600	50	52
Ethyleneimine	1	0.02	50
Heptachlor	0.5	0.01	50
Chloroprene	90	2	45
Vinyl chloride	1300	30	43
Methyl methacrylate	410	10	41
Cyclopentadiene	200	5	40
Methylcyclohexane	2000	50	40
Hydrogen cyanide	11	0.3	37
Dioxane	360	10	36
Propylene dichloride	350	10	35
Ethylene chlorohydrin	16	0.5	32
Butyl alcohol	300	10	30
Tetranitromethane	8	0.3	27
Aldrin	0.25	0.01	25
Dieldrin	0.25	0.01	25
Ethylmercaptan	25	1	25

Source: Ekel, G.J., Teichner, W.H. An Analysis and Critique of Behavioral Toxicology in the USSR. DHEW Publ. NIOSH 77-160, 1976.

Note: The MACs in the table are for work areas. In most cases the American MACs are weighted average concentrations for an 8-hr shift, while the Soviet MACs are the ceiling values. This makes the true ratios even higher than listed in the table.

12.2.1. Unconditioned Responses

12.2.1.a. Elicited (Reflex) Responses

Elicited responses include reflexes such as the constriction of the pupil to light, the knee jerk to a gentle tap, salivation to food, or paw withdrawal to a footshock. Although important, they constitute a small portion of an animal's total behavior. They occur regularly and quickly when the eliciting stimulus is presented. Under normal conditions, the response is generally stimulus specific. The reflex response depends on the properties of the eliciting stimulus (duration, intensity, and frequency of presentation), and is quantified by its latency of onset, its amplitude, and the intensity of the stimulus necessary to induce it. Elicited responses have been employed widely to assess the analgesic effects of a drug or drug specificity (i.e., whether a drug will affect other behavior at a dose that does not affect reflex responses).

The usefulness of elicited responses in toxicological work depends in part on the organism tested. Aquatic toxicologists studying an important estuarine food web may find it difficult to use a key species such as a larval crustacean in experimental learning situations. However, crustacean reflex behavior may serve as a sensitive indicator of the effect of thermal or chemical pollution. Alterations in the phototactic reflexes, also associated with the shadow reflex, of crab and grass shrimp larvae may subject these and similar species to greater predation. As these species mature, their responses to sudden light changes often decrease; consequently, early larval stages are most appropriate for studying this elicited behavior. Selected elicited responses may also be useful in screening tests for toxicological studies involving mammals.

12.2.1.b. Emitted (Spontaneous) Responses

Unlike elicited responses, emitted responses are not induced by an identifiable stimulus. Instead, many variables, both exogenous and endogenous, affect the spontaneously emitted behavior of the organism; e.g., the amount of swimming activity of a goldfish placed in an aquarium slowly but characteristically decreases with time. The time of day, nutritional state, reproductive season, and water temperature and chemistry, as well as the fish's previous experience in the aquarium, influence the characteristics of the habituation. The specific eliciting stimuli are not easily recognized unless one controls the specific enviornmental stimuli responsible for the emitted behavior of the fish. The use of spontaneously emitted behaviors in evaluating a toxic agent requires detailed observational methods that permit the recording of all definable elements of behavior. Toxicological field studies of this sort are almost nonexistent; however, studies of spontaneous activity and social behavior in undisturbed residential laboratory settings continue to be developed.

The interaction between reflexive and spontaneous responses may be complex in natural behavioral patterns. Much social behavior (particularly reproductive behavior) initially is dominated by spontaneous behavior. Slowly, however, specific eliciting stimuli cause reflexive behavior to appear in sequence, so that the final result (fertilization) is controlled via autonomic nervous reflexes. Often, this sequence is predictable and stereotyped and may serve as a behavioral unit for study in toxicology. Such studies are needed because these complexes of behavior that occur in nature are relatively unchanged in the laboratory; consequently, they reflect a truer picture of animal behavior as it occurs in nature.

12.2.2. Conditioned Responses

Reflexive and spontaneous responses may be modified by two types of conditioning, classical (or Pavlovian) and operant; reflexive responses are best modified classically and spontaneous responses operantly.

12.2.2.a. Classical Conditioning

In classical or Pavlovian conditioning, a neutral stimulus (one that does not normally elicit a response) is presented with an eliciting stimulus that produces a response. Several paired presentations of these two stimuli create a condition wherein the neutral stimulus alone may elicit the response. One example is that of a dog that salivates when meat is placed in its mouth. If a buzzer is sounded with the presentation of meat, after several trials the dog may salivate in response to the buzzer alone. At this time, the buzzer is called the conditioning stimulus and salivation is the conditioned response. The meat is called the unconditioned stimulus, and the salivation is called the unconditioned response. The rate of acquisition of a conditioned response depends on factors such as the intensity of and time period between the conditioning and unconditioned stimulus. Classical conditioning increases the number of stimuli capable of controlling a response, and it is restricted to responses that have an initial unconditioned response.

The classically conditioned subject is very sensitive to slight changes in the experimental environment or procedure, and therefore behavior can be disrupted easily. However, when conditions are constant, a strong consistent conditioned response can be maintained for years. Classical conditioning has been useful in determining sensory thresholds when the intensity of the neutral stimulus is varied. These techniques may be useful in alerting behavioral toxicologists to signs of sensory dysfunction. Such methodologies are time consuming and costly, and they require highly skilled individuals to conduct the tests. Methodological refinements are needed that will preserve or increase the sensitivity of behavioral assessments of sensory functions and concurrently lower the cost of this high-priority research.

12.2.2.b. Operant Conditioning

Our complex behavior develops as a result of past experience. Operant conditioning deals with processes by which the consequences of present behavior determine future behavior. Unlike classical conditioning, operant paradigms are not concerned with modification of the eliciting condition for behavior. For example, if a food-deprived pigeon is placed in a sound and light-attenuating operant chamber containing an illuminated response key and a mechanical food dispenser, the response key would not be considered a normal eliciting stimulus. However, when the bird is given free access to food presented several inches below the response key, the probability that the bird will peck the key by chance is increased. One accidental key peck (the response) followed by brief food presentation (reinforcement) increases the likelihood of future responses.

Subsequent responding further increases the probability of future responses when the reinforcement immediately follows the response. A positive reinforcement refers to the presentation of pleasant events (food, water), while a negative reinforcement would involve the removal of unpleasant events (shock, loud noise); both types of reinforcement, although opposites, increase responding for reasons too complex to describe here.

The value of operant procedures may also be observed when studies are conducted comparing the stable operant behavior of animals dosed prior to behavioral training with those dosed after the animal has acquired a stable baseline of behavior. Such comparisons enable researchers to determine whether the rate and pattern of the training process is more or less affected by toxins than the maintenance of the ongoing stable behavioral baseline. The reproducibility of operant behavioral techniques is beneficial to toxicologists since there are few simple stereotypic natural behaviors that can be easily and objectively measured in laboratory test animals.

12.3. Variables Influencing Behavioral Effects

Numerous exogenous and endogenous factors enhance or mask the behavioral effects of toxic substances. In this section emphasis is placed on the dilemma confronting toxicologists in attempts to conduct controlled experiments that relate the variables of age, nutrition, previous diseases, medical history, genetics, and agent interaction.

12.3.1. Endogenous Factors

12.3.1.a. Age

Clearly, age is an important factor predisposing organisms to behavioral effects of toxins. Nervous systems are inherited, develop, and reach some optimal functional state that is closely related to the number and maintenance of neurons; and nervous systems begin to degenerate, often well before senility is evident. Moreover, behavioral dysfunctions, at any age, are not necessarily correlated with pathological biochemical, or physiological changes. There is mounting evidence that exposure to chemicals while immature is more likely to produce detrimental effects than exposure as an adult. During the period of embryonic development an animal is particularly vulnerable because of its excretory capacity, the blood–brain barrier, the binding capacities of serum and tissue proteins, the proportion and distribution of tissues, and the differences in tissue concentration of the chemical. The developing organism often does not have the same capacity as the adult to metabolize and detoxify toxic chemicals.

The placenta is no longer recognized as the protective barrier between mother and fetus, as was once believed. The prenatal organism is highly vulnerable to congenital malformations and severe functional deficits resulting from prenatal exposure to drugs (e.g., thalidomide), X-rays, or organic forms of mercury. However, prenatal exposure to a chemical at a concentration ordinarily encountered in the human environment is not likely to produce clinically evident birth defects. Without obvious impairment, subclinical dysfunctions may exist that will become apparent only on aging.

The techniques of behavioral teratologists, who measure subtle functional disturbances in organisms exposed to foreign substances while immature (zygote through puberty), may well be some of the most sensitive indicators of chemical toxicity. Much research in behavioral teratology has focused on heavy metals (e.g., methylmercury) and psychotherapeutic drugs. In these studies behavioral effects often did not appear until maturity. This is not surprising for several reasons. First, there is a lack of neuronal mitosis after birth. A brief toxic exposure involving the central nervous system may inflict permanent damage. Second, behavioral dysfunction may not appear until later in life when the reserve capacity of the nervous system has been reduced by natural aging processes. Humans between the ages of 60 and 80 lose roughly 50,000 neurons/day, and there is an increase in the size of the ventricles, reduced cortical convolutions, and a clearing of the meninges during this period. Third, the brain may influence the pace at which aging occurs in other tissues; consequently, neuronal damage at any age, but particularly during senescence, may trigger a wide range of systemic effects. Much research is needed to relate the dynamics of the life cycle to specific critical periods of exposure to toxins. Whether laboratory animals or humans are studied, time-consuming longitudinal studies are essential. Such studies involve following specific individuals, controlling or monitoring genetic background, controlling or monitoring prenatal and post-natal influences, and periodically assaying systemic and behavioral functions throughout the life of the organism.

12.3.1.b. Genetic Factors

It is possible that genetic determinants may directly or indirectly predispose exposed animals to behavioral dysfunctions. Mutagenic processes and genetic metabolic diseases have been expressed by behavior in humans and higher mammals. Since mutagenic effects may first be expressed by altered forms of behavior, multigenerational studies involving behavioral measures should be conducted in conjunction with those procedures used by behavioral teratologists.

12.3.1.c. Previous Diseases

Very few toxicological studies have examined the interaction of current or previous diseases with exposure to toxic substances. Pharmacological studies have pointed out the need to correlate these variables. For example, meningitis alters the blood–brain barrier such that responses to psychoactive drugs are affected. Diseases of the nervous system may reduce neuronal cell reserves to numbers that cannot mask the nervous system damage from earlier exposures to toxins. The interaction of toxins such as carbon disulphide, lead, mercury, and manganese in subjects already exhibiting forms of psychopathologies can be complex and potentially lethal, for these agents alone may induce psychoses. Since psychotropic drugs lead other drugs in both sales and abuse, behavioral toxicologists are justified in conducting studies that link ordinary diseases and psychopathologies with exposure to toxins.

12.3.2. Exogenous Factors

12.3.2.a. Agent Interactions

Reports of the synergistic effects of two or more toxins are increasing. With hundreds of new chemicals being synthesized and released into a market already containing an astounding list, the number of possible combinations and permutations of agents is too enormous for combined study. Chemicals whose behavioral effects occur by a common mechanism often have an additive effect. On the other hand, ethanol can mask some of the motor symptoms of inorganic mercury poisoning; or additive behavioral effects may be seen in humans who consume ethanol while being treated for neurotic anxiety with minor tranquilizers such as diazepam and chlordiazepoxide.

12.3.2.b. Nutritional Factors

Little research has related dietary factors to the behavioral effects of toxic agents. Calcium deficiency magnifies lead toxicity and may be a factor causing lead pica (the craving for unnatural foods). Likewise, protein deficiency affects toxicoses in a multifaceted manner. Both micronutrient and macronutrient deficiencies can influence the onset of diseases that enhance the effects of toxic chemicals. On the other hand, a typical human diet may include chemicals that aggrevate existing psychiatric conditions such as depression. Soft cheese foods containing tyramine, when eaten by patients treated with monoamine oxidase inhibitors, may cause a dangerous hypertensive condition. Dietary deficiencies are particularly important in developing and postreproductive organisms. Certain agents may reduce the nutritional quality of milk in treated nursing mothers, thereby complicating the behavioral effects that arise from transplacental exposure during prenatal periods. If the milk from treated nursing mothers is not examined for nutritional constituents (in addition to being examined for the toxin), the effects seen in growth, maturation, and functional deficits may be assigned to an inappropriate mechanism of action.

12.3.2.c. Stress and Other Factors

Although there are numerous other factors that may enhance the behavioral effects of toxins, factors such as stress, reproductive physiological condition, and environmental and energetic aspects of seasonal migratory behaviors are worth noting.

Many organisms show marked hormonal and other physiological and behavioral changes during reproductive seasons. Often, courtship rituals involving physical struggles for dominance and opportunity to mate, or fasting during long nursing periods increases stress and lowers stamina such that exposure to toxins during these periods may disrupt normal behavior and/or prove lethal. Migratory behaviors may precipitate toxicological crises in organisms such as Mexican free-tailed bats, which carry DDE in their fat. The blood–brain levels of DDE increase greatly in bats that are food deprived and even more so when they are exercised. Their energetics and altered feeding habits during migratory periods mobilize body fats and may be responsible for the decline in the number of free-tailed bats since bats with high DDE blood–brain levels show classic signs of pesticide intoxication (convulsions and tetanus).

12.4. Future Needs

12.4.1. Methods and Strategies

The lack of acceptable research approaches for studying the behavioral and neurological effects of toxic and potentially toxic chemicals became evident when legislators included "behavioral" measures in the Toxic Substances Control Act of 1976. Government and private institutions found themselves inundated with hundreds of chemicals to evaluate. New and more efficient strategies for assessment are needed.

A strategy proposed by Bernard Weiss of the University of Rochester consists of three phases. The first is a nonspecific or screening phase during which a search for central nervous system effects is conducted. Simple techniques are employed because, with some chemicals, any nervous system effect prohibits use, or because the aim may be to estimate the relevant range of dose levels. Observations include gross locomotor activity, exploratory activity in an open field test, swimming tests (which have been useful in studies on methylmercury), gross coordination, and body weight as an indication of hyperphagia, adipsia, inanition, or pica.

In the second phase specific functions are examined such as sensory and motor function and complex discriminative processes. These techniques usually involve highly trained animals skilled in performing operant tasks that incorporate specific visual and/or auditory cues. Special instrumentation, computers, and a neuropathological work-up after testing are usually involved.

The third phase, the most difficult, centers on human susceptibility and its parameters. Laboratory tests similar to those used to assess the effects of alcohol on the psychomotor skills involved in driving are applicable. In other tests, similar to those conducted on monkeys exposed to mercury vapors, humans with a known history of exposure to mercury may be examined for signs of tremor. This paradigm requires the subject to depress a strain gauge with one finger so that the force applied is maintained between 10 and 40 g. The upper and lower limits are evident to the subject by the illumination of two different signal lights.

Field tests on humans are more difficult when dealing with relatively nonspecific complaints associated with early intoxication. Questionnaire instruments such as Goldberg's General Health Questionnaire or the Symptom Distress Check List are employed. More recently, clinical field performance studies have shown promise in the detection of nervous system dysfunction of workers exposed to lead. Scores on the Block Design Test, Digit Symbol Test, Embedded Figures Test, and the Santa Ana Dexterity Test were significantly correlated with blood lead and zinc protophyrin levels.

Optimal strategies for the selection of behavioral tests for safety evaluation are needed. One method would be to subject known behavioral toxins to batteries of behavioral tests. Recently, Hugh Tilson and Patrick Cabe of the National Institute of Environmental Health Sciences reported a strategy for assessing neurobehavioral consequences of environmental factors. They proposed that test validation in animal models may be accomplished by evaluating known neurotoxins in a battery of tests chosen to assess a wide range of effects based upon reported human toxicosis symptomatology. Measurements include ongoing home cage motor activity, food and water consumption (and the diurnal cycling of these), neurological/physiological indices (reflexes, autonomic signs, equilibrium/gait, balance, tremor, reactivity, muscular strength), and aspects of cognitive and associative behavior involving both endogenous and exogenous (sensory) control of responding. The procedure involves testing during 90 days of chemical treatment and 30 days of postdosing recovery. By comparing the results of these animal models with the predicted effects based on reported human symptoms, a decision concerning the validity of each procedure can be made. Validated neurobehavioral tests should help identify toxin-induced changes in neurochemical and neurophysiological function and assist in the search for neuropathology in a specific region of the nervous system.

12.4.2. Some Dosing and Testing Problems

The manner in which organisms and humans are exposed should be mimicked closely in laboratory studies. When the mode of entry of an agent is by human inhalation, it serves little purpose to administer the agent to a laboratory animal by intraperitoneal injection or by some other unlikely route. Likewise, the magnitude and duration of exposure should be realistic; consequently, if the organism in nature is likely to be exposed briefly but at high concentrations, then that model of exposure (acute dosing) should be examined first in the laboratory. On the other hand, chronic exposure at low doses may be the pattern in which human industrial workers are exposed to specific agents. These statements need some qualification since laboratory animals may be more or less sensitive to specific agents than humans. For example, humans tend to be substantially more sensitive to the effects of psychotropic drugs than test animals. Furthermore, rats may show effects, while cats may not. Consequently, toxicologists test more than one species.

One final problem is related to the capacity of portions of the brain to compensate for lesions that occur in adjacent areas. For example, animals given gradually larger cortical lesions in successive operations show little disruption in their performance within a maze. However, animals given a large lesion in one operation show gross disruptions in maze performance with many days required for recovery. Presumably, animals given progressively larger lesions have the opportunity to relearn between operations since unaffected areas of the brain can assume the function. This phenomenon is applicable in behavioral toxicology since chronic exposure to neurotoxins, with simultaneous behavioral testing, may result in a gradually increasing lesion without measurable behavioral changes.

The techniques, equipment, theory, and previous experiences of behavioral pharmacologists combine to provide an exciting prognosis for rapid development in this reemerging discipline of behavioral toxicology. As is true of all developing scientific disciplines, a period of descriptive studies will dominate initially, soon to be followed by the investigations that point to mechanisms of action and the neurochemical correlates of neurotoxicoses.

Suggested Reading

Bignami, G. Behavioral pharmacology and toxicology. Ann. Rev. Pharmacol. Toxicol. 16:329, 1976.

Ekel, G. J., Teichner, W. H. An analysis and critique of Behavioral Toxicology in the USSR. DHEW Publ. NIOSH 77-160. Washington, D.C., 1976.

Goldberg, D.P. The Detection of Psychiatric Illness by Questionnaires. London: Oxford University Press, 1972.

Spyker, J. Assessing the impact of low level chemicals on development: Behavioral and latent effects. Fed. Proc. 34:1835–1844, 1975.

Valciukas, J. A., Lilis, R., Eisinger, J., et al. Behavioral indicators of lead neurotoxicity: Results of a clinical field survey. Int. Arch. Occup. Environ. Health 41:217–236, 1978.

Weiss, B. Behavioral methods for investigating environmental health effects. International Symposium of Recent Advances in the Health Effects of Environmental Pollution, Paris, 1974.

Weiss, B., Laties, V. Behavioral Toxicology. New York: Plenum Press, 1975.

Xintaris, C., Johnson, B. L., deGroot, I. Behavioral toxicology: early detection of occupational hazards. DHEW Publ. NIOSH 74-126 Washington, D.C., 1974.

John R. Bend
Margaret O. James
John B. Pritchard

13

Aquatic Toxicology

13.1. Introduction

The aquatic environment, inlcuding streams, rivers, lakes, estuaries, and oceans, serves as a reservoir for tremendous quantities of foreign organic chemicals, or xenobiotics. These compounds, many of which are toxic to both aquatic and mammalian species, enter our waterways by diverse routes. Atmospheric fallout of air-borne particles associated with smog, runoff of applied herbicides and pesticides from agricultural areas, release of concentrated industrial and urban wastes into rivers and streams, spillage (both accidental and intentional) that occurs during shipping, and natural seepage of petroleum hydrocarbons from submarine oil fields are major sources of marine pollution.

The contamination of waterways with chemicals has been well documented in the scientific literature. Recent examples in North America include PCBs in the Hudson River and the Great Lakes, mirex in the Great Lakes, chlordecone (Kepone) in the James River, and benzo[a]pyrene in marine mussels in selected areas of the Pacific Northwest. The potential for harm as a result of this aquatic pollution is at least twofold. First, populations of aquatic vertebrate and invertebrate species can be affected directly, with potentially disastrous effects on localized ecosystems (e.g., estuaries). Moreover, aquatic animals consumed as foodstuff represent a source of human exposure to toxic xenobiotics, including proximate carcinogens and mutagens. Due to the ability of many fish and invertebrate species to bioaccumulate trace amounts of xenobiotics in water to high tissue concentrations, and to the possible formation and storage of proximate toxicants in tissues of these animals, pollutant exposure by this route can have a substantial impact on human health. Since man will probably depend more and more upon protein from marine sources in the future, the fate of these xenobiotics in aquatic animals is of importance. This chapter is concerned with the ability of these animals to biotransform and excrete foreign chemicals. The use of selected aquatic species as sentinel or early warning indicator systems for the presence in water of chemicals toxic to humans is also considered.

13.2. Biotransformation and Toxicity

13.2.1. Effect of Metabolism on Toxicity

In general, lipophilic organic molecules present in an animal must undergo biotransformation to more polar derivatives before they can be excreted. The first step is usually oxidation at one or more carbon atoms in the molecule. The oxidized xenobiotic may then react with small endogenous molecules such as water, glucuronic acid, sulfate, single amino acids, glutathione (GSH), or other small peptides. This general sequence was proposed from studies using mammalian species and has been verified with several marine species. Since the excreted metabolite is usually less toxic than the parent compound, the overall sequence may be considered a detoxication or deactivation. However, individual reactions in the sequence may also give rise to metabolic intermediates that are more toxic or biologically active than the parent compound (toxication or activation), as shown in the following examples.

Chemically reactive alkene and arene oxides are formed by oxidation of many xenobiotics. Under certain circumstances some of these epoxides react with critical cellular macromolecules and initiate changes resulting in mutagenesis and carcinogenesis. For example, the mycotoxin, aflatoxin, is a hepatocarcinogen in several species, including rainbow trout and the rat. Pure aflatoxin was less mutagenic to a *Salmonella* strain in the Ames' assay than aflatoxin that had been incubated with rat or trout hepatic microsomes fortified with NADPH in the presence of the bacteria, suggesting that an oxidized metabolite of aflatoxin (such as the 2,3-oxide) is the ultimate mutagen, and probably the ultimate carcinogen.

For many years, conjugation reactions were thought of solely as deactivation reactions. However, sulfate esters of both *N*-hydroxy-2-acetylaminofluorene and *N*-hydroxyphenacetin are very reactive chemically and can bind covalently to cellular macromolecules. Similarly, the glucuronide of *N*-hydroxyphenacetin has been shown to react covalently with protein. Recently, glutathione conjugation was reported as an activation pathway in ethylene dichloride toxicity. An incubated mixture of GSH *S*-transferase, GSH, and ethylene dichloride was shown to contain a more active mutagen in the Ames' assay than ethylene dichloride alone.

The examples emphasize the point that biotransformation of xenobiotics may result in the formation of more active or toxic derivatives. However, it is still true that for most xenobiotics the overall result of biotransformation is metabolic deactivation, since after oxidation and/or conjugation most xenobiotics are readily excreted from the body.

13.2.2. Oxidation

13.2.2.a. Reaction Mechanisms

Studies performed in the 1950s were the first to demonstrate that the microsomal fraction of rat liver homogenate could oxidatively metabolize chemicals. Several years later (mid 1960s), similar enzyme activities were reported in the liver of some fresh-water and marine fish. Since then the mechanism of xenobiotic oxidation has been studied extensively in hepatic microsomes from a few mammalian species, mainly the rat, mouse, and rabbit. Microsomes arise from the endoplasmic reticulum of hepatocytes during homogenization of liver and contain one or more of a family of hemoproteins, cytochromes P-450. Based on our present knowledge the following sequence of interactions represents a generally accepted scheme for mixed-function oxidation of foreign chemicals. Initially, the oxidized (ferric) form of cytochrome P-450 interacts with the substrate to form a hemoprotein–substrate complex. Subsequently, a one-electron reduction occurs, leading to a reduced (ferrous) cytochrome P-450–substrate complex. The electron is normally donated by NADPH–cytochrome P-450 reductase. However, since NADH can support low rates of mixed-function oxidation in the absence of NADPH, it appears that electrons can be transported by an alternative route, which involves cytochrome b_5 and NADH–cytochrome b_5 reductase. The reduced cytochrome P-450–substrate complex then combines with molecular oxygen to form an unstable oxygenated reduced-cytochrome P-450–substrate complex, which accepts an electron via NADPH–cytochrome P-450 reductase or NADH–cytochrome b_5 reductase and decomposes to hydroxylated product, oxidized cytochrome P-450, and water.

13.2.2.b. Mixed-Function Oxidases in Marine Species

Substrate oxidation in vitro. In most species studied to date, the liver or an equivalent organ, such as the hepatopancreas, has the highest specific and total enzyme activity for oxidation of xenobiotics. Thus, preliminary studies in species about which little is known usually utilize the hepatic system. The hepatic mixed-function oxidase system of every marine and fresh-water fish studied requires NADPH and molecular oxygen for maximum oxidase activity and is localized in the microsomal fraction, although some activity is often found in mitochondrial fractions, probably due to sedimentation of large fragments of endoplasmic reticulum with mitochondria. NADH can substitute for NADPH as cofactor in those few fish species tested, but much lower activities are achieved.

Cytochrome P-450 has been measured in hepatic microsomes from a wide variety of marine and freshwater fish species and the specific content usually ranges from 0.1 to 0.5 nmole/mg microsomal protein, or less than one-half the amount found in rat or rabbit hepatic microsomes (Table 13.1 shows mean values for a few representative species). Hepatopancreatic microsomes from some crustacean species studied also contain cytochrome P-450. One crustacean, the spiny lobster (*Panulirus argus*), has about the same specific content (nmole/mg microsomal protein) as the rat.

Certain xenobiotics interact with cytochrome P-450 in mammalian hepatic microsomes in such a way that characteristic spectral changes are observed. Type 1 spectral changes (peak near 385–390 nm, trough 418–427 nm) are produced by the addition of substrate molecules, such as drugs, fatty acids, and steroids, and have been demonstrated in several fish and crustacean species, with benzphetamine used as a ligand. However, not all fish species studied exhibited type 1 difference spectra with benzphetamine or other ligands even though these species were able to oxidize benzphetamine—an interesting difference from the mammals studied. Type 2 spectral changes (peak near 425–435 nm, trough 390–405 nm) are produced by the interaction of cytochrome P-450 with basic amines and have been observed in hepatic microsomes from fish and crustacea after the addition of aniline or pyridine.

Table 13.1 Hepatic Microsomal Cytochrome P-450 Content, NADPH–Cytochrome c Reductase Activity, and Mixed-Function Oxidase Activities in Selected Marine Species Compared with the Rat and the Rabbit

Species	Cytochrome P-450 content (nmoles/mg microsomal protein)	NADPH–cytochrome c reductase activity (nmoles product/min/mg protein)	Benzo[a]pyrene hydroxylase activity (fluorescence units/min/mg protein)	7-Ethoxycoumarin O-deethylase activity (nmoles product/min/mg protein)	Benzphetamine N-demethylase activity (nmoles product/min/mg protein)
Rat	1.04	70.0	3.2	—	—
Rabbit	1.52	48.0	5.0	3.5	6.5
Sheepshead	0.29	56.0	3.2	0.19	1.0
Winter flounder	0.17	—	2.5	0.32	0.59
Mullet	0.47	53.0	3.0	0.15	2.78
Stingray	0.43	49.0	0.78	0.08	0.74
Little skate	0.32	60.0	0.17	0.32	1.1
Spiny lobster	0.88	4.6	0.03	<0.001	0.07
Blue crab	0.18	5.2	<0.01	<0.001	0.02

Source: Rat and rabbit data from Philpot, R. M., Bend, J. R. Life Sci. 16:985–998, 1975. Marine species data from James, M. O., Khan, M. A. Q., Bend, J. R. Comp. Biochem. Physiol. 62C:155–164, 1979. Pergamon Press, Ltd.

Another necessary component for mixed-function oxidation, NADPH–cytochrome P-450 reductase, has also been found in hepatic microsomes from the few marine fish tested, but this enzyme was not active in hepatopancreas microsomes from spiny lobster or blue crab (*Callinectes sapidus*). NADPH–cytochrome *c* reductase, which in mammals is very similar to cytochrome P-450 reductase, has been found in hepatic microsomes from several marine and fresh-water fish at activities comparable to those found in mammals (Table 13.1), whereas hepatopancreatic microsomes from crustacea contain only one-tenth the cytochrome *c* reductase specific activity found in fish and mammals.

Optimum conditions for in vitro assay of mixed-function oxidation of a variety of substrates (e.g., benzo[a]pyrene, 7-ethoxycoumarin, benzphetamine, amino-pyrine, aniline, dieldrin, parathion) appear to be similar to those reported in the rat and rabbit, except that the temperature optimum is usually lower than 37°C for fish species. The optimum temperature for in vitro oxidative activity in hepatic microsomes from fresh-water trout found in cold northern lakes is 26°C, from marine fish found in the North Atlantic, about 30°C, and from marine fish found in warmer waters off the Florida coast, about 35°C. Incubation at higher temperatures appears to cause denaturation of enzyme activity.

Oxidation of xenobiotic substrates has been detected in most of the fish species tested. Activities in some representative species are shown in Table 13.1. Wide inter- and intraspecies variability is found, especially with substrates such as benzo[a]pyrene. Hepatic microsomes from some fresh-water trout have higher benzo[a]pyrene hydroxylase activities than those found in rat hepatic microsomes, while this activity is very low in hepatic microsomes from a marine teleost fish, the King of Norway (*Hemitripterus americanus*). Hepatopancreatic microsomes from a few crustacean species catalyzed xenobiotic oxidation at very low rates compared with mammals and most fish. The data shown in Table 13.1 represent the lowest values that can be accurately measured in the assays used. If substrate and hepatopancreatic microsomes are incubated in the presence of sodium periodate or cumene hydroperoxide instead of NADPH, oxidation occurs much more rapidly. In this reaction, the cytochrome P-450–substrate complex is directly oxidized, bypassing the steps involving NADPH–cytochrome P-450 reductase.

Xenobiotic oxidation has been measured in some extrahepatic organs of aquatic organisms, but with a few exceptions (e.g., renal activity in some elasmobranch fish), the rates are much lower than those found in hepatic microsomes.

Substrate oxidation in vivo. The literature contains very few systematic in vivo studies of xenobiotic metabolism by marine species. Some of these investigations have shown that oxidative metabolism of aromatic and aliphatic hydrocarbons occurs in marine and fresh-water fish, some crustacea, and very few lower invertebrates. More recent studies suggest that extremely sensitive assay proce-dures are required to detect xenobiotic biotransformation in aquatic inverte-brates such as the mussel (*Mytilus edulis*), but that it does occur. Oxidized metabolites of aromatic and aliphatic hydrocarbons and PCBs are usually excreted more slowly by aquatic species than by mammals; this is especially true for crustacea and lower invertebrates. The extent and rate of metabolism and excretion vary with chemical structure. In general, aquatic species metabolize and excrete aliphatic hydrocarbons more rapidly than aromatic hydrocarbons. Highly substituted aromatic hydrocarbons, including some PCB isomers, are metabolized and excreted only very slowly.

13.2.3. Hydrolysis

Two main classes of foreign chemicals, esters and epoxides, are metabolized by hydrolytic pathways. A number of herbicides and pesticides are esters, or are applied as esters; for example, 2,4-D is often applied as its butyl ester. The hydrolysis of carboxylic and organophosphoric acid esters has been studied in several fish species. Liver, kidney, and intestine had esterase activity, and the in vivo hydrolysis of butyl-2, 4-D was demonstrated in fresh-water mosquitofish (*Gambusia affinis*), rainbow trout (*Salmo gairdneri*), bluegill (*Lepomis macrochirus*), and fathead minnow (*Pimephales promelas*).

Epoxides are formed in vivo by metabolism of organic chemicals with unsaturated carbon–carbon bonds. In addition, some stable epoxides, e.g., dieldrin, are used as pesticides. Most epoxides formed in vivo can be further metabolized by hydrolysis, catalyzed by epoxide hydrase. Epoxide hydrase activity has been measured in hepatic and extrahepatic organs of several marine fish, crustacea, and molluscs. The general order of activity in hepatic microsomes is crustacea > fish > molluscs. In most species liver or hepatopancreas had the highest epoxide hydrase activity, although all other tissues assayed, including gill, kidney, ovary, and testis, also had enzyme activity.

13.2.4. Conjugation

Xenobiotics that have chemically reactive functional groups usually must combine with low molecular weight endogenous molecules, which increases their polarity, before they can be excreted in urine or bile. These biotransformations have been termed conjugation reactions and they generally involve cofactors. Depending on the substrates, either the xenobiotic or the endogenous molecule reacts with the cofactor to form an activated intermediate. When this activated intermediate reacts with the second substrate, the cofactor is regenerated.

13.2.4.a. Glucuronic Acid Conjugation

Phenols, alcohols, amines, and carboxylic acids are all potential substrates for conjugation with glucuronic acid, at least in mammalian species. A family of enzymes found in the microsomal membrane, the uridine diphosphate (UDP) glucuronyltransferases, catalyze the transfer of glucuronic acid from uridine-5'-diphospho-*D*-glucuronic acid to the xenobiotic.

UDP glucuronyltransferase activity has been found in the liver of marine and fresh-water fish, and also in the kidney and intestine. The difference between UDP glucuronyltransferase activity in rainbow trout and sea lamprey (*Petromyzon marinus*) is one of the factors that accounts for the greater susceptibility of lamprey to 3-trifluoromethyl-4-nitrophenol (TFM). TFM is used as a lampricide in the Great Lakes and is detoxified by glucuronidation. A paucity of information is available concerning in vitro enzyme activity in crustaceans and lower invertebrates. Several investigators have shown that fish species excrete glucuronide metabolites in urine and/or bile after administration of xenobiotics with carboxylic acid or phenolic functional groups. Some of these xenobiotics were first metabolized to derivatives with suitable functional groups. Glucuronide metabolites have not yet been identified in any crustacean or lower invertebrate species.

13.2.4.b. Glutathione Conjugation

Conjugation with GSH is the first step in the formation of mercapturic acids (N-acetylcysteine conjugates). No cofactor is involved, and many electrophilic compounds are substrates for the reaction, which is catalyzed by a family of cytosolic enzymes, the GSH S-transferases.

GSH S-transferase activity has been found in cytosol fractions from liver and extrahepatic organs of all marine fish, crustacea, and some invertebrates assayed. The substrates used were epoxides and chloronitrobenzenes. Activity was usually highest in liver, but varying amounts of transferase activity were also present in gill, intestine, gonads, and kidney (fish) or green gland (crustacea). The subsequent reactions that lead to mercapturic acid formation in mammals have not been investigated in marine species.

13.2.4.c. Amino Acid Conjugation

A number of nonnutritive carboxylic acids and other xenobiotics are conjugated with an amino acid before they are excreted in urine. This biotransformation is especially interesting from a comparative viewpoint because the amino acid used varies with species. In mammals glycine, glutamine, and sometimes taurine are used, whereas in fish taurine is most commonly used. Amino acid conjugation takes place in the mitochondria of liver and kidney cells. First, the carboxylic acid is converted to the coenzyme A (CoA) derivative, which then reacts with the amino acid to form the conjugate, and CoA is regenerated.

Taurine N-acyltransferase activity has been measured in the liver and kidney of several marine fish and hepatopancreas and green gland of some crustacean species, with phenylacetyl-CoA used as the acyl donor. Activity is usually highest in the kidney but is also found in the liver of fishes. Activity in the hepatopancreas or green gland of the crustacea studied was low or undetectable.

Those fish species studied in vivo, excrete phenylacetic acid, 2,4-D, 2,4,5-T, and (2,2-bis[p-chlorophenyl]acetic acid (DDA), mainly as taurine conjugates, although varying amounts of unchanged acid are excreted by some species, depending on the structure of the carboxylic acid administered. Apparently, crustacea do not excrete taurine conjugates, although they are able to metabolize some carboxylic acids to derivatives with the properties of amino acid conjugates. The amino acid or peptide portion of the metabolite excreted by crustacea has not yet been identified.

13.2.4.d. Sulfate Conjugation

Xenobiotic phenols and alcohols (which are also substrates for glucuronyl-transferases) may be excreted as sulfate conjugates. The sulfotransferases are found in the cytosol fraction and catalyze the reaction of 3'-phosphoadenine-5'-phosphosulfate (PAPS) with the hydroxyl group. Sulfate conjugates have been tentatively identified as metabolites of l-naphthol and of pentachlorophenol in fish, and S-transferase activity with 4-nitrophenol has been found in liver cytosol from some marine fish, but the pathway has not been extensively investigated in aquatic species.

13.2.5. Induction

In most mammalian species, exposure of an animal to certain foreign organic chemicals or drugs for a period of time increases the rate at which the animal can metabolize that chemical and/or structurally related compounds. Mixed-function oxidation is the biotransformation pathway most frequently affected by exposure to inducing agents, but hydrolysis and conjugation pathways are sometimes induced. Superficially, it would seem that the phenomenon of induction should benefit the animal, since polar metabolites that are readily excreted are formed more quickly. However, since certain xenobiotics are metabolized by mixed-function oxidases to more toxic intermediates, an increase in the rate of oxidation may in some cases adversely affect an animal, especially if pathways for further metabolism and elimination of the toxic intermediate are not also induced.

Hepatic mixed-function oxidases of marine and fresh-water fish are readily induced by polycyclic aromatic hydrocarbons and related chemicals but seem to be less markedly affected by phenobarbital-like compounds.

13.2.5.a. Effects of Hydrocarbon Administration

3-Methylcholanthrene, dibenz[a,h]anthracene, weathered crude oil, and an uncharacterized mixture of used crankcase oils were all effective in inducing benzo[a]pyrene hydroxylase activity in different fish species, whereas hexadecane, an aliphatic hydrocarbon component of petroleum, was not. All of these compounds are found in water near marinas or in tar balls in the ocean after oil spills. Where studied, 7-ethoxycoumarin O-deethylase activity was also induced by those hydrocarbons that increased specific benzo[a]pyrene hydroxylase activity. The effect on hepatic microsomal cytochrome P-450 content was usually slight, but cytochrome P-448 (which is induced by polycyclic aromatics in the rat) has been isolated from livers of little skates treated with dibenz[a,h]anthracene, suggesting similarities between the fish and the mammalian systems. None of these hydrocarbons affected benzphetamine N-demethylase activity, epoxide hydrase activity, or GSH S-transferase activity in fish liver.

13.2.5.b. Effects of Administering Polyhalogenated Aromatic Compounds

A number of industrial chemicals and pesticides, such as PCBs, induce xenobiotic metabolism in mammals and in fish, and in mammals the induction is often referred to as "mixed type" since cytochrome P-450– and cytochrome P-448–dependent oxidation is induced, as well as other pathways of xenobiotic metabolism. In many cases, different isomers present in a mixture induce different pathways of metabolism. Marine species are often exposed to these compounds in polluted rivers and estuaries. Arochlor 1254 (a mixture of PCBs), Firemaster FFl a mixture of polybrominated biphenyls (PBBs), (2,3,7,8-

tetrachlorodibenzo-*p*-dioxin) (TCDD), 5,6-benzoflavone, and DDT all induce hepatic benzo[a]pyrene hydroxylase activity in different fish species. 7-Ethoxy-coumarin *O*-deethylase activity, benzphetamine *N*-demethylase activity, and epoxide hydrase activity are also induced in some fish species by Arochlor 1254, Firemaster FFl, and TCDD, although because of high individual variation, the increases in benzphetamine *N*-demethylase and epoxide hydrase activities are not always statistically significant. There is no effect on GSH *S*-transferase activity.

13.3. Excretion

13.3.1. Bioconcentration and Biomagnification

As discussed in preceding chapters, bioconcentration within a given animal and biomagnification along a food chain are determined by many factors, including the persistence of a chemical, its availability, and its absorption by animals and plants. Excretion, too, plays a major role in determining whether or not a given chemical is preferentially sequestered in living organisms. For example, even a highly persistent, widely distributed chemical will not accumulate in a given organism if its metabolism and excretion are more rapid than its uptake from the environment. Conversely, another equally persistent chemical present at very low levels in the environment will be effectively accumulated if its excretion is limited. The factors that determine the rate of excretion of foreign chemicals by aquatic organisms are described below.

13.3.2. Role of Metabolism

While much of the discussion below will center on the ways in which the physical and chemical properties of each chemical interact with the physiological processes responsible for their elimination, it is important to remember that it is not solely the characteristics of the parent chemical that determine the site and effectiveness of its excretion. The metabolic conversions described previously are in many cases the primary determinant of excretory route and rate. For example, in mammals benzoic acid is excreted almost exclusively as its glycine conjugate, hippuric acid, which has a far higher affinity for the renal organic anion transport system than benzoic acid. Comparable examples of the conversion of relatively apolar xenobiotics to more water-soluble derivatives that may be more readily excreted by the liver and/or kidney were described earlier in this chapter. Finally, it should be noted that since these metabolic events may greatly alter the rate of excretion, those chemicals that induce xenobiotic-metabolizing enzymes may greatly increase their own excretion rate as well as that of other compounds.

13.3.3. Routes of Excretion

Three major routes are available for excretion of foreign chemicals by aquatic organisms. First, compounds may leave the body by diffusing across the integument into the surrounding water. In practice, however, due to the low permeability of the skin, such exit is restricted to the respiratory surfaces of the gills, where the permeability barriers are reduced to permit efficient gas exchange. The second route is via the digestive tract, where the secretions of the digestive organs, notably the liver, may carry xenobiotics or their metabolites from the body. However, the effectiveness of this route may be limited by subsequent absorption from the gastrointestinal tract. Finally, many small molecules (<400–500 daltons) may be eliminated via the kidneys through filtration, tubular secretion, or both. Specific examples presented below demonstrate the characteristics of each system and the types of compounds that may be excreted.

13.3.3.a. Gill

The role of the gill in the excretion of molecules such as CO_2 and NH_3 is widely appreciated. A unique set of physical properties permits these molecules to utilize the gill surfaces for exit. Not only are both molecules sufficiently lipid soluble to diffuse readily through the epithelium of the gill, they are also water soluble enough to enter the aqueous environment around the gill. To date, few xenobiotics have been shown to possess the necessary solubility in both lipophilic and aqueous media. The notable exception is the anesthetic tricaine methane sulfonate (MS222), which has been shown to be well excreted across the gills of the dogfish shark (*Squalus acanthias*). MS222 is a weak acid, like CO_2 and NH_3, and in its un-ionized form it is lipid soluble; in an aqueous enviornment it dissociates, rendering it water soluble. In contrast, in the same experimental system DDT did not enter the water across the gills, even though it was very lipid soluble and entered the epithelium of the gill. Similarly, more polar xenobiotics were equally lacking in significant gill clearance (Table 13.2). Thus, current evidence indicates that gill clearance is of limited importance in the excretion of most xenobiotics or their metabolites. Even those weak acids and bases physically capable of utilizing this excretion route may be more effectively eliminated by active transport at the kidney or liver, where excretion rates may greatly exceed those possible by diffusion at the gill (see below).

13.3.3.b. Liver

The liver of aquatic vertebrates plays a significant role in the excretion of foreign compounds, just as it does in mammals. In fact, it has been suggested that the bile of teleost fish might be used to assess water quality since many pollutants

Table 13.2 Excretion of Foreign Compounds by the Gill

Compound	pKa	Partition $CHCl_3$: H_2O at pH 7.4	Gill clearance (ml/hr)
Benzolamide	3.2	0.0003	2
Sulfanilamide	10.4	0.08	4
Ethoxyzolamide	8.1	27	84
Antipyrine	1.4	28	84
Tricaine methane sulfonate	3.5	312	540
DDT		Very High	0

Source: DDT data from Dvorchik, B. H., and Maren, T. H. Comp. Biochem. Physiol. 42A: 205-211, 1972. All other data from Maren, T. H., Embry, R., Broder, L. E. Comp. Biochem. Physiol. 26:853–864, 1968. Pergamon Press, Ltd.

are concentrated there. The excretory role of the hepatopancreas and other accessory digestive organs in crustacea, molluscs, and other invertebrates has been less well studied, but in general seems limited.

The liver plays two major roles in the excretion of xenobiotics. Its metabolism converts foreign compounds to more readily excreted metabolites, and the transport systems associated with bile formation facilitate their entry into the bile. Based on mammalian studies there appear to be three major transport systems important in hepatic xenobiotic excretion. First, an organic anion (acid) system, mediates transport of the bile salts, bilirubin, and many conjugated metabolites of xenobiotics. Similar systems for organic cations (bases), particularly quaternary amines, and for neutral organic compounds (including ouabain, steroids, and certain drugs) are also important. Certain heavy metals (e.g., lead, copper, and manganese) may also be actively transported into bile. Wide species variations may occur even in mammals, but those aquatic species that have been studied appear to follow these patterns. As with mammals, polar compounds of molecular weight in the range 400–500 and above are primarily eliminated in the bile, while those of lower molecular weight are excreted in the urine. Once secreted into the bile, xenobiotics must traverse the intestine before being eliminated in the feces. Often intestinal reabsorption occurs, particularly of lipid-soluble compounds or those hydrolyzed by intestinal flora (particularly the glucuronides). Upon absorption by the gut, the compounds are returned to the liver via the portal vein and then are cleared and resecreted into the bile. This phenomenon called enterohepatic circulation, may severely limit biliary excretion of certain compounds, including the heavy metals.

13.3.3.c. Kidney

The basic processes involved in urine formation are filtration and tubular transport. Therefore, two types of compounds are found in the urine: (a) those molecules small enough to pass through the membrane ultrafilter at the glomerulus for which no special excretion mechanism exists and which consequently are eliminated slowly; and (b) those, such as hippuric acid, that are very rapidly eliminated by virtue of effective tubular secretion. The availability of a given xenobiotic for renal excretion may also be severely limited by binding to plasma macromolecules, which lowers the free concentration available for filtration or tubular secretion. The net rate of elimination of some substances may be further reduced by passive reabsorption across the tubular epithelium (particularly lipid-soluble compounds, weak acids or bases, or small water-soluble molecules such as urea). Still other compounds, such as sugars and amino acids, may be actively reabsorbed by specific transport systems.

Until recently very few studies focused on the mechanisms of renal xenobiotic excretion. However, such studies have provided a great deal of insight into the handling of xenobiotics and the basis for the bioaccumulation of pollutants. For example, compare the distribution and excretion of DDT with its polar metabolite, DDA. After equal doses in vivo, DDA was excreted into the urine nearly 250 times as rapidly as DDT by the winter flounder (*Pseudopleuronectes americanus*). Associated with this excretion was extensive renal accumulation of DDA. Plasma binding was similar for both compounds (>97%). In vitro studies using isolated renal tubules showed extensive energy-dependent uptake of DDA, which could be inhibited by other organic anions. Autoradiography confirmed that uptake represented intracellular cytoplasmic accumulation. Thus, it appeared that DDA was accumulated by the renal organic acid transport system responsible for the secretion of hippuric acid in vivo. In vivo clearance studies in the flounder confirmed the importance of such secretory organic acid transport in DDA excretion.

These results emphasize the importance of fundamental renal physiological principles in determining the effectiveness of renal xenobiotic excretion by marine organisms. DDA excretion is favored by its water solubility, its low molecular weight, and its affinity for secretory transport. It is limited by its extensive plasma binding, against which the transport system must compete. The importance of plasma binding can be demonstrated by comparing the clearance of the herbicide 2,4-D, which is only 70% bound, with that of DDA (> 95% bound). In vivo 2,4-D clearance was nearly 10 times as rapid as DDA clearance (Figure 13.1), even though isolated renal tubules transported these compounds similarly in the absence of protein binding. DDT, on the other hand, was extensively bound; it is not a substrate for active transport, and it is highly lipid soluble. Its lipophilicity means not only that any filtered DDT is passively reabsorbed from tubular fluid, but also that much of the DDT is sequestered in lipid-rich tissues, where it is not available for excretion or for metabolism to the more readily excreted DDA. Thus, the persistence and bioconcentration of DDT in the flounder becomes readily explicable in terms of the interactions of its physical and chemical properties with the physiological processes governing excretion.

Figure 13.1 Renal clearance of the herbicide 2,4-D and the polar DDT metabolite DDA by the winter flounder *(P. americanus)*. Results are expressed as the clearance ratio, i.e., the clearance of the xenobiotic (C_x) divided by the glomerular filtration rate (GFR). A clearance ratio greater than 1 indicates that the compound is excreted more rapidly than it is filtered, i.e., it is secreted by the renal tubules. Higher clearance ratios indicate greater net tubular secretion.

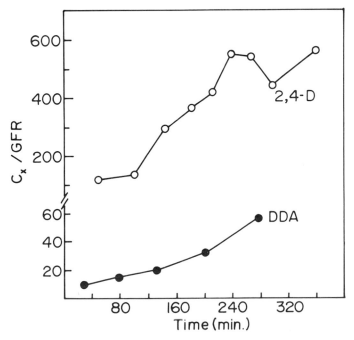

13.4. **Human Health Implications**

Protein derived from aquatic animals will almost certainly play a prominent role in feeding an ever increasing human population. Since many fish and shellfish bioconcentrate lipophilic compounds from surrounding water and, to a less extent, from their food, meat from these animals may contain substantial amounts of chemical poisons. Consequently, it is important to understand those processes such as distribution, metabolism, and excretion that help to determine the site (i.e., tissue), chemical form(s), and amount of toxin accumulated. The fact that PCBs, chlordecone (Kepone), mirex, DDT, DDE, and benzo[a]pyrene have all been found in aquatic animals of North America that are used as food sources emphasizes the potential for harm. Another important aspect of the same problem is the presence of carcinogenic or mutagenic compounds in potable water, whether or not these chemicals are formed during water purification.

13.4.1.   Aquatic Species as Sentinel or Early Warning Indicator Systems

Since all fish that have been studied in detail have hepatic and extrahepatic mixed-function oxidase activities, it is not surprising that some of these animals develop neoplasms when exposed to procarcinogens. In fact, aflatoxin was first shown to be a hepatocarcinogen in fish, where this mycotoxin is metabolically activated to an ultimate carcinogen. Other chemicals, including some polycyclic aromatic hydrocarbons, are also carcinogenic to fish. Data such as these suggest that certain aquatic species may serve as sentinel systems in nature for chemical carcinogens and mutagens. Obviously, the fact that aquatic animals bioconcentrate those lipophilic chemicals present in the water is relevant in this context. It should also be pointed out that cancer is not the only end point that should be considered. Any other pathological, physiological, or biochemical alteration that can be *specifically* attributed to a chemical compound or class will serve the same purpose.

It may be possible to use enzyme induction as an indicator for selected environmental contaminants. The hepatic microsomal mixed-function oxidase system of all fish species tested so far is induced following exposure to polycyclic aromatic hydrocarbon-type (type II) inducers, including the PCBs, PBBs, and dioxins, whereas this enzyme system does not respond noticeably to phenobarbital-type inducing compounds. Since almost all type II inducing agents have proven or suspected human toxicity, it seems reasonable to assume that induction of hepatic mixed-function oxidase activities in wild fish may represent exposure to dangerous chemicals. However, caution must be exercised in this approach. It is necessary to use only those species that have been thoroughly studied in the laboratory prior to field studies. Thus, although this approach has considerable potential, more detailed investigations are required before it can be successfully applied in nature.

13.4.2. Aquatic Species as Experimental Animals

There is a real need for inexpensive test systems to evaluate both the acute and chronic toxicity of a large number of industrial chemicals, as evidenced by the recent passage of the Toxic Substances Control Act. Certain aquatic species have characteristics that make them suitable for experimentation, including the ability to produce large numbers of genetically homogeneous offspring, the ability to live at high population densities, and the fact that in the proper location costs associated with long-term experimentation are moderate. Considerations such as these, coupled with the fact that disposition, metabolism, and excretion processes are generally very similar in aquatic vertebrates and mammals, are likely to lead to the development of selected aquatic animal test systems for the evaluation of xenobiotic toxicity.

Suggested Reading

Bend, J. R., James, M. O. Xenobiotic metabolism in freshwater and marine species. In Malins, D. C., Sargent, J. R. (Eds.) Biochemical and Biophysical Perspectives in Marine Biology, Vol. 4. New York: Academic Press, 1978, pp. 125–188.

Brown, E. C., Jr. Biochemical aspects of detoxification in the marine enviornment. In Malins, D. C., Sargent, J. R., (Eds.). Biochemical and Biophysical Perspectives in Marine Biology, Vol. 3. New York: Academic Press, 1976, pp. 320–403.

Corner, E. D. S. The fate of fossil fuel hydrocarbons in marine animals. Proc. R. Soc. Lond [Biol.] 189:391, 1975.

Guarino, A. M., Pritchard, J. B., Anderson, J. B., et al. Tissue distribution of [^{14}C]-DDT in the lobster after administration via intravascular or oral routes or after exposure from ambient sea water. Toxicol. Appl. Pharmacol. 29:277, 1974.

Klassen, C. D. Biliary excretion. In Lee, D. H. K., Murphy, S. D. (Eds.). Handbook of Physiology,—Section 9. Reactions to Environmental Agents. Bethesda, Md.: American Physiological Society, 1977. pp. 537–553.

Kraybill, H. F., Dawe, C. J., Harshbarger, J. C., et al. (Eds.). Aquatic pollutants and biological effects with emphasis on neoplasia. Ann. N. Y. Acad. Sci. 298:1, 1977.

MacLeish, W. H. (ed.). Marine biomedicine. Oceanus 19:2, 1976.

Pritchard, J. B., Karnaky, K. J., Guarino, A. M., et al. Renal handling of the polar DDT metabolite DDA(2,2-bis(p-chlorophenyl)acetic acid) by marine fish. Am. J. Physiol. 233:F123, 1977.

Statham, C. N., Melancon, M. J., Jr., Lech, J. J. Bioconcentration of xenobiotics in trout bile: A proposed monitoring aid for some waterborne chemicals. Science 193:680, 1976.

Woodwell, G. M. Toxic substances and ecological cycles. Sci. Am. 216:24, 1967.

John E. Hobbie
B. J. Copeland

14

Estuarine Ecosystems

14.1. Introduction

In all aquatic systems, nutrients are important raw materials supporting a basic biological activity, primary production. Estuaries, which are open ended and subject to tidal flushing, are highly dependent upon a continuous input of nutrients to maintain their productivity. Under circumstances of an oversupply of nutrients, however, the normal rate of primary productivity is altered and changes in the structure and function of the ecosystem result.

The most obvious symptom of increased nutrient input is the often cited bloom of certain types of algae. This is usually manifested by the rapid growth of the few species capable of rapid utilization of the incoming nutrients. The result is the competitive exclusion of many species present under more normal conditions. When these imbalances in the primary producers occur, entire food chains may also be altered and the secondary production prized by man may decrease.

Algal blooms may also lead to more subtle changes in the ecosystem. Decomposition of the dying and sinking bloom organisms results in low oxygen conditions, especially in areas of slow flushing, which lead to fish kills and the destruction of benthic populations. Some algae prominent in blooms are little utilized by consumer organisms and may also clog gills of animals. Shading occurs in bloom conditions and the photosynthetic activity of bottom plants is affected.

Estuarine waters are a mixture of sea and fresh water. As sea water contains large amounts of salts, most of the salts necessary for plant growth, such as potassium and sodium, are plentiful. There is no lack of trace elements (e.g., molybdenum and cobalt), which often limits photosynthesis in oligotrophic lakes. Two nutrients that are low in concentration in both sea and fresh water, nitrogen and phosphorus, have been shown to control productivity in estuaries. Consequently, only phosphorus and nitrogen are considered in the discussion of nutrients.

14.2. Sources of Nutrients

Estuaries receive nutrients in both dissolved and particulate forms. Almost all of these nutrients enter the estuary in streams and rivers; a small amount is received from precipitation and from the ocean. Relative proportions are different in different reaches of an estuary; at the mouth, for example, most of the nutrients may have come from sea water. In their dependence on outside sources of nutrients, estuaries resemble lakes and rivers.

Many of the nutrients entering the fresh water streams and rivers of the United States come from sewage and agricultural wastes. Nutrients in sewage arise from human wastes, detergents, street runoff, and industrial wastes. There are a number of detailed studies of the amounts contributed by each source; for example the average conditions in Central Europe are presented in Table 14.1 and those in the Potomac Estuary are shown in Table 14.2. The actual concentrations of nutrients in a given river vary according to such factors as volume of flow, number of cities, amount of forest, and type of agriculture. High concentrations of nutrients are added by point sources, such as domestic sewage and industrial wastes. The concentrations of nutrients from nonpoint sources, such as farms and forests, is low, but the total amount added often equals or exceeds that from point sources (Table 14.1). Thus, a lightly fertilized pine forest may receive 2 kg P/ha and 26 kg N/ha each year, while heavily fertilized farmland may receive 37 kg P/ha and 340 kg N/ha; 10–25% of the nitrogen and 1–5% of the phosphorus will enter the streams from this fertilized land.

Sea water is also a source of nutrients in estuaries. It is usually considered that the reverse is true, and little thought is given to input from the ocean. As will be discussed later, however, there are a number of processes in estuaries that concentrate nutrients from water; even the nutrient-poor ocean water may lose

Table 14.1 Amounts of Nitrogen and Phosphorus (kg/ha/year) in Runoff from an Average Area

Source	N	P
Sewage		
Human wastes	6.6	0.8
Detergents		0.4
Street runoff	0.7	0.1
Industrial wastes	0.7	0.1
	8.0	1.4
Agricultural and forest runoff		
Arable land[a]	2.3– 5.8	0.1–0.5
Meadows and grasslands[a]	4.3–13.3	0.1–0.5
Forests	1.0	0.1
	8.6–20.1	0.3–1.1
Total	16.6–28.1	1.7–2.5

Source: Vollenweider, R.A. Technical Report of Organization for Economic Cooperation and Development, DAS/CSI/6827. Paris, 1968.
[a]The range for farmlands and meadows and grassland reflects different amounts of fertilizer reaching the streams.

Table 14.2 Summary of Nutrient Sources (kg/day) in the Upper and Middle Reaches of the Potomac Estuary, Washington, D.C.

Nutrient	Land runoff	Waste-water discharges	Air–water interface
Low-flow conditions			
(33.98 m³/sec)			
Carbon	77,100	72,600	431,000
Nitrogen	3,040	27,200	726
Phosphorus	454	10,900	0
Median-flow conditions			
(184.06 m³/sec)			
Carbon	159,000	72,600	431,000
Nitrogen	18,100	27,200	726
Phosphorus	2,400	10,900	0

Source: Jaworski et al. *In* Likens, G.E. (Ed.). Nutrients and Eutrophication. Special Symposium, Vol. I. American Society of Limnology and Oceanography, Lawrence, Kansas, pp. 246–273, 1972.

some phosphorus and nitrogen to estuaries. In the Ythan Estuary in Scotland 70% of the phosphorus and 30% of the nitrogen that flow into the estuary are marine in origin, but the amounts of the phosphorus and nitrogen retained have not been measured.

14.3. Transport of Nutrients

After the nutrients enter streams and rivers, some fraction may be lost due to various processes before they finally reach the estuary. One process is absorption by plants and bacteria; another is absorption by sediments. The total quantity absorbed is difficult to determine; it is also possible that some of the absorbed material eventually reaches the estuary (e.g., by washout during exceptionally high discharge). In the Upper Potomac Basin 38% of the phosphorus entering the surface waters is retained in the channel. The high nutrients in the water and the rich sediments cause a dramatic increase in aquatic plants.

Another factor causing loss of nutrients in streams is adsorption onto particulate matter. More than 20% of the reduction of phosphates measured during peak flows can be attributed to adsorption followed by sedimentation of the particulate.

Nitrogen in land runoff enters the rivers and streams mostly as nitrates; however, the nitrogen from waste water enters mostly as ammonia. This nitrogen is taken up by algae and other plants, deposited on the bottom (as organic nitrogen after death of the algae and plants), and oxidized to nitrite and nitrate by nitrifying bacteria. In the Potomac River nitrification is the dominant reaction and most of the nitrogen is converted to nitrate.

14.4. Processes Affecting Nutrient Concentration

There are a number of distinct processes that change the concentrations of nutrients in estuaries. Most of these act simultaneously in most cases, but at times one process predominates.

14.4.1. Physical and Chemical Processes

14.4.1.a. Dilution

Circulation of estuaries causes a continual inflow of sea water and continual mixing with fresh water. If this were the predominant mechanism changing the concentrations of the nutrients, their concentrations would decrease in direct proportion to the increase in salt concentration.

One estuary where dilution is important is Charlotte Harbor, on the west coast of Florida. Water from the Peace River contains 0.6 mg P/liter. This phosphorus (as phosphate) comes from phosphate mines and there are no accompanying high amounts of nitrogen. Therefore, there are no algal blooms and the phosphate remains in the water.

14.4.1.b. Adsorption and Complexing

Some of the nutrients entering estuaries are attached to particulate materials in the rivers. This is particularly true for phosphate and, to a lesser extent, ammonium. When phosphorus is added to stirred suspensions of estuarine sediment, one-half of the phosphorus is adsorbed to the particulate matter within 15 sec. Much of the particulate matter is clay and silt and the adsorptive properties of clay are well known. There is evidence that some of this phosphorus may be released or displaced by competing ions, such as chloride or sulfate, when the particulate matter reaches brackish water.

There also appears to be a good correlation between the amount of phosphorus and the amount of extractable iron in estuarine sediments; this leads to the hypothesis that phosphorus can also be bound to particulate matter as a part of a phosphorus-iron-solids complex.

14.4.1.c. Coagulation and Sedimentation

When nutrient-rich river water reaches the upper parts of the estuary, the current slows as the river broadens. As a result, there is a rapid sedimentation of particulate matter and the phosphorus complex mentioned above. This sediment is very rich in phosphorus.

Some of the particulate matter is colloidal. Typically, these colloidal particles are clays with an electrical charge. In fresh water, the particles are kept from aggregating by repulsive forces, but when the particles move into brackish water the ions affect the particles and flocs are formed. The size and settling velocity of these flocs may be several orders of magnitude larger than those of the individual particles. In the Pamlico Estuary of North Carolina the decrease in phosphorus in the downstream sediments possibly is caused by the coagulation and release of some of the phosphorus when the salinity of the water increases.

Although coagulation undoubtedly occurs in estuaries, it is a process that is easy to demonstrate in the laboratory and difficult to study in the field. In natural waters, organic colloids are present in addition to the clay colloids, as well as mixtures of the two. In addition, the adsorption sites on the clays in nature may be filled with a variety of both organic and inorganic ions. Thus, natural particulate material does not absorb low molecular weight organic compounds. Finally, other processes may be acting that obscure the coagulation effects. In the Pamlico Estuary, for example, large populations of clams in the upper parts of the river may be just as effective in removing the particulate matter from suspension as the coagulation process.

Regardless of the exact mechanism, a large amount of nutrient is deposited in the sediments of an estuary. In upper Chesapeake Bay, for example, a loss of some 45 μg-atom nitrate nitrogen/liter (610 μg NO_3-N/liter) was measured during the late spring and summer (450 mg-atom/m^2 at the mean water depth of 10m). Annual sedimentation rate of 1 mm/year would add 500 mg-atom N/m^2 to the sediments.

14.4.1.d. Equilibrium Between Sediments and Water

Particulate matter and estuarine sediment remove phosphorus from solution and also release phosphorus back into the water. Surface sediments may act as a giant buffer or reservoir for phosphates (Table 14.3). When the phosphorus in the water is less than about 0.9 μg-atom/liter (28 μg P/liter), phosphorus is released from the sediments into the water. Thus, these particular sediments are in equilibrium with water containing 0.7–0.9 Mg-atom P/liter.

Although it is likely that many of the same reactions and processes occur with nitrogen compounds, these interactions of nitrogen and sediment have never been investigated in detail.

14.4.1.e. Estuarine Nutrient Trap

There is upstream movement of sea water or diluted sea water in estuaries; otherwise there could be no salty water in the upstream areas. In certain estuaries with a high fresh-water runoff, a shear zone is maintained for long periods, with fresh water or low salinity water on top moving downstream and more saline water on the bottom moving upstream. If nutrients are moving vertically from the top to the bottom layers, by sinking or migration of the organisms, then the bottom waters will be enriched with nutrients that otherwise would be lost from the estuary. The bottom waters will also be enriched by decomposition of organic particulate matter in the surface sediments.

A good example of this countercirculation is found in the Gulf of Venezuela. The sea water, containing about 0.5 μg-atom P/liter, moves into the shallow waters of the gulf. As it does so, it accumulates phosphorus (up to 1.0 μg-atom P/liter). Although the nutrient trap certainly exists in estuaries, its importance in the annual nutrient budget has not yet been clarified.

14.4.2. Biological Processes

14.4.2.a. Biodeposition

A number of biological processes also remove particulate matter and its associated nutrients from solution. This biodeposition may be even more important than the physiochemical processes already discussed. Dense populations of molluscs filter clay from the water and produce pellets and flakes that behave like sand grains. Organic detritus also traps clay particles and the resulting flocs settle faster than those formed by coagulation.

The biodeposition rate of the oyster is approximately 1.5 g dry weight/ individual/week. If the amount of suspended solids is 5 mg/liter, this represents a minimum of 300 liters water filtered per week. Certainly, a tremendous

Table 14.3 Influence of Suspended Sediments on Estuarine Water of Varying
Phosphate Content (μmoles/liter)

Initial PO_4^{3-} of water	Final PO_4^{3-} of water[a]	PO_4^{3-} in sediment (μg PO_4^{3-}/g dry sediment)	n
0	0.72 ± 0.03	− 1.0	7
0.5	0.73 ± 0.02	− 0.4	4
1.0	0.90 ± 0.07	+ 0.6	8
2.5	0.89 ± 0.05	+ 7.6	8
4.3	0.87 ± 0.002	+ 11.0	8
8.4	1.61 ± 0.22	+ 30.9	3

Source: Pomeroy, L.R., et al. Limnol. Oceanogr. 10:167–172, 1965.

[a]Mean ± 1 SEM.

amount of water is processed by an oyster bed; when this oyster filtering is added to the activity of other filter feeders, it is enough filtering activity to process the whole volume of an estuary in a matter of days or a few weeks.

The large-rooted plants of estuaries also act as traps for the sediments, both by catching fine sediments and by providing protection (e.g., mangroves), so that the sedimentation rate is increased in the calm water. Various invertebrates and even diatom algae also secrete mucus or slime that traps sediment.

The net result is that estuaries in general, and marshes in particular, act as giant filters to remove particulate materials from the water. The vegetation of the marshes also stabilizes the sediment and thus reduces the turbidity. The importance of these processes is illustrated by the rapid siltation that took place in many harbors in southeastern England when the marshes were first diked and filled.

14.4.2.b. Uptake by Organisms

There are four main types of photosynthetic organisms in estuaries: rooted plants, attached algae, phytoplankton algae, and sediment algae. The obvious plants are the marsh grasses and rushes (e.g., *Spartina* and *Juncus*). These plants take up nutrients only from the sediments and are not in active competition with other primary producers for nutrients. Their presence creates conditions favoring sedimentation and biodeposition (e.g., the mussels in salt marshes). These plants also tie up a tremendous quantity of nutrients. For example, the annual production of organic matter in a Georgia *Spartina* marsh is 1600 g/m².

In some areas, submerged eelgrass (*Zostera*) may provide as much as 64% of the total production of phytoplankton, *Spartina*, and eelgrass in shallow estuaries.

Attached algae are not important generally in estuaries because the soft substratum and the tidal flooding of the marshes do not offer a suitable habitat. Permanently submerged plants, on the other hand, accumulate a thick layer of attached algae (reds and browns) that show a photosynthesis rate equal to that of the *Zostera*.

Microscopic algae also live in the upper layers of the mud. In extensive mud flats, such as in the Georgia salt marshes, the primary production may be as high as 420 g C/m²/year.

Phytoplankton algae are not abundant in many estuaries because there is rapid flushing and high turbidity. However, they may be the most important food for zooplankton and invertebrate larvae. In very large estuaries, such as Chesapeake Bay, there is adequate time for the algae to develop and primary production may reach several hundred g C/m²/year.

The well-known efficiency of algae in taking up nutrients from even very nutrient-poor waters makes them an agent for removing nutrients from the water of the estuary. The removal of the algae can result from their dying and sinking to the sediments, from the filtering action of benthic worms and molluscs, from their being eaten and carried away by migrating fish, or from washout from the estuary when strong tides are present.

Green plants are not the only organisms removing nutrients—bacteria are also important. *Spartina* has extremely small amounts of nitrogen and phosphorus relative to carbon, while bacteria need a C:N:P ratio of 200:10:1 for their growth. Thus, bacteria decomposing the *Spartina* must get the additional nitrogen and phosphorus they require from the surrounding water.

14.4.2.c. Nutrient Cycling

Once nutrients reach the estuary and are either transported to the sediments or taken up by the biota, they can cycle through various compartments before being locked into the sediments or flushed out of the estuary. For example, *Spartina* is tall near the creek banks, where fresh sediments are continually deposited, but short farther from the creek; this effect was traced to nitrogen deficiencies in the sediments away from the creeks. Once the nutrients are taken up into the plant, part is used for growth, part is excreted or otherwise lost from the plants, and part is eventually released during decomposition.

The general pattern of the nitrogen cycle in the estuary is for nitrate to enter the estuary and be rapidly removed from solution. Since ammonia is continually being formed (by decomposition processes and nitrate reduction) and taken up its concentration does not change very much. Organic nitrogen excretion and decomposition products are also continually cycled through the sediments and water. In the Pamlico River Estuary, it was found that urea was recycled every 1.4 days in the summer and every 200 days during the winter. The budget for nitrogen in this estuary (Table 14.4) indicated that during a winter month the nitrogen assimilated during photosynthesis was balanced by the nitrogen

Table 14.4 Some Contributions to the Net Increase in Inorganic Nitrogen (t N/day) That Occurred Within the Pamlico River Estuary, N.C.

Net increase[a]	Increase		Decrease	
Feb. 1972: 6.91	Sediment release	0.52	N assimilation	6.68
	Rainfall	0.11		
		0.63		
Aug. 1972: 0.10	Sediment release	3.43	N assimilation	231.65
	Rainfall	0.71		
		4.14		

[a]Calculated from inputs minus output.

(mostly nitrate) left in the estuary as the water flowed through (a net increase of 6.91 tons). The budget is badly out of balance during the summer, however, and it is likely that ammonia recycling in the water column and coming from the sediment made up the discrepancy of 227.5 tons/day.

Nitrogen may be lost from the estuaries, and particularly from the marshes, by denitrification. This is an anaerobic bacterial process that requires nitrate, and the energy for bacterial growth comes from organic molecules. Both denitrification and the opposite process, nitrogen fixation, occur in estuaries but their importance has not been clarified.

14.4.3. Estuarine Responses to Nutrient Additions

In a review of the literature on estuaries that receive sewage wastes, it has been concluded that hydrographic conditions, particularly the rate of flushing, is the most important factor determining the response of the ecosystem. An estuary with rapid flushing can handle tremendous amounts of added nutrients as long as they are quickly transported away and quickly diluted with low-nutrient ocean water.

14.4.3.a. Moriches Bay and Great South Bay, Long Island, New York

Duck farms around Moriches Bay formerly fed wastes into the bay. These nutrients reached Great South Bay, which has a retention time of 1 month. This bay formerly had a good stock of fish and shellfish but the fishery began to decline in the early 1940s as the duck population increased. Laboratory and field tests showed that the algae were actually limited by the low nitrogen, which was assimilated almost as soon as it entered the estuary. The damage to the oysters came from a shift of phytoplankton from a mixed group of species dominated by diatoms to two small forms, *Nannochloris* and *Stichococcus*. Although oysters eat these forms, these algae are nutritionally inadequate. Another factor adversely affecting the oysters was the large production of serpulid worms, which were able to overrun the oyster beds and competitively exclude the oysters.

14.4.3.b. Pamlico River Estuary, North Carolina

The cities on the Tar River, the main influence, are relatively small but a great deal of nutrient enters the Tar from agricultural runoff, presumable from heavily fertilized tobacco, potato, corn, and soybean fields. The total phosphorus entering the estuary ranges from 2.4 to 6.3 μg-atom/liter (74–195 μg/liter), while the reactive phosphorus ranges from 0.4 to 4.1 μg-atom/liter (12.4–127 μg/liter). There is adequate phosphorus in the estuary and there is also enough ammonia. In the winter months (January until April), in the middle reaches there are tremendous blooms of dinoflagellates (especially *Peridinium triquetrum*); this occurrence is apparently triggered by the winter influx of nitrate nitrogen into the estuary.

The ecological effect of these blooms has been slight thus far. The estuary still harbors a commercial blue crab and shrimp industry and the benthic biota are diverse. This estuary has reached a high level of production but the species are unchanged. The only effect has been an indirect one: there is increased oxygen uptake by the sediment during periods of low flow and calm conditions.

14.5. Control Mechanisms

14.5.1. Control at the Source

The potentially most successful and least harmful means of control of nutrient inputs to estuaries is to control the nutrients at their sources. Technology is available to institute control mechanisms for most point sources, but in some cases the costs outweigh the benefits. In cases of nonpoint sources of nutrient pollution the technology for control has not become feasible. In these situations, effective nutrient control is possible through change in land use, cultural practices, environmental manipulations, economics, and other management schemes.

14.5.1.a. Sewage Treatment

Since nitrogen and phosphorus concentrations in domestic sewage are rather high, sewage effluent constitutes an important source of nutrient material. Recent developments in technology, however, have made it economically possible to control the nutrient emissions from sewage treatment plants. In most instances these technologies have not been utilized, and large nutrient inputs are still contributed by sewage treatment plants.

Through the utilization of treatment technology and the enforcement of regulations, nutrient inputs from sewage treatment facilities can be controlled. Nutrient control at the sewage plant should be done on a case basis and be dictated by the location of the treatment facilities and the nature of the receiving waters.

14.5.1.b. Fertilization and Agricultural Practices

About one-third to one-half of the food and fiber production in the United States is attributed to the use of fertilizers in agricultural practices. Studies have shown, however, that 10–25% of the nitrogen fertilizer applied to cultivated crops leaves the field in drainage water.

Through changes in agricultural practice and technological breakthroughs it may be possible to control this source of nutrient input. One possibility is the use of cover crops during the noncropping seasons to hold the fertilizer in the soil layers. Other possibilities include adjustments of the timing and rates of fertilizier applications, repeated small applications, and the development of new crops. One measure with high potential for control of nutrient transport is the control of water drainage from fields by catchment basins, with repercolation back into the fields between plowings. The very recent development of chemicals to control nitrifying bacteria and to prevent conversion of ammonia to nitrate, offers great hope for reducing nitrogen loss from fields.

Animal production techniques are changing from small producers with several types of animals on a pasture to intense production of one species in feed lots. Confinement has allowed increased and more economical production, but it has also resulted in point sources of nutrient materials for surface waters. Although these materials are disposed of in liquid systems because they are convenient and economical, land disposal is considered to be another feasible method of terminal disposal.

The most likely means of immediate control of this nutrient source is in the practices of disposal. Some feasible alternatives include deep well injection, controlled land application, or recycling through newly devised feed preparation systems. This area of activity, however, probably presents one of the more serious disposal problems facing present-day technology.

In large metropolitan areas adjacent to coastal waters the practice of the surburban dweller "keeping up with the neighbors" and overfertilizing his lawn presents a real nutrient input problem. The main control mechanism available at the present time is to cycle these materials through municipal treatment plants.

14.5.1.c. Industrial Waste Treatment

Industrial wastes represent another large source of nutrients for surface waters for which treatment technology is available for control. The problem has been in instituting complete and proper waste control facilities in existing industrial complexes.

The runoff of nutrient materials from the surface areas of industrial complexes presents a separate problem in the control of nutrient sources. Mechanisms need to be developed for channeling this runoff through treatment or filtering systems to reduce nutrient inputs and drainage.

14.5.1.d. Runoff

One of the most difficult sources to control is the runoff of materials from watersheds. This represents a very diffuse, highly variable, and important source of nutrient materials. The major methods of controlling nutrients from runoff involve watershed management. Carefully controlled foresty practices, reforestation, protection of uncovered areas, road maintenance, controlled drainage, vegetated filter strips, and contour plowing are management techniques currently available for erosion control.

14.5.1.e. Ground Water

Ground water as a source of nutrients for estuaries is not very well understood. Drainage of nutrient materials from septic tanks into ground water has been documented in several situations, particularly on the Barrier Islands along the U.S. seashore. The best means of control in these situations is the central collection of waste waters and channeling through waste treatment facilities on a regional basis.

A problem that must be dealt with is the physical manipulations that allow alterations in ground water drainage patterns. Dredging of deep channels in estuarine systems may enable ground water percolation to bring in a new source of materials from outside the estuarine system.

14.5.2. Control of Transport Mechanisms

Control of nutrient inputs through manipulation of transport processes has little potential. These measures may have little beneficial effect on the receiving system downstream because detrimental side effects may be greater than any benefit from nutrient control (e.g., reduction of vital fresh-water inputs).

14.5.2.a. Stream Flow

Once nutrient materials reach the streams flowing into estuaries, institutional controls offer little benefit. There is considerable evidence of a decrease in nutrient concentrations downstream from sources due to deposition, biological cycling, etc., but additional control of nutrient inflows is not now technologically feasible.

Reservoirs on streams may offer some control benefits. Selective release of water through reservoir dam structures can be used to regulate nutrient concentrations downstream.

14.5.2.b. Channelization

The increase in channelization of natural streams in recent years for the purposes of increased drainage and agricultural activities has changed normal stream flow mechanisms. The creation of faster flowing streams has minimized the natural loss of nutrients as water meanders downstream. Channelization also allows the water to move downstream rapidly, thus avoiding the natural cleansing action by swamp soils around these streams where water normally percolates.

14.5.2.c. Denitrification

Denitrification offers the best possibilities for the control of nitrogen during transport. Considerable reduction of nitrogen can be achieved if conditions are properly maintained over a period of time. Drainage water from agricultural lands, for example, could be held and maintained under conditions favorable for denitrification. Small reservoirs and low-level dikes in some stream situations could be utilizied for denitrification. Sewage holding ponds have long been used to achieve reductions in nitrogen concentrations in effluents.

14.5.3. Control Within the Estuary

Control mechanisms for nutrient reduction within estuarine systems probably have the least potential for effective reduction in nutrient concentrations. The worst problems include detrimental side effects, high costs, and interference with normal cycling procedures within the ecosystem.

14.5.3.a. Selective Harvesting

Since certain organisms take up large amounts of nutrients, selective harvesting of these species could serve as a means of removing the nutrients from the system. This technique, however, offers little hope for effectively removing nutrient materials from estuarine waters since the cost and engineering of such harvesting systems would be large. Natural means of doing this have been tried in several cases by culturing species of algae-consuming fish, by using manatee to harvest underwater grasses in Florida, by culturing species of clams and oysters, etc., all with limited success.

14.5.3.b. Diversions

The creation of canals to divert nutrient-laden water around estuarine systems is an unlikely means of control because of the obvious side effects. There are several examples in the U.S. coastal area where large regional sewage interceptors are diverting large amounts of waste waters around estuaries for offshore disposal—an expensive and disruptive procedure.

14.5.3.c. Zoning

Estuaries in each state might be zoned so that some receive added nutrient input while others are protected. This means of control, however, assumes that correct decisions can be made concerning which estuaries receive added nutrients and which do not.

14.5.3.d. Impounding

The construction of impoundments at the heads of estuaries offers some possibility for selective control of nutrient inputs into the large estuarine expanse. Impoundments offer the advantage of trapping water, allowing time for denitrification and deposition of phosphorus materials into the sediments, and selected withdrawal of water from the impounded area. This type of control, however, has serious side effects in that the normal flushing activity of fresh-water inputs would be altered, possibly leading to severe changes in the estuarine system.

14.5.3.e. Regeneration of Marshes

The marsh system, with its grasses, algae, and accumulated organic muds, acts as a filtering system to reduce the nutrient content of the surrounding water; this is one of the beneficial roles of marshes as part of the estuarine system. It is possible to plant marsh grasses and generate new marsh area around estuarine shores.

Suggested Reading

Chabreck, R. H. (Ed.). Proceedings of the Coastal Marsh and Estuary Management Symposium. Division of Continuing Education, Louisiana State University, Baton Rouge, 1973.

Cronin, L. E. (Ed.). Estuarine Research, Vols. 1 and 2. New York: Academic Press, 1975.

de la Cruz, A., Brisbin, I. L. (Eds). Towards a Relevant Ecology. Athens, Ga.: University of Georgia Press, 1971.

Eutrophication: Causes, Consequences, Correctives—Proceedings of a Symposium. Washington, D.C.: National Academy of Sciences, 1969.

Likens, G. E. (Ed.). Nutrients and Eutrophication. Special Symposium, Vol I. American Society of Limnology and Oceanography, Lawrence, Kansas, 1972.

Nelson, B. W. (Ed.). Environmental Framework of Coastal Plain Estuaries. Boulder, Colo.: Geological Society of America, 1972.

Odum, H. T., Copeland, B. J., McMahan, E. A., (Eds). Coastal Ecological Systems of the United States, Vol. 3. Washington, D. C.: Conservation Foundation, 1974.

Jerome J. Perry

15

Oil in the Biosphere

15.1. Introduction

World petroleum production during the period 1975–1978 exceeded 2.5×10^9 t per year. In addition, more than one-half the petroleum (the term crude oil can be used interchangeably) was produced in a country other than that in which it was refined and consumed. The refined petroleum products are generally transported from the refinery to the point of consumption by ship, barge, or pipeline. It is inevitable that a considerable amount of the refined petroleum transported in this manner will be spilled into the environment by accident, mechanical failure, or negligence. The accidental spillage of oil in huge quantities has had a dramatic impact on people throughout the world. Some major spills of recent years are listed in Table 15.1. Although these spills had considerable short-range effect, it is evident that more significant damage can result from chronic petroleum pollution of the environment. However, the short-term environmental consequences of major petroleum spills are more apparent and more readily quantitated than the long-term toxicological effects of chronic pollution, and much of our present knowledge of toxicity related to petroleum has come from such studies. The two most thoroughly studied spills occurred near marine research institutes, and the personnel were able to assess effects of the spillage over an extended period of time. These were the *Torrey Canyon* disaster, which occurred at Milford Haven, England, near the Marine Biological Association Laboratories, and the *Florida* spill at West Falmouth, Massachusetts, only a short distance from the Woods Hole Oceanographic Institute.

Petroleum contains five principal classes of hydrocarbons: normal paraffins, branched-chain paraffins, cycloparaffins, aromatics, and asphaltics. The distribution of the various hydrocarbons may differ in a crude oil and depends on the origin. Paraffin-base crudes are predominantly paraffinic hydrocarbons, whereas asphalt-base crudes are lower in paraffinics and contain more high boiling point asphaltic hydrocarbons. Crude oil also contains oxygen (generally

Table 15.1   Some Major Oil Spills in Recent Years

Year	Ship	Site	Cargo	Oil spilled (t)
1957	*Tampico Maru*	Baja, Mexico	Diesel oil	8000
1967	*Torrey Canyon*	Milford Haven, England	Kuwait crude oil	115,000
1969	*Florida*	West Falmouth, Mass.	No. 2 fuel oil	700
1969	*Well A-21*	Santa Barbara Channel, Calif.	Crude oil	4,500
1970	*Arrow*	Chedabucto Bay, Nova Scotia	Bunker C crude oil	10,000
1974	*Metula*	Strait of Magellan, S.A.	Arabian crude oil	52,000
1976	*Argo Merchant*	Nantucket Shoals, Mass.	No. 6 fuel oil	20,000
1978	*Amoco Cadiz*	Brittany Coast, France	Crude oil	220,000

less than 3%), nitrogen (less than 1%) and sulfur (0.1–10%). There are varying amounts of heavy metals (i.e. vanadium, nickel, iron, and copper) in crude oil. Refining operations separate the petroleum into a number of fractions for commercial purposes (Table 15.2). Generally, long-term toxic effects result from spillage of crude oil, residual fuel oil, and lubricants. Gasoline, distillate fuel oil (low boiling point), and kerosene evaporate quickly on spilling and are less of a problem. High boiling point residual tars are insoluble and, as used for road surfaces, roofs, etc., would not be considered a significant problem in the environment.

The presence of petroleum or refined petroleum products in aquatic systems is generally harmful for physical reasons (coating, smothering, etc.), or because water-soluble fractions of the oil are toxic to the biota. Crude oil causes more physical damage and fuel oil is generally more toxic.

The results presented in Table 15.3 suggest that more petroleum pollution of the sea results from activities on land [3.30 million metric tons per annum (mta)] than from operations at sea (2.813 mta); there is a marked difference, considering that the latter figure includes 0.60 mta from natural offshore seeps.

Table 15.2   Production of Crude Oil and Relative Demand for Major Products During 1974

Product	Amount ($\times 10^6$ barrels)
Crude oil	20,537.7
Residual fuel oil (ship and industrial fuel)	4,525.8
Gasoline (motor and aviation)	4,163.4
Distillate fuel oil (home, etc.)	3,695.2
Kerosene and jet fuel	1,126.6
Lubricants	153.7

Source: Adapted from Symposium on Sources, Effects and Sinks of Hydrocarbons in the Aquatic Environment. Washington, D.C.: American Institute of Biological Sciences, p. 8, 1976.

Table 15.3   Estimated Annual Input of Petroleum Hydrocarbons into the Ocean

Origin	Input (mta)
Terrestrial	
River runoff	1.60
Atmospheric origin	0.60
Urban runoff	0.30
Municipal wastes (coastal)	0.30
Industrial wastes (coastal, nonrefining)	0.30
Coastal refineries	0.20
Total	3.30
Marine	
Tankers	1.08
Dry docking	0.25
Terminal operations	0.003
Bilges and bunkering	0.50
Tanker accidents	0.20
Nontanker accidents	0.10
Offshore production	0.08
Offshore seeps	0.60
Total	2.813

Source: Adapted from *Petroleum in the Marine Environment,* page 6, with the permission of the National Academy of Sciences, Washington, D.C.
Note: Data were obtained during 1970–1973 but are considered representative.

The estimated 6.1 mta entering the marine environment surpasses the amount of hydrocarbon entering the ocean each year from planktonic activity. This total figure for hydrocarbon generated from natural sources is derived by measuring total biological productivity and considering that 0.01–0.02% of all living cells is hydrocarbon. The hydrocarbons of biological origin are generally of relatively simple structure, e.g., *n*-alkanes. They are of broad distribution and are readily degraded by the indigenous microbial population.

A major problem of petroleum hydrocarbon pollution is that most occurs near land, in sounds, bays, and coastal areas where maximum toxic effects are realized. The petroleum spills that occur in confined areas, e.g., bays, are particularly harmful, as the level of toxic material remains high for longer periods than when spillage occurs where rapid dispersion can take place.

Some of the major factors involved in the spillage of oil can be considered according to the origin (as outlined in Table 15.3).

15.2. Marine Origin

15.2.1. Tankers

The cargo compartment of tankers involved in the transport of crude oil contains significant quantities of oil after unloading. The bottom of the tank, walls, inside beams, and structural recesses retain about 5% of the total load. This oil was washed into the sea during earlier times, but the more modern tankers incorporate "load on top" (LOT) procedures that minimize this discharge by accumulating tank washings and oily water ballast in one compartment of the tanker, allowing the oil–water to separate, and incorporating the oil fraction into the next shipment. The oil–water remaining in the bottom of the tank is generally discharged into the sea on completion of the return voyage. It is estimated that the LOT tankers (80% of total tankers) discharge approximately 0.31 mta, and the ships not equipped for this procedure (the remaining 20%) discharge 0.77 mta. The total amount of crude oil transported by sea is in the range of 1100–1200 mta.

15.2.2. Dry Docking

All tankers undergo maintenance and inspection at intervals (generally within 18 months) and must be clean and gas free prior to this operation. Facilities to handle the washings from these tankers are not available at many dry dock sites, and the total washings from the vessel are therefore dumped at sea. The world tanker fleet of 180 dead weight tons would discharge about 0.25 mta.

15.2.3. Terminal Operations

The routine handling of oil in ports results in a spillage rate in the range of 0.00015%. Since much of the oil is handled when unloaded into the refinery and again after refining, the total world-wide loss during these procedures has been estimated to range between 0.0015 and 0.005 mta, with a generally accepted value of 0.003 mta.

15.2.4. Bilges and Bunkering

There is an estimated loss per ship of about 10 t/year either in bilge water or leaks from bunkers. This would apply to all ships at sea and would result in an estimated total discharge of 0.50 mta.

15.2.5. Tanker Accidents

During the period 1969–1973 there were 3183 recorded accidents that occurred with tankers larger than 2000 gross tons, and 452 of these accidents resulted in oil spillage. The average loss per vessel was 2110 t oil. The major cause of accidents during the period was structural failure, with grounding and collision following in frequency of occurrence.

15.2.6. Natural Seeps

The amount of petroleum discharged into the sea by natural seeps is considerable, but the total quantity is open to question. If the estimates given are reasonably valid for geological time, then 50–100 times more oil has seeped into the biosphere than now exists in reservoirs.

15.2.7. Offshore Production

There is a loss of petroleum associated with normal drilling and production operations. In addition, there are blowouts, ruptures of gathering lines, and other occurrences that result in significant spillage of petroleum. The estimated loss of petroleum from this source is 0.014% of the offshore oil produced and would be approximately 0.2 mta in the early 1980s.

15.3. Terrestrial Origin

15.3.1. Coastal Refineries

Since loss from terminal operations was considered previously, only the dispersed oil discharged in the waste water from seaboard refineries will be mentioned here. Water usage in oil refineries occurs at an estimated rate of 3000 m³ water/hr/mta petroleum refining capacity. Separation of the oil from water involved in refinery operations by gravity separation results in an effluent with 20 ppm oil. This level is sufficient to cause a considerable discharge problem. However, pressure from governmental agencies with more stringent waste water standards has resulted in the addition of facilities for further treatment of effluent water and/or recirculation of the cooling water. This has considerably reduced the level of oil in effluent water, and the estimated 0.20 mta discharge may be unrealistically high.

15.3.2. Atmosphere

The total world-wide influx of petroleum hydrocarbons into the atmosphere from transportation, stationary fuel combustion, industrial processes, gasoline and solvent evaporation, etc. has been estimated to be 60–70 mta. Approximately two-thirds of this atmospheric petroleum-derived material emanates from internal combustion engines involved in transportation, and one-half of these products of combustion are reactive in the atmosphere. It is believed that virtually all of the reactive material and most (90%) of the nonreactive fraction is converted to other products after combining with particulate matter in the air and these do not return to the earth as petroleum. The amount of petroleum, therefore, entering the oceans through rainfall or dry fallout would be about 10% of the total entering the atmosphere.

15.3.3. Coastal Municipal and Industrial Wastes

Results reported from studies conducted in California indicate that municipal waste water contains approximately 4 g petroleum hydrocarbon per capita per day. This would include discharges from households, gas stations, and garages, and a wide variety of wastes in the municipal sewer system. Considering the number of people in the coastal zone (68×10^6 in the United States), there is a discharge of 0.3 mta from this source world wide. The input from industrial operations in coastal areas not involved with petroleum refining probably equals the total petroleum discharged in domestic waste water.

15.3.4. Urban Runoff

Urban areas receive significant amounts of petroleum hydrocarbons from oil heating systems, automobiles, road oiling, etc. These petroleum products are carried into storm drains and local waters, and eventually much of the material flows into the ocean. It is estimated that the total amount of oil and grease from urban runoff is between 0.1 and 0.6 mta. This total depends to a great extent on climatic conditions and the amount of automobile traffic, and the world-wide best estimate from storm drainage is 0.3 mta.

15.3.5. River Runoff

The Mississippi River is considered a representative river for the United States; it contains a minimum of 0.085 mg/liter of extractable petroleum hydrocarbon. Using this figure for the total river flow in the United States gives an estimated 0.53 mta petroleum flowing into the ocean from U.S. rivers. This figure multiplied by 3 (ratio of world to U.S. petroleum utilization) gives a world-wide input of about 1.6 mta petroleum.

15.4. Environmental Effects of Oil

The impact of oil pollution on the environment can be divided into two major categories: (a) acute effects observed when major spills occur (e.g., the *Torrey Canyon* spill), with immediate consequences to the biota and to the entire coastal recreation area; and (b) chronic pollution of the entire marine ecosystem caused by constant spillage or drainage of petroleum into the environment. The chronic effects can occur when petroleum or its derivatives flow into the biosphere at a constant rate or at consistent intervals such that the flora and fauna have an insufficient time to recover between exposures to the petroleum. Activities associated with the petroleum industry can also damage aquatic organisms. Dredging operations in port areas with the accompanying filling of marshes alters the habitat and spawning areas for marine animals. Modifications of the marine ecosystem brought about by chronic pollution and other activities of the petroleum industry can alter populations through changes in the rate of birth, longevity, and distribution of species, causing an imbalance in the entire community.

The overall effects of petroleum hydrocarbons in the marine environment may be summarized as follows:

1. The introduction of high concentrations of selected hydrocarbon fractions can be lethal to seafood species. At sublethal levels, the seafood can contain hazardous concentrations of petroleum hydrocarbons or be tainted such that taste or aroma renders the food unfit for human consumption. This is of considerable consequence to the commercial seafood industry.
2. Oil slicks on water or oil deposited on beaches are unsightly, and tar lumps carried by the tides onto beaches adjacent to major shipping lanes (Florida Coast, Bermuda) are undesirable from an aesthetic standpoint.

3. A decrease in diversity and/or productivity of a species can bring about modifications that can have long-range deleterious effects on the entire marine ecosystem.
4. Extensive damage to wildlife, generally caused by large spills or blowouts in offshore drilling, can significantly decrease populations of seabirds and marine mammals.

The ocean is a remarkably stable environment with relatively constant pH, temperature, and chemical composition. The level of dissolved oxygen resulting from photosynthesis by planktonic organisms, at depths to which light can penetrate, and its solution from the atmosphere is sufficient to support a vast biomass. All living species in the ocean are interdependent; some known effects of petroleum on the flora and fauna of the marine environment will now be considered.

15.4.1. Fish and Fisheries

It is probable that fish swim away from heavy oil pollution and particularly from oil spills, where the oil layered on the ocean causes a decrease in photosynthesis and consequently a lowering of oxygen levels in the water. The slimy mucus on the gills of fish make them somewhat resistant to oil. However, there is much evidence that fish are adversely affected by both spilled petroleum and chronic pollution by refined petroleum products. There were significant fish kills (of at least 10 species) following the oil spill from the *Ocean Eagle* in the harbor at Puerto Rico, and spilled heavy fuel oil at Wake Island and West Falmouth, Massachusetts, also resulted in the death of many fish. Fuel oil is apparently more toxic than crude oil.

Fisheries are adversely affected by chronic petroleum pollution, and the catch of fish off the coast of Louisiana has decreased concomitantly with the development of the petroleum industry. Tainting of commercial species of fish by oil and the resulting unsalable catches can be a serious problem. Mullet caught in Australian coastal waters in the vicinity of port and refinery facilities are frequently contaminated with petroleum hydrocarbons. Analysis of these hydrocarbons by gas–liquid chromatography indicates that they are similar in composition to kerosene. Generally, fish and other marine organisms nonspecifically accumulate the entire range of hydrocarbons to which they are exposed.

The greatest harm to fish life from petroleum hydrocarbons from both spillage and chronic pollution is the effect on eggs, larval stages, and fry. The destruction of young fish can have serious long-term consequences. In many cases in which significant amounts of emulsifier are employed in cleanup operations, it is difficult to distinguish between the harmful effects of the petroleum and those of the more toxic emulsifying agents. After the *Torrey Canyon* accident, for example, 50–90% of the eggs of pilchards in Cornish waters were dead. Larval fish concentrate at the ocean surface, where they are subject to entrapment and the toxic effects of the petroleum hydrocarbons. Fish eggs are often laid at the ocean bottom, but fry immediately swim to the surface. Herring fry exposed to 5 ppm dissolved fraction of hydrocarbon have a mortality of 70–100% within 4 days. Eggs that hatch after exposure to crude or fuel oil yield deformed larvae. Turbot eggs exposed to 0.1 ppm water-soluble fraction of crude oil hatched at a 50% rate, and many of the larvae hatching from these eggs were distorted.

15.4.2. Birds and Mammals

The oiling of birds in the marine environment has received considerable publicity and is a serious problem associated with oil spills and oil slicks emanating from washing of tankers. These oilings can be catastrophic for a population as migratory activity can bring a major proportion of a bird species to a confined area. Oil fouling of birds can cause a disruption in the insulating capacity of feathers and result in death from pneumonia or it can cause a loss in buoyancy and subsequent drowning. The loss of insulation also brings about an elevated metabolic rate and "accelerated starvation." Oil ingested during preening by the oiled birds causes an inflammation of the digestive tract, and this factor along with the increased metabolism results in death to most oiled birds. Birds and mammals have a relatively impervious skin but can breathe toxic components of both oil and emulsifiers. These have serious physiological effects when ingested during preening, grooming, or feeding. Diving birds suffer inordinate mortality, whereas sea gulls, shearwaters, and some other species avoid oil. Unfortunately, some birds, e.g., the long-tailed duck, settle preferentially on oil slicks. Auks, puffins, razorbills, guillemots, and sea ducks apparently are attracted by the physical appearance or aroma of petroleum and swim into the slick of their own volition.

It is difficult to ascertain precisely the number of birds killed by petroleum pollution, although counts of oiled birds on the shore have been made. In estimating the total, the number that reach land is considered to be 5–15% of those killed. The estimated numbers of birds that died as a result of typical spills are as follows: *Torrey Canyon*, 40,000–100,000; Santa Barbara blowout, 3600; San Francisco Bay spill, 7000; and stranding of the *Gerd Maersk* in the Elbe Estuary, 250,000–500,000. The oil spilled following the collision between the *Fort Mercer* and the *Pendleton* off Chatham, Massachusetts (1952), reduced the wintering population of eider ducks from 500,000 to 150,000. The Santa Barbara incident killed 64% of the loons and grebes in that area, which represented 7–10% of the total bird population. The jackass penguin, restricted to South Africa, faces extinction because it is gradually being killed off by floating oil from tankers rounding the Cape of Good Hope. An estimated 150,000–450,000 birds are killed each year in the North Sea–North Atlantic by chronic oil pollution.

Although a bird may not be affected directly by oil, some bird species, if oiled, do not lay eggs or eggs that are laid may not hatch. Gannets are unaffected by floating oil as they only dive on visible prey but foul themselves and their eggs by collecting oiled seaweed as material for building nesting mounts. The hatch rate of oiled eggs is generally low as oil reduces the permeability of the egg shell with an apparent adverse effect on the embryo.

The pinnipeds—walruses, sea lions, and seals—occupy coastal marine habitats and are potential victims of oil pollution. Whales and dolphins are powerful swimmers and apparently avoid oiled areas. At the time of the year at which the Santa Barbara incident occurred in 1969, the gray whale usually migrates through that channel but avoided the polluted area that year.

Oil can cause suffocation of pinnipeds, and poisoning from oil ingestion during preening. There have not been reports of significant numbers of these animals killed by petroleum pollutants, but cases of severe eye irritation have been documented. Gray seals have been observed in Nova Scotia lost in the forests unable to see because of eye inflammation caused by oiling.

The sea otter on the U.S. West Coast, now struggling back from near extinction, would be seriously affected by oil spillage in that area, and muskrats in coastal wetlands of Louisiana have been decimated by oil pollution from production fields.

15.4.3. Bentnic Organisms

Organisms living in the sea bed (e.g., clams, abalone, starfish, sea urchins, shrimp, snails, lobsters, etc.) are of limited mobility. The introduction of toxic materials into their environment can have serious consequences. Benthic organisms tend to accumulate petroleum hydrocarbons in their tissue, and the hydrocarbons are retained as long as the animal remains in polluted water.

Fuel oil is apparently more toxic than crude oil to animals living in the sea bed. A massive kill of benthic animals resulted from the No. 2 fuel oil spill off West Falmouth, and waves of dead animals, including lobsters, were washed ashore. During subsequent months the oil moved from shallow water to deeper areas, accompanied by a high degree of animal mortality. Animals were virtually eliminated from the heavily oiled bottoms, and in peripheral areas the more susceptible amphipods and crustaceans were selectively killed. There was a marked difference in the resistance of animal species to oil; the quahog survived at West Falmouth, whereas the razor clam was decimated by the fuel oil pollution. After 4 years significant areas of the bay at West Falmouth remained polluted (even the readily biodegradable n-alkanes persisted) and the ban on harvesting of shellfish was retained. The level of oil in water that can give a discernible odor and/or taste is quite low; 0.01 ppm fuel oil renders mussels and oysters unfit for human consumption.

The *Tampico Maru* was stranded and broke up across a cove along the coast of Mexico, and diesel oil flowed into a confined area. There was extensive mortality of Pismo clams, abalone, starfish, and other benthos. The persistence of the oil resulted in an ecological imbalance as grazers and predators were decimated and did not recolonize rapidly enough to control the growth of seaweeds and algae. The cove had not completely recovered ecologically after 7 years. Divers at the site of the *Torrey Canyon* spill found extensive areas with moribund and dead clams, snails, crustaceans, and echinoderms. As oil dispersants were used, it would be difficult to determine which caused more problems, crude oil or emulsifiers. The French Government added 3000 t chalk to sink the crude oil drifting from the *Torrey Canyon* toward the coast of France. Masses of oil subsequently fouled fishing gear in that area, and catches of fish were contaminated by the oil.

Studies on ecological alterations at the site of the Santa Barbara incident were fruitful as an extensive survey of benthic animals in the channel had been made 10 years prior to the blowout. There was a considerable decrease in total biomass after the oiling of the area, and some species, e.g., echinoid worms, which were in dense beds prior to the incident, were decimated.

Many sessile animals can be smothered by oil, and some (e.g., limpets) are washed away as the oil disrupts their holdfast. An exceedingly low level of oil in water can cause problems for benthic animals: 10 ppb of the soluble fraction of crude oil will disrupt the reproductive behavior of the shore crab and the offspring of the sea urchins and sea star are abnormal if the animals are placed in sea water over weathered tank sludge. The emulsifiers used in cleanup operations are also toxic at low levels: the sea urchin is unhealthy at 1 ppm and the tubeworm is killed at 2.5 ppm. Shrimp tend to ingest crude oil when hungry, and this adheres to the foregut and reduces the rate of feeding. It also lowers the specific gravity of the animal, making it more susceptible to predators.

15.4.4. Plankton, Pleuston, and Neuston

Many species of plants and animals live on or near the surface of the ocean. Among the neuston are the plankton that serve as a major source of energy in the sea since they capture energy from the sun and are an indispensible initial stage in the food chain. The phytoplankton, being more sensitive to petroleum hydrocarbons than zooplankton, were decimated to a greater extent by the oil from the *Torrey Canyon*. Water extracts of crude oil, fuel oil, and dispersants inhibit the growth of phytoplankton and decrease the rate of photosynthesis. Fuel oil added to sea water at 100 ppb will depress photosynthesis in these organisms by 60%. Diatoms are killed by 24-hr exposure to 100 ppm fuel oil or kerosene. While zooplankton are more resistant to the lethal effects of oil, oil readily accumulates in these organisms. Following the spillage of bunker C oil in Chedabucto Bay, about 10% of the total oil in the water column was found in the zooplankton. Incorporation of oil at this level could lead to considerable biomagnification in the food chain. The larvae of fish and benthic species spend time as zooplankton and are more susceptible to the toxicants in oil than are adults.

The effect of petroleum hydrocarbons on the *Sargassum* community is not well understood, although the location of this group at the ocean surface would render it susceptible to the toxic effects of oil pollution. There are reports that petroleum hydrocarbon contamination of plants and animals in the *Sargassum* community has occurred. Oil slicks cause considerable damage to pleustonic animals, although our knowledge is limited to scattered eyewitness accounts. The pleuston—jellyfish, Portuguese man-of-war, goose barnacle, purple snail, and other floating animals—are, like the plankton, passively carried by the ocean currents.

15.4.5. Intertidal Organisms

Oil spillage from tanker accidents, oil released by negligent handling, river runoff, and other petroleum ultimately end up in intertidal areas. Floating oil and the thick "mousse" that is generated by emulsification of oil on the surface on the ocean often wends its way to this sector and has an undesirable aesthetic and lethal effect. The sessile barnacles, surf grass, kelp, algae, and other biota are harmed considerably by all forms of petroleum pollution. Evaporation of petroleum on rocky shores results in a heavy coating of the shore and prevents recolonization by barnacles and other sessile organisms. However, the long-term toxic effect of oil on muddy and sandy beaches is more severe.

Oil has a nontoxic lethal effect on intertidal organisms by smothering and fouling, or in the case of mobile species (e.g., snails) the presence of oil causes behavioral problems that result in death of the animal. The snail retracts into its shell when oil is present, and the animal is swept from the habitat by ocean currents. This occurs with many molluscs. Thick oil can also cement organisms in place, and the inability to graze results in starvation. There is considerable evidence that components of petroleum are lethally toxic to many intertidal organisms. The breakup of the *Tampico Maru* in a sheltered cove on the coast of Mexico resulted in devastating kills of all intertidal organisms in the cove. The only survivors were a few anemones. The fuel oil spill at West Falmouth killed all intertidal organisms with the exception of a few highly resistant polychaete worms. Both of these catastrophes involved fuel oil, which, as previously stated, is apparently more toxic than other forms of petroleum.

Giant kelp are not seriously affected by crude oil, nor are organisms with a natural coating of mucilage or mucus, e.g., macroalgae and anemones. Surf grass, a vascular plant, suffered great losses in the Santa Barbara incident. Oil-resistant large algae, which are important intertidal primary producers on rocky shores, often become coated with oil and are torn from the matrix to which they are attached. Oil adhering to algae is ingested by grazing invertebrates and can have a deleterious effect on these organisms. The reproductive ability and relatively short generation time of algae permits rapid recolonization of these species but can present problems in the total recolonization of an affected area, particularly if herbivorous invertebrates are destroyed. Rapid growth of algae produces a "green phase," which is replaced by brown fucoid algae. The fucoid algae are not grazed, and the thick cover inhibits the reestablishment of mussels, barnacles, limpets, and other organisms.

15.4.6. Wetlands

The wetlands are an unappreciated part of the oceanic ecosystem, as witnessed by man's destruction of these resources by channeling and draining. These areas are among the most productive on earth, with a food web based on detritus. They support the living systems found in the estuary. Overall, they serve as a habitat, feeding, and nesting ground for all species of shore and ocean-going birds and a breeding ground for fish and many other animals.

A small amount of oil on marsh plants is not excessively harmful, but repeated application is lethal. Large doses can devastate shoots and plants, but generally roots are not killed by oil. The extent of damage is dependent on the type of oil, the plant species involved, and the time of year. Weathered oil with few low molecular weight aromatics is less toxic than fresh oil or light fuel oil. Oil tends to interfere with flowering, seed development, and vegetative reproduction in underground root systems. Consequently, annuals that develop from seeds are more sensitive than perennials that regenerate from roots.

The West Falmouth spill killed salt-marsh cord grass and marsh plants. Spills in Puerto Rico and Panama caused the death of mangrove trees and associated animals. Much of a marsh near a refinery effluent in Southampton, England, was denuded by chronic low-level pollution. The consequent rapid erosion of the marsh bank caused considerable inconvenience and expense.

15.4.7. Polar Regions and Coral Reefs

The toxic effects of oil spilled in polar regions are of growing concern as crude oil produced and transported from the North Slope in Alaska increases in volume. The low evaporation rate at polar temperatures means that toxic lower molecular weight aromatic compounds remain for a longer time than they would in temperate climates. The rate of weathering and biodegradation is also considerably reduced. The marine biota of polar regions are long-lived and of low reproductive potential, and they generally do not have wide-ranging dispersal stages. Hence, a large oil spill in the Arctic would have considerable immediate effect and would persist and remain toxic over an extended period of time. Recovery and recolonization of the contaminated area would occur at an exceedingly slow rate.

Coral reefs generally found in tropical oceans are an environment of enormous biological diversity, complexity, and productivity. The branched corals are particularly sensitive to oil, and markedly so while exposed to air, and many reefs in the Pacific Ocean and Indian Ocean protrude far above the water surface at low tide. An important part of a living coral reef community is dead rubble, which is a porous limestone, and it would be harmful to the reef if significant quantities of toxic petroleum were absorbed into this integral part of the biosystem.

Suggested Reading

Baker, J.M. Marine Ecology and Oil Pollution. New York: Wiley, 1976.

Boesch, D. F., Hershner, C. H., Milgram, H. H. Oil Spills and the Marine Environment. Cambridge, Mass.: Ballinger, 1974.

Malins, D. C. (Ed.). Effects of Petroleum on Arctic and Subarctic Environments and Organisms. Vol. 1., Nature and Fate of Petroleum. Vol. II, Biological Effects. New York: Academic Press, 1977.

Nelson-Smith, A. Oil Pollution and Marine Ecology. New York: Plenum Press, 1973.

Petroleum in the Marine Environment. Workshop on Inputs, Fates and the Effects of Petroleum in the Marine Environment. Washington, D. C.: National Academy of Science, 1975.

Sources, Effects and Sinks of Hydrocarbons in the Aquatic Environment. Proceedings of a Symposium. Washington, D. C.: American Institute of Biological Sciences, 1976.

William T. McKean

16

Pulp and Paper Industry

16.1. Introduction

Output of the pulp and paper industry traditionally parallels population growth and the industry is the 10th largest in the United States, with about 63.5×10^6 tons of products generated in 1976. Figure 16.1 shows the distribution of pulp production by process and product type. Population and industrial growth of all types during the past two decades have focused attention on environmental matters. Along with various governmental agencies, the pulp and paper industry has acted to identify the impact of its manufacturing operations and to take appropriate measures to minimize the effect on the atmospheric and aquatic environment. As long as several decades ago, waste-water treatment systems were installed to limit BOD, suspended solids, and in some locations color emissions. More recently, increased concern about toxic substances has resulted in a review of manufacturing operations from a new viewpoint. After a major effort the main toxic substances have been identified. It is becoming clear that most toxic substances in pulp and paper effluents respond to a large extent to the waste treatment systems originally developed for BOD control. In order to illustrate the quantity of substances and their response in waste treatment systems, in the following sections a description of the industry is given in terms of raw material characteristics, processing, and product type.

The pulp and paper industry is essentially forest based, and almost any tree species in the softwood or hardwood category can be used for pulping. Regardless of the species, wood is comprised of cellulose, hemicellulose, lignin, and extractives. While relative composition varies with species, typical softwood and hardwood compositions are shown in Figure 16.2. Some discussion of the nature of these components is essential since each behaves differently during processing, and toxicity of raw waste is influenced by the specific wood composition and degradation products.

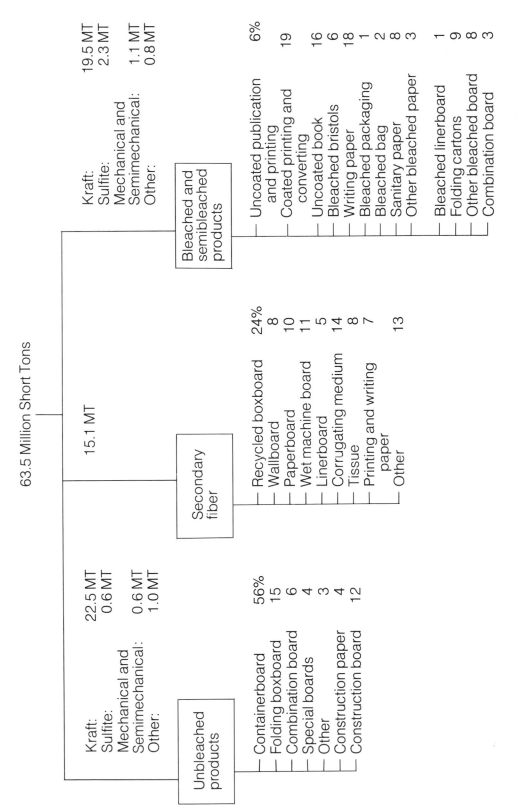

Figure 16.1 Total pulp production in the United States, 1976. (From Bureau of Census, U.S. Department of Commerce. Current Industrial Reports, Series M26A, Pulp, Paper and Board, 1976.)

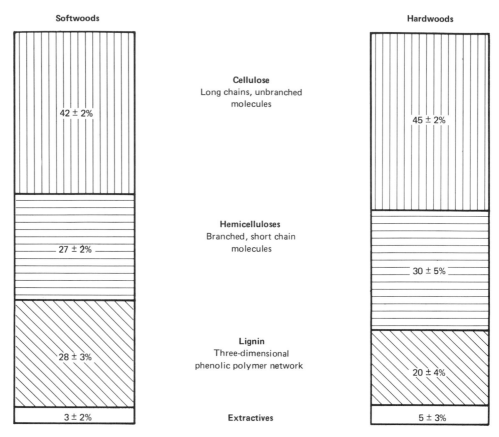

Figure 16.2 Typical composition of softwoods and hardwoods.

1. *Carbohydrates:* These are the major constituents in plant tissue. Cellulose is a linear polymer of glucose with a chain length sufficiently large to be insoluble in water, acids, or alkali at room temperature. Even at temperatures up to about 175°C it is fairly resistant to the action of pulping chemicals. Hemicelluloses also are polymers, but with shorter chain length and a greater degree of branching than cellulose. There are a variety of hemicelluloses which are differentiated by the sugar moieties included in the polymer, the degree of branching, and the types of substitution. In general, this class of polysaccharide is more soluble and less resistant to degradation in pulping and bleaching than cellulose. The degradation of wood polysaccharides that does occur during pulp processing leads mainly to low molecular weight sugars and sugar acids, which, if they enter receiving water, exert an environmental effect measured primarily by the BOD.

2. *Lignin:* The main noncarbohydrate material in plants, lignin is a high molecular weight, three-dimensional polymer with a variety of types of cross-linking bonds. Substances resulting from lignin degradation in pulp and paper processes vary in exact composition and character with the type of process, however, they are generally phenolic in nature and generally somewhat water soluble. If they enter the receiving waters their impact may be measured in terms of BOD, color, and toxicity.

3. *Extractives:* These are low molecular weight compounds of various types which can be removed from wood by water, organic solvents, or pulping solutions. Substances in this category that are of toxicological interest include resin acids, fatty acids, and a variety of terpenes and polyphenolic substances (tannins).

Wood is comprised of cells called fibers. The polysaccharides described above are located almost totally in the fiber walls, while the space between fibers is called the middle lamella and is composed mainly of lignin, which acts as a type of bonding agent to hold the wood in dimensionally stable form. Lignin is also distributed as a matrix in the fiber wall between and around the polysaccharides. Between 25 and 45% of the lignin resides in the cell walls and the remainder in the middle lamella.

The environmental impact of discharges depends on the type of mill process and the extent to which discharges are retained and reused in the mill or treated by external waste treatment systems. Common practices are illustrated in the sections that follow.

16.2. Pulp and Paper Manufacture

The objective of pulping is to separate the wood substance into discrete fibers. Paper mills then reaggregate the fibers into new patterns, sometimes in combination with papermaking chemicals to make a variety of paper products. In some cases, bleaching is done before papermaking to remove colored substances and to make white fiber. Figure 16.1 shows that about equal quantities of unbleached and bleached pulps are generated by the U.S. pulp and paper industry and lists typical types of products as percentages of the parent pulp category.

Depending on the requirements of the paper products, varying amounts of the wood constituents are dissolved during fiber separation steps. The three broad classes of pulping methods are mechanical, chemical and semichemical, and the yields of these are normally in the range of 85–95%, 40–55%, and 50–85%, respectively, based on the original amount of dry wood. One can readily see that high-yield processes are attractive from an environmental point of view, since much of the wood substance is retained in the pulp fibers. The use of these pulps is growing; however, product requirements limit the use of high-yield mechanical pulps to the amounts shown in Figure 16.1.

16.2.1. Mechanical Processes

In the manufacture of mechanical pulps, wood fibers are separated by mechanical action that results in high yield since very little of the wood becomes dissolved during the process. Regardless of the exact form of the equipment, fibers are torn from the wood by the friction generated by a moving surface. A high yield makes mechanical pulps attractive but also limits their use. Most of the original wood substances are retained in the fibers and the residual lignin causes color reversion when exposed to light, so that papers prepared from mechanical pulps do not retain their brightness as long as lower yield pulps. Furthermore, mechanical separation results in greater damage to fibers, so that the paper products are inherently weaker than those obtained by milder chemical treatments. Consequently, these pulps are used alone or mixed with stronger chemical pulps for nonpermanent papers, such as newsprint, catalog, magazine, and tablet papers, and in tissue, wrapping paper, wallpaper, and some paperboard products.

Mechanical pulps often require some brightening to improve the eye appeal of papers and boards. To retain high yields achieved by the mechanical processes, agents such as hydrogen peroxide or hydrosulfite are used since these do not remove wood substances, but alter their optical properties. Consequently, very little pollution loading is associated with bleaching these pulps. Most of the pollutants are released from the wood during the grinding/refining operation and are primarily related to the extractives. Extractive quantity and quality vary with species, but the toxicity of raw, untreated effluents is generally greater with softwoods and resinous species than with hardwoods and nonresinous species.

16.2.2. Chemical Processes

Chemical processes convert wood chips to fibers using one of several chemical solutions to dissolve the lignin and allow fibers to be easily separated from each other: soda pulping uses sodium hydroxide; the sulfite process uses acid bisulfite solutions; and the kraft process uses mixtures of sodium hydroxide and sodium sulfide for pulping.

Figure 16.1 shows that the kraft process dominates the U.S. pulp capacity and much of the following discussion is restricted to that process. Figure 16.3 illustrates schematically the relationship of major pulp streams, aqueous streams, and chemical streams in the process and shows the major sources of aqueous effluents. A large degree of water reuse is practiced within and between the major sections of the mill to minimize the volume of waste streams that enter waste treatment. Process water reuse, omitted from Figure 16.3 for clarity, is a major part of the chemical recovery and waste control strategy of pulp and paper mills. This tends to reduce the volume and loading of raw, untreated, sewered wastes. The response of the waste streams to waste treatment processes is described in Section 16.4.

16.2.2.a. Unbleached Pulp Mill

Logs are debarked and chipped either in the mill vicinity or at remote locations, and wood chips are loaded into batch or continuous digesters with pulping liquor. The temperature is raised to about 170°C by directly adding steam to the digester or by circulating heated pulping liquor, which removes most of the lignin. Then the wood residue is discharged to a blow tank, where shear and impact forces generated by blowing the chips to atmospheric pressure fiberize the pulped chips.

The fibers are then washed nearly free of used pulping chemicals and dissolved wood substances and screened to separate unfiberized wood residue. Clean wash water is added to the last of a series of washing stages and the effluent from each wash stage is used for washing in the preceding stage. In this way 96–98% of the dissolved wood constituents are recovered in the effluent from the first wash stage. This effluent is termed black liquor and is burned for steam and power generation and to recover its inorganic content for reuse in

215

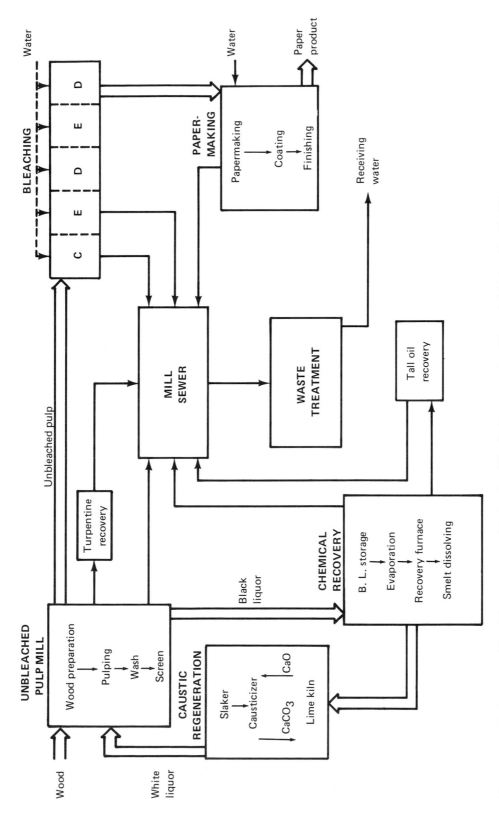

Figure 16.3 Kraft process. Bleaching stages are chlorination (*C*), alkaline extraction (*E*), and chlorine dioxide (*D*).

pulping. Normally almost no effluent enters the raw waste sewer from this part of the process. During nonsteady state periods of operation, spills and overflow occur and mills often use spill containment systems to segregate the spill from the sewer and return liquids to the process.

The pulp lignin content varies depending on the type of products desired. For unbleached products, pulps contain 8–14% lignin (about 33–50% of the original wood lignin) at about 48–55% yield. The pulp is sent to a paper machine after screening and cleaning, and the residual lignin causes typical brown colors associated with boxes, brown paper, shopping bags, and similar unbleached paper and paperboard products. To produce bleached products, pulping is extended to 4–6% lignin content (about 10–20% of the original wood lignin) at 44–46% yield. Further purification by bleaching is described later.

The screen room is more commonly a source of aqueous effluent than the pulping and washing areas. Depending on the design of the mill, effluent volume from this source may range from 0 to about 10,000 gal/ton pulp. Internal modifications are being installed in many mills to minimize effluent from this source. Extractive related materials emitted from this part of the mill can contribute a substantial part of the toxic loading of the total mill.

The process for turpentine recovery may generate small amounts of effluent that contains some toxicity. When wood chips are heated in the initial stages of pulping, the volatile portion of wood extractives evaporates and condenses outside the digester. Small quantities of aqueous condensate containing unrecovered terpenes and volatile sulfur compounds are sewered to waste treatment.

16.2.2.b. Chemical Recovery

One of the reasons for the predominance of the kraft process is the associated chemical recovery system. Black liquor containing dissolved wood substances and used pulping chemicals is concentrated by evaporation and burned. The recovered inorganic chemicals are recycled in the caustic regeneration area to make more pulping liquor.

The major raw waste flow from the recovery area originates from the multiple-effect evaporator, where large volumes of contaminated condensates are generated. A large part of these condensates are reused in various parts of the mill that may need hot water, but often a small part of the stream is sewered. Methyl mercaptan, dimethyl sulfide, dimethyl disulfide, and small amounts of hydrogen sulfide make up most of the toxic load of this stream under normal operating conditions. In addition, when foaming occurs in the evaporators, some resin and fatty acids may also carry over into the condensate and contribute to the toxicity of raw waste.

16.2.2.c. Pulp Bleaching

The objective of pulp bleaching is to produce white or lightly colored pulps and retain strength properties that are characteristic of chemical pulps. The method of bleaching varies depending on the source of the pulp and its intended end use.

Chemical pulps are purified to a higher brightness by lignin-removing bleaching agents. In general, this is accomplished in multiple stages, several of which employ chlorine-containing agents with intermediate alkaline extractions. Chlorination (C) promotes degradation of lignin, and in the process generates lower molecular weight chlorine-substituted phenolic materials. Alkaline extraction (E) neutralizes acids formed during chlorination and dissolves degradation products. Normally bleached yields drop to about 41.5% based on wood compared to 45% unbleached yield. About 80% of that shrinkage occurs in the combined CE stages. Consequently, measured in terms of nearly all pollution parameters, these first two bleaching stages are the major sources of loading in the bleach plant.

The remaining bleach stages remove less material and produce less toxicity. Chlorine dioxide (D) or hypochlorite (H) is used as a polishing step followed by alkaline extraction, a second D stage, and sometimes hydrogen peroxide treatment to finish pulp purification and reach high brightnesses.

The volume of effluent from the bleach plant is directly influenced by the configuration of bleaching sequences. The minimum volume would be achieved by adding wash water on the final bleaching stage and using the effluent as dilution and wash water sequentially in the preceding stages. This full counterflow washing would tend to minimize water and effluent and concentrate dissolved substances in the single effluent from the C stage. However, this approach is limited to special situations because of problems with equipment corrosion and excess bleach chemical consumption. A variety of partial counterflow systems and improved bleach processes can limit effluent volume from the bleach plant to 4000–12000 gal/ton pulp depending on particular mill constraints. Even when effluent volume is minimized, the bleach plant remains the major source in the pulp and paper mill in terms of volume and loading. In contrast to the pulp mill, bleach plant effluents cannot be processed internally by a conventional recovery system. If the effluents were concentrated in the recovery system, the chloride would accumulate in the closed cycles and at some point cause unacceptable corrosion of the process equipment. The alternatives are (a) to sewer the effluents to waste treatment, as presently practiced, or (b) to design alternative bleaching systems or recovery systems at large capital investment. The industry is devoting a great deal of effort to the development of alternative systems.

16.2.2.d. Papermaking

In papermaking, pulp fibers are reaggregated to produce the desired products. Pulp fibers are diluted to a ratio of about 1:200 with water and flow onto a moving, continuous wire to form a sheet. Water passes out of the fiber mat through the wire and is reused. Further dewatering devices decrease the fiber/water ratio to about 1:25. Excess water is evaporated by passing the fiber mat over steam-heated cylinders.

A variety of inorganic and organic additives are added to the water slurry of fibers to improve paper and board properties and these substances can contribute to toxic loading of the pulp and paper mill raw wastes.

The sources of sewered raw wastes shown in Figure 16.3 are normal in a modern well-run mill operating at steady-state conditions. However, spills, leaks, and overflows occur during startup and shutdown and unexpected equipment failures that cause temporary changes in the effluent flows. Consequently, many mills employ spill containment systems that allow for segregation of spills and metering back into the process. At mills lacking such control systems, sizable liquor spills may result temporarily in substantial surge loading on the waste treatment system.

16.2.3. Semichemical Pulping

The term semichemical pulping implies a combination of the features of mechanical and chemical processes. In principle, all processes in the semichemical pulping category involve a mild chemical treatment to soften lignin partially, followed by mechanical refining to complete the defiberization. Yields are intermediate between those produced by mechanical and chemical processes because only a portion of the lignin and polysaccharides dissolves. The mild chemical pretreatment requires less chemical than full chemical processes and results in lower refiner power consumption, decreased fiber damage, and greater strength than mechanical processes. However, these pulps are still generally weaker than full chemical pulps. In general, they are stiff and are used for corrugating medium in shipping cartons. They are not useful in fine papers since yield losses and bleach costs to remove the large amounts of residual lignin are excessive.

Waste pulping liquor washed or pressed out of the pulped chips before refining contains extractive-, lignin-, and carbohydrate-related materials. Usually this liquor is concentrated and burned in an adjacent kraft mill; pollution loading is due mainly to spills occuring during upset conditions. The higher resin acid content of softwoods may cause greater toxic loading in raw waste than found when hardwood species are pulped.

16.2.4. Secondary Fiber

Reclaimed fibers from wastepaper products contribute about 20% of the total fiber supply. This source of fiber is available primarily in metropolitan areas where supplies of newspapers, magazines, wrapping paper, and similar materials from residences and commercial firms are concentrated enough to operate collection systems economically. The main steps in secondary fiber recovery include segregation, repulping, cleaning, refining, and papermaking. Segregation eliminates nonfibrous solids such as plastics, metal, and other extraneous material. This is done at the collection site and by centrifugal devices after repulping. After centrifugal cleaning, large fiber bundles are refined to individual fibers and the stock is formed on paper or board machines similar to those used in papermills previously described.

In general, secondary fibers are used in the manufacture of coarse industrial papers, roofing, felts, sheathing, and related building board products. Substances associated with secondary fiber effluents can originate from the recycled fiber or from manufacturing steps in the production of the secondary product. In the first case, substances are used to prepare the original paper product for its intended use and are inherited by the secondary fiber plant when it receives wastepaper products for recycling. The only substances in this category that have been identified as possible toxicants are PCBs used in the manufacture of carbonless papers. Since these are no longer used, the quantity found in secondary fiber will decline. The main potential toxic materials from secondary fiber processing are detergents used in deinking.

16.3. Toxicity of Raw Pulp and Paper Wastes

It is known that raw, untreated pulp and paper wastes are toxic to aquatic fauna, although by most standards the impact is limited. The majority of studies have been based on acute or lethal bioassay techniques. Acute toxicity to fish is usually expressed in terms of 96-hr LC_{50}—this indicates the effluent concentration in percent by volume (based on undiluted waste) at which 50% of the test fish population survive after a 96-hr exposure to the diluted waste. Some toxic streams in pulp mills may have a 96-hr LC_{50} of 1–10% by volume. Thus, the undiluted stream is toxic and must be diluted to 1–10% of its original concentration to reach the 50% kill level after 96 hr. After dilution by the large volumes of nontoxic effluents, the 96-hr LC_{50} for total, raw mill waste is commonly 25–50% by volume.

An alternative method for comparing toxicity of waste streams and known toxic substances employs toxic units (TU):

$$TU = \frac{\text{Actual concentration of waste or substance}}{\text{96-hr } LC_{50}}$$

This approach has been used by a number of investigators but is not standardized in its use by the pulp and paper industry.

A wide range of substances at various concentrations contribute to toxicity, and this unit provides a convenient method for comparing the characteristics of the range of toxic effluents. One TU can be considered the lethal threshold, i.e., the toxic waste concentration at which 50% of the assay organisms survive. Typically, the least toxic pulp and paper wastes vary from 1 to 5 TU and the most toxic from 30 to 50 TU. Full use of the TU concept will require that 96-hr LC_{50} values and concentrations be known for all waste streams and ultimately all compounds in the wastes. Since that information is only partially available, in the following discussion toxicity is given in terms of 96-hr LC_{50}, and TU when available.

The range of concentrations in pulp and paper effluents is partly a result of the wide range of water usage (Table 16.1) and partly due to nonstable operations

Table 16.1 Typical Water Usage for Pulp and Paper Production

Process	Water (gal/ton pulp)
Hydraulic debarking	500–10,000
Mechanical processes	6,000–12,000
Neutral sulfite semichemical	3,000–15,000
Kraft pulping	10,000–20,000
Sulfite pulping	15,000–25,000
Bleaching	10,000–20,000
Papermaking	5,000–20,000

that cause occasional upsets and spills that enter the sewer. In the past decade the industry has succeeded in reducing total mill effluent volumes from 50,000–70,000 gal/ton pulp to 20,000–30,000 gal/ton by employing new processes and improving existing processes. In many cases these efforts do not reduce the amount of toxic material in the same proportion, so that concentrations may fluctuate. Furthermore, the discharge volumes still remain large.

16.3.1. Wood Preparation Wastes

The concentration and loading of toxic substances in effluents from wood preparation depends largely on the wood species and the amount of water used. Mills with dry debarking processes produce no effluent. Water usage in hydraulic debarkers varies widely from mill to mill (Table 16.1) and extensive reuse can reduce the volume to very low levels, although loading of toxic substances is not necessarily reduced in the same proportion.

The toxicity of wood room wastes is directly dependent on the type of wood extractives. For example, debarking of hardwoods results in effluents with a 96-hr LC-$_{50}$ of 40–50% by volume, while with softwoods it is 1–10% by volume. The high toxicity of softwood wood room effluents is primarily caused by the high resin acid content of the bark. Effluents from debarking of eastern and southern softwoods typically contain 30–50 mg/liter of resin acids and 10–20 mg/liter of fatty acids, terpenes, and terpene-related substances. The corresponding values for less toxic effluents from western softwoods are about 1.5 and 0.5 mg/liter, respectively. The results in Table 16.2 show that substances in the extractives category are among the most toxic measured by 96-hr LC-$_{50}$ and have the greatest impact on mill toxic load as measured by TU. Unsaturated fatty acids and terpene alcohols are much less toxic than the resin acid fraction. In general, the sodium salts of resin acids are about twice as toxic as the parent resin acids, so black liquor and crude tall oil spills can have a serious impact on waste treatment systems that receive the effluent.

16.3.2. Mechanical Pulping Waste

Mechanical pulping is applied to both hardwoods and softwoods, but effluents from the latter are more toxic than those from the former due to the higher resin acid content of softwoods. Typical 96-hr LC-$_{50}$ values for softwood barking effluents range from 4 to 10% by volume.

16.3.3. Kraft Mill Wastes

The toxic character of wastes sewered from kraft mills is significantly different in the pulp mill recovery area than in the bleach plant area. Wastes originating from washing and screening of pulps include unrecovered spent pulping chemicals as well as dimethyl sulfide, dimethyl disulfide, methyl mercaptan, resin acids, and fatty acids. Although these substances are all toxic, their concentrations are reasonably low, and 96-hr LC-$_{50}$ values range from 10 to 100% by volume. About 80% of that toxicity has been attributed to the resin acid fraction and the remainder to the classes of compounds listed above. Lignin-related materials contribute to the toxicity only to a small extent. As discussed

Table 16.2 Toxicity and Toxic Units for Some Identified Substances in Kraft Pulp and Paper Wastes

Compound	96-hr LC_{50}	TU^a
Resin acids		10–30
Abietic	0.7	
Dehydroabietic	1.1	
Isopimaric	0.4	
Palustric	0.5	
Pimaric	0.8	
Sandaracopimaric	—	
Chlorinated resin acids		1–5
Monochlorodehydroabietic acid	0.6	
Dichlorodehydrabietic acid	0.6	
Unsaturated fatty acids		1–10
Oleic	<9	
Linoleic	<9	
Linolenic	<9	
Palmitoleic	<9	
Unsaturated fatty acid derivatives		5–20
Epoxystearic acid	1.5	
Dichlorostearic acid	1.5	
Dipertene alcohols		1–5
Pimarol	0.3	
Isopimarol	0.3	
Abienol	1.8	
Dehydroabietol	0.8	
Chlorinated phenolics		10–20
Trichloroguaiacol	0.72	
Tetrachloroguaiacol	0.32	
Volatiles		5–10
Hydrogen sulfide	0.3–0.7	
Methyl mercaptan	0.5–0.9	
Sodium sulfide	1.0–1.8	
Sodium hydroxide	10–27	
Sodium carbonate	33–58	
Chlorinated catecols		10–20
Tetrachlorocatecol	0.8	
Dichlorocatecol	2.9	

Source: 96-hr LC_{50} data from Leach, J. M., Thakore, A. N. The Isolation of the Toxic Constituents of Kraft Pulp Mill Effluents. CPAR Rep. 11–4. Canadian Forest Service, Ottawa, Ontario, 1974.

^{a}Ranges in concentration lead directly to ranges in TU.

earlier, efficient recovery of wood solids is a primary feature of kraft mills; despite this, the wash and screen areas are generally the source of the largest volume of waste to the raw waste, pulp mill sewer.

Evaporator condensates contain volatile sulfur compounds and terpenes mentioned earlier. The extent of toxic load from this source depends on the volume of condensate sewered and the efficiency of steam stripping systems which are sometimes used to concentrate and burn volatile substances.

Effluents from crude tall oil recovery are highly acidic and toxic, however, since they are low in volume, their contribution to total mill toxic load is negligible.

Bleach plant effluents are a major source of toxicity in the raw waste since all material generated in the bleach plant is sewered and has some inherent toxicity. The largest amount of organic material is removed in the C and first E stage, while remaining bleach stages mainly decolorize (brighten) the pulp. Consequently, the first E stage effluent is commonly the most toxic in the bleach plant, followed by C stage and the final bleaching stages.

Toxic substances identified in bleach effluents include trichloro- and tetrachloroguaiacol and dichloro- and tetrachlorocatechol, all produced from chlorination of lignin. In addition, mono- and dichlorodehydroabietic acid, epoxy stearic acid, and dichlorostearic acid are formed from parent resin and fatty acids that are not washed from the pulp before bleaching. The concentrations of these compounds range from 0.25 to about 2 mg/liter, which, combined with the 96-hr LC-$_{50}$, yields the range of toxic units shown in Table 16.2. These substances are considered to account for 50–80% of the total raw bleach plant toxicity load. The remainder of the load is contributed by small amounts of terpenes and terpene alcohols and other unidentified substances.

In kraft mills the approximate contribution to total raw waste toxicity is 40% from E_1 filtrate, 30% from pulp mill recovery–related operations, 15% from C stage filtrate, 5% from other bleach stages, and 10% from paper mill and minor sources.

16.3.4. Sulfite Mill Wastes

In general, sulfite mill wastes are considered less toxic than kraft mill wastes because greater degradation of toxic substances takes place during sulfite pulping. Furthermore, the resinous softwood species with high concentrations of resin acids are not pulped by the sulfite process. The 96-hr LC-$_{50}$ values typically range from 8 to 60% by volume depending on the particular mill design and pulping chemicals. Phenolic compounds and resin acids each contribute about 25% of the total toxicity and the source of the remainder has not yet been determined.

16.3.5. Secondary Fiber

The major source of toxicity associated with secondary fiber processes appears to be detergents that aid in deinking the waste paper. Typical 96-hr LC-$_{50}$ values range from about 10 to 40% by volume. There are probably a number of unidentified substances in effluents that originate from the waste source and more characterization needs to be done.

16.3.6. Papermaking

A variety of additives are employed in papermaking, some of which add somewhat to total mill toxicity. The types of additives used are extremely variable depending on the paper product and particular mill problems. The classes of substances include slimicides, scale corrosion inhibitors, pitch control agents, and defoamers to control those problems in the water system. These materials disperse between pulp and water but are primarily intended to be retained in the paper machine area by remaining dissolved in the water. Any water that is sewered will carry dissolved additives.

On the other hand, dyestuffs, flocculating agents, sizing agents, and various coatings are used to modify the character of the paper product, and every effort is made to retain them on the sheet. However, small amounts of these materials can enter the water system and eventually are sewered. As mentioned earlier, the contribution of these materials to total toxic loading of the mill probably does not exceed 5–10%.

16.3.7. Toxicity Material Balance

The extent to which toxicities of separate waste streams are additive varies with the sources. For example, when the toxicity of bleaching wastes in fish is expressed as TU, the toxicities are additive. This means that toxic loading (toxicity × volume) may be calculated for the total raw bleach effluent from information about the separate waste streams originating in the bleach plant.

However, material balances are less successful when applied to the total mill, and particularly those wastes associated with the pulp mill cause difficulties. Within normal biological limits, small changes in pH have a large synergistic effect on the toxicity of resin acids in fish. For example, solutions of resin acids are much more toxic when adjusted to pH 6.6 than at pH 7.5. Consequently, pH adjustments that occur in the total mill sewer after mixing of various wastes could lead to lower toxicity than expected from analyses of the various pulp mill effluents. Since the flow and pH of mill wastes is variable, pH monitoring and control by the addition of appropriate chemicals would be necessary to provide a predictable reduction in toxicity.

Success in accounting for total mill toxicity also depends on the assay organism. In some cases lower food chain members, such as phytoplankton, respond to pulp and paper wastes such that toxic effects of various waste sources are additive and total raw sewer toxicity can be calculated from the various input streams.

Table 16.3 summarizes in a semiquantitative fashion the contribution of each class of toxic compounds. Clearly, substances included in the extractives category and chlorinated phenolics contained in bleach plant effluents contribute to the major toxicity of total raw pulp and paper mill effluent. A wide range of substances contribute variable but smaller amounts of toxicity. One might expect that the diversity in types of toxic materials may lead to a variable response in waste treatment systems, which is the subject of the following section.

16.4. Response to Waste Treatment Processes

Waste treatment systems are in widespread use in the pulp and paper industry. These were developed originally for BOD reduction and suspended solids removal, but in many cases are effective in reducing the toxicity of pulp and paper mill effluents. The systems can be classified as biological and physicochemical processes.

Table 16.3 Toxic Compounds in Pulp and Paper Effluents

Class of compounds	Toxic contribution		
	Major	Intermediate	Minor
Resin acids	KSMD	—	—
Chlorinated resin acids	CE	—	—
Fatty acids	—	K	—
Fatty acid derivatives	—	CE	—
Lignin related phenols	—	S	M
Chlorinated phenols	K	S	—
Papermill additives	—	KSM	—
Volatile substances	—	—	KS

Note: K, kraft; S, sulfite; R, recycle; M, mechanical; D, debarking; P, papermaking; E, E filtrate; C, C filtrate.

16.4.1. Biological Processes

Biological processes used by the pulp and paper industry include aerated lagoons, normally with about 5-day retention, and single- or two-stage air- or oxygen-driven activated sludge systems with 8–16 hr retention. Rotating biological disc treatments have not traditionally been used by the industry but are receiving more attention now because of their low maintenance and power requirements and their ability to absorb toxic shock loadings that occur when upset conditions in the mill cause pulp mill liquor and condensate spills to be sewered.

In general, aerated lagoons with normal retention times successfully remove a large part of the toxicity from effluents originating in mechanical and unbleached and bleached chemical processes. Substances in the resin and fatty acid categories are normally removed with 90% or greater efficiency except when liquor spills impose shock loads on the waste treatment system. Chlorinated resin and fatty acids and phenolics originating in the bleach plant are more resistant to biological reduction. This is reflected in the more variable performance of aerated lagoons on bleached effluents and the fact that some treated effluents contain small amounts of chlorinated substances. These quantities are detectable, but are normally in the range reported for many municipal drinking waters (2–150 ppb).

The performance of activated sludge systems has been less consistent than that of aerated lagoons. These difficulties are related to at least two problems: First, in some installations sludges do not settle and thus cannot be recycled. The system behaves as a flow-through reactor with inadequate retention time. Decreased system temperature improves settling and performance. Second, activated sludge systems do not easily handle toxic shock loadings caused by liquor spills. The performance can be improved substantially by installation of scum removal or foam fractionation systems ahead of the activated sludge plant. These physicochemical systems are described in the next section.

In unbleached mills, both aerated lagoons and activated sludge systems remove more than 98% of the toxicity. In bleached mills these systems remove about 90% of the toxicity. Rotating biological discs have given equivalent or better performance in testing at several mill sites.

16.4.2. Physicochemical Processes

Adjustment of waste pH, primary clarification, lime precipitation, foam fractionation, activated carbon treatment, ultrafiltration, and reverse osmosis are all processes that are in use or have been tested alone or in combination with biological systems for BOD, suspended solids, color, and more recently toxicity removal. Primary clarification by itself has little or no effect on raw waste toxicity, indicating that toxic materials are not associated with suspended solids. Surge equalization also is not effective by itself, but provides a way to collect large-volume surges resulting from unexpected liquor spills. Metering to the sewer from surge containment allows efficient toxic removal by the waste treatment system. Foam fractionation tends to reduce toxicity by concentration of toxic materials in a small quantity of foam at the surface of the waste; it provides another approach to protect biological processes from surges of toxic materials. The performance of activated sludge systems has been improved substantially by installing surge equalization and/or foam fractionation ahead of the activated sludge system.

Lime and alum precipitation is very efficient at removing substances in the resin and fatty acid categories and toxicants generated in the bleach plant. Activated carbon by itself can totally detoxify pulp and paper wastes and in combination with alum and polyelectrolyte treatments can reduce BOD and color loadings. In laboratory and pilot plant units reverse osmosis has been used to totally eliminate resin and fatty acid constituents of waste streams and a large proportion of the bleach effluents. Ultrafiltration systems are less efficient. Because of their high capital and operating costs, these systems are more generally applicable for polishing treatment to remove residual quantities of pollutants.

Lime precipitation installed as a color removal unit totally eliminated toxicity of unbleached waste, and alum treatment in combination with activated sludge removed over 98% of the toxicity. A reverse osmosis installation efficiently removed toxicity from the waste of a neutral sulfite semichemical mill. Ultrafiltration pilot plants located at the mill site were ineffective at treating bleach effluents of toxicity.

Pulp and paper processing, like any manufacturing operation, has potential for emitting substances deleterious to the environment. A large effort has been expended to identify and to quantify potentially toxic substances, and it is clear that well-designed and controlled processes coupled with maximum use of internal recovery and recycling of process streams can limit the quantity of potentially toxic substances in raw, untreated waste streams. With secondary waste treatment systems, the amount of these substances entering receiving waters can be maintained at very low levels.

Suggested Reading

Easty, D. B., Borchardt, L. G., Wabers, B. A. Wood derived toxic compounds: Removal from mill effluents by waste treatment processes. TAPPI. 61 (10):57, 1978.

Leopold, B. Pulp mill of the future—Environmental and raw material considerations. American Chemical Society Symposium Series 49, 1977, p. 239.

MacDonald, R. G. (Ed.). Papermaking and Paperboard Making. New York: McGraw-Hill, 1970.

Rydholm, S. A. Pulping Processes. New York: Interscience, 1965.

Sarkanen, K. V., Ludwig, C. H. (Eds.). Lignins: Occurrence, Formation, Structure and Reaction. New York: Wiley Interscience, 1971.

Walden, C. C., Howard, T. E., Mueller, J. C. Toxicity of pulp and paper mill effluents. Can. Pulp Paper Assoc. Annu. Meeting (Montreal) 62B:217, 1976.

Lenore S. Clesceri

17

Case History:
PCBs in the Hudson River

17.1. Introduction

In many respects the case of polychlorinated biphenyls (PCBs) in the Hudson River is a classic one with regard to the impact of uncontrolled technology on natural waters. The Hudson River, which originates in the Adirondack Mountains in New York, has been a significant commercial and sport fishery for years, but today commercial fishing has dropped by 60% and sport fishing is completely restricted along certain sections of the river due to the high levels of PCBs found in the tissues of fish. The Hudson is a drinking water reservoir for many riverside communities. PCB levels exceeding federal guidelines for drinking water standards are found in certain areas as a result of the discharge of PCBs into the river over the past 25 years.

Although the most notorious, the Hudson River is certainly not the only body of water suffering from PCB pollution. The temporary tolerance limit for fish tissue of 5 ppm placed by the Food and Drug Administration (FDA) is exceeded by the larger trout and salmon in the Great Lakes, catfish and carp in the Ohio River, and trout in New York's Finger Lakes, to mention a few. PCBs have been found in marine animals as well as terrestrial animals throughout the world. This ubiquity as well as the toxic and persistent nature of PCBs is the basis for the concern over their presence in the environment.

17.2. Characteristics of PCBs

Early investigations into chlorinated hydrocarbon pesticides found in the environment revealed high levels of chlorinated hydrocarbons in the tissues of animals dependent on aquatic environments. Many investigators also reported the presence of organochlorine compounds not identifiable as the chlorinated pesticides or their metabolites. In 1966, Jensen, while studying chlorinated hydrocarbons in fish and wildlife, identified these unknown compounds as polychlorinated biphenyls, or PCBs, and directed attention to them as a possible environmental hazard.

Later chemical studies of these compounds revealed that they are a class of compounds having the generalized structure shown in Figure 17.1, in which an *x* denotes the positions that may be occupied by either chlorine or hydrogen atoms. There are a total of 210 combinations possible, but probably only 102 actually exist, if one assumes a range of five to eight chlorine atoms per molecule and the number in each ring differing by no more than one.

The similarity to the chlorinated hydrocarbon pesticides (Figure 17.1) in structure and, therefore, properties accounts for the confusion between PCBs and pesticide residues in studies of environmental samples before 1966. Analyses of samples of fat and eggs of birds, both before and after PCB separation, showed ranges of actual pesticide levels from 0 to 100%. The magnitude of the PCB component varies according to the trophic level studied and the distance from urban to industrial areas.

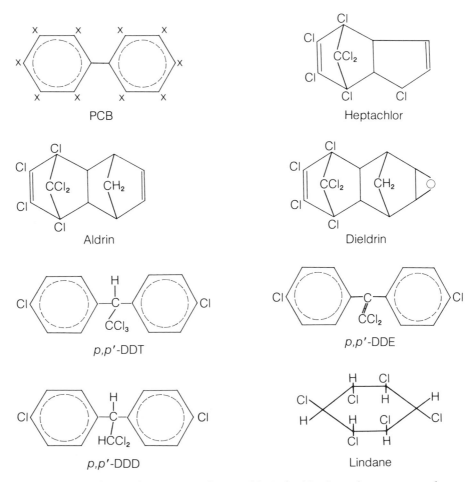

Figure 17.1 Chemical structures of some chlorinated hydrocarbon compounds.

The chemical properties that make PCBs valuable industrial materials are their excellent thermal stability, strong resistance to attack by acids and bases, and general chemical inertness. Among the most important physical properties of the PCBs are their low vapor pressures, extremely low water solubilities, and high dielectric constants. They are miscible with most organic solvents and compatible with many types of polymers. Their physical state ranges from liquid to resinous to crystalline as the degree of chlorination increases.

Because of their many forms and properties, PCBs have been used in a multitude of diverse applications, e.g., in the manufacture of capacitors, as plasticizers, and in hydraulic fluids, adhesives, and printing products, to list only a few of their many uses.

The occupational hazards to workers in industries manufacturing or using PCBs have been known for years. Repeated or prolonged contact can cause chloracne. Systemic poisoning can induce jaundice, nausea, vomiting, weight loss, edema, abdominal pain, and liver lesions.

One of the most spectacular examples of acute PCB poisoning occurred in Japan and has come to be known as the Yusho (rice oil disease) incident. In 1968 this disease, which affected more than 1000 Japanese, was traced to PCB contamination of rice oil during manufacture. Levels of 2000 ppm PCBs in the rice oil produced disease symptoms including eye discharges, severe acne, ulcers of the uterus, and darkening of the skin. Miscarriages and stillbirths were produced and surviving infants suffered from abnormal pigmentation as the result of transplacental transmission of PCBs.

Acute toxicity of PCBs to both vertebrates and invertebrates, however, is relatively low (lower than that of DDT by up to two orders of magnitude) and inversely proportional to the degree of chlorination. A range of LD_{50} values from 250 to 1300 mg/kg has been found in the literature for rats in feeding experiments with the 1254 isomer. The lower vertebrates are much less susceptible than mammals to PCB poisoning.

The problem of chronic toxicity by PCBs is a much more serious problem than that of acute toxicity. The environmental PCB hazard is one of long-term, low-level poisoning. The wide dispersal of these persistent compounds poses a serious threat to the environment.

Chronic PCB toxicity to chickens was found quite accidentally and reported in 1970. Gustafson at the University of Missouri observed that chickens were dying after being placed in a feeding house that had been freshly painted with an epoxy paint. The investigation that followed revealed that the toxic factor was the PCB, Aroclor 1242, which was used as a binder in the paint.

The pathology of chronic effects of sublethal dosing of PCBs is different in mammals than in birds. The only site of action in mammals seems to be the liver tissue, whereas in birds detrimental effects are seen in the pericardial sac, the kidneys, and the spleen, as well as the liver.

PCBs have been found to interfere with two pathways that affect the shell thickness of birds' eggs. Since they are powerful inducers of steroid hydroxylases, they are instrumental in lowering the level of the steroid hormone estrogen, which in turn regulates the calcium reserve in birds. PCBs also reduce the availability of calcium by interfering with the carbonic anhydrase system, which controls the flow of calcium in the blood stream to the oviduct.

The toxicity of PCBs to aquatic organisms is more subtle due to the limited solubility of these compounds. In natural systems the complexity is compounded by intricate food web dynamics.

Recent reports of various metabolic effects produced by PCBs in different organisms range from the promotion of dioxin toxicity and vitamin A deficiency to an antitumor effect of Aroclor 1254. The toxicology of PCBs on the cellular level is complex and remains to be clearly defined. A summary of the various effects produced by PCB exposure can be found in the EPA Criteria Document for PCBs and in a report published by the United States Department of Health, Education and Welfare, cited in "Suggested Reading."

17.3. Sources of PCB Pollution

PCBs have been manufactured in the United States since 1929 exclusively by the Monsanto Company. It is estimated that Monsanto has produced about 400,000 tons of PCBs during the period 1948–1973. The company produces about one-half of the world's PCBs. They have also been made in Japan, Great Britain, France, Germany, Italy, Spain, Czechoslovakia, and the Soviet Union. In 1971, Monsanto voluntarily announced that it would restrict sales to "closed cycle" systems in transformers and capacitors.

PCB usage by the General Electric capacitor manufacturing facilities at Hudson Falls and Fort Edward on the Hudson River in upstate New York (Figure 17.2) has been both extensive and long-standing. Between 1966 and 1974 these facilities purchased 78×10^6 lb of PCBs, representing about 15% of U.S. domestic sales of PCBs during that time. PCBs had been used as the primary capacitor dielectric for the past 25 years at General Electric. Although the use of PCBs in capacitors and transformers does not result in environmental damage (except when these items become corroded or broken when discarded), the process of manufacturing them results in large volumes of PCB-laden aqueous discharges.

Although elevated levels of PCBs were first observed in Hudson River biota in 1969, their importance was not widely recognized. In 1971, the New York Bureau of Fisheries learned that striped bass from the Hudson River had 11 ppm PCBs in their eggs and 4 ppm in their flesh. In December 1972, General Electric applied to the EPA for a discharge permit stating that its two plants were discharging an average of 30 lb/day of chlorinated hydrocarbons. The permit became effective on January 31, 1975.

Until late summer 1973, the PCB discharge was retained by the old Fort Edward Dam. The state granted permission for removal of the dam in October 1973. This mobilized massive volumes of sediment that had collected behind the dam. Later it was found that they were heavily contaminated with PCBs. (To compound the problem, in April 1976, a record flood in that region washed more of the PCB-laden sediment downstream.) It was in 1975 that extensive sampling of sediment and fish from the Hudson River finally and clearly implicated General Electric's capacitor manufacturing facility as the point source for the major quantity of PCBs in the Hudson.

Acting on this information, the New York Department of Environmental Conservation brought charges against the General Electric Company for polluting the Hudson River with the toxic PCBs. In September 1976, a settlement

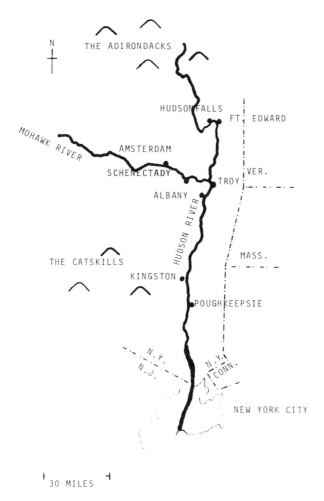

Figure 17.2 Hudson River Basin.

between the two parties was finalized. The hearings that resulted in the final settlement found both parties guilty: corporate abuse on the part of General Electric and regulatory failure on the part of New York State. General Electric was required to reduce PCB discharges to 1 lb/day beginning September 1976, to 1 g/day by May 1977, and to cease using PCBs by July 1977. Both General Electric and the State of New York have shared in the costs of extensive studies since then to monitor the presence and levels of PCBs in the Hudson, to investigate the need for remedial action, and to implement such action if necessary.

Although a point source was clearly shown to be the major contributor to the PCB problem in the Hudson, several other sources have also been identified. PCBs enter the environment from municipal wastes, through leaching from dumps and landfills, and from the burning of refuse. They are then transported via waterways and the atmosphere. Deposition from the atmosphere occurs as dryfall, rain, and snow.

17.4. Persistence and Effect in River Biota

The persistence of PCBs in the aquatic environment results partially from the fact that they are readily adsorbed onto particulate matter that rapidly settles out of the water column to become part of the sediment of the river. There, oxygen is a limiting factor for most microorganisms and the process of microbial biodegradation is severely curtailed. Many microorganisms have the ability to metabolize PCBs, but the conditions for growth must be suitable.

The result of this settling is the accumulation of PCBs in benthic organisms in proportion to their lipid content. PCB levels in macroinvertebrates that attach to an artificial surface were studied along the length of the Hudson River. Mostly midge larvae (Chironomidae) were collected, with the next most abundant organism being oligocheate worms. During the sampling period, June 1976 to August 1977, the data that were collected showed consistently higher PCB concentrations in the organisms from the Upper Hudson below Fort Edward than anywhere else in the river. PCB levels in the fish and sediments were also highest in this region. The macroinvertebrates that were collected in the Hudson River Estuary (below Troy) contained levels well above background, but less than in the Upper Hudson.

PCBs have been found to accumulate in phytoplankton and macrophytes as well. They have been shown to reduce the growth of some aquatic vegetation at levels less than 5 ppm. A marine diatom (*Cylindrica closeterium*) has been shown to accumulate Aroclor 1242 to a cell concentration 1100 times that of ambient levels. RNA synthesis was sharply inhibited over a period of 2 weeks during the long-term PCB exposure. This delay in growth of microorganisms was also observed for many species of marine bacteria.

Fish that feed upon these lower organisms subsequently accumulate PCBs in their tissues. The 5 ppm tolerance limit for edible fish set by the FDA is exceeded by all species sampled below Hudson Falls except for American shad, large sturgeon, and goldfish. The shellfish fishery in the Hudson River Estuary is completely closed, representing a multimillion dollar loss to the New York fishing industry.

17.5. PCB Disposal on Land

It is estimated that about 50% of the PCBs in the Hudson River Basin are presently in landfills and dredge spoil sites in the Upper Hudson Basin. About one-quarter of this amount is associated with dredge spoil sites that are immediately adjacent to the river. They contain the sediments dredged out of the river by the state of New York for normal maintenance of the river for transportation. Measurable quantities of PCBs leach or erode away from these sites. Although PCBs are only slightly volatile, these sites also emit PCBs to the air.

Several different species of terrestrial plants were examined in the areas adjacent to the disposal sites. Concentrations of PCBs on or in these plant tissues vary widely from 2770 ppm (dry weight) to less than detection. The plants with the highest levels are goldenrod, aster, and grasses. Taller plants that have sticky surfaces, such as staghorn sumac, also have high levels. The dust associated with these plants is the major source of the PCBs rather than systemic transport. Effects of PCBs on terrestrial plants is minimal. Even at high concentrations, no abnormalities or signs of chlorosis appear. However, the grazing of animals on these PCB-laden plants poses a serious threat to the environment.

17.6. Distribution of PCBs in the Hudson River

Since 1974 more than 1300 sediment samples have been taken from the length of the Hudson River for PCB analysis. Sampling density was greatest in the section of the river just south of Fort Edward.

It was found that sandy and gravelly sediments are low in PCB content, whereas sediments that have a high organic content typically have PCB concentrations greater than 50 ppm and seldom less than 25 ppm in the Upper Hudson. In addition, fine-textured sediments have higher levels than coarse-textured sediments. The surface sediment ranges in PCB concentration from 100 ppm at Fort Edward, to 60 ppm at Albany, to 6 ppm at New York Harbor. At a depth of 30 cm into Upper Hudson sediment cores, a higher concentration band is seen, (Table 17.1). The eight dams between Fort Edward and Troy provide for

Table 17.1 PCB Profiles in Sediment Cores

Depth in core (cm)	Mean PCB concentration (ppm)	No. of samples
Old Fort Edward Dam to Thompson Island Dam (5-mile stretch)		
0–8	93	87
8–16	112	57
16–30	120	103
30–46	133	63
46–70	75	27
70–91	69	9
91	5	7
Thompson Island Dam to Northumberland Dam (5-mile stretch)		
0–8	102	47
8–16	153	23
16–30	130	51
30–46	48	22
46–70	6	11
70–91	3	1
Northumberland Dam to Federal Lock at Troy (30-mile stretch)		
0–8	22	48
8–16	47	25
16–30	49	62
30–46	14	22
46–70	5	6
70–91	3	1
New York City Harbor		
0–10	4	
10–20	6	
20–30	7	
30–60	6	
60–80	Not detectable	

Source: Adapted from New York State Department of Environmental Conservation Technical Paper 51, 1978.

a change in elevation of 36 m. Sediment collects behind these dams. When the Fort Edward dam was removed, massive deposition of PCBs along the river followed. The covering of that band with newly deposited sediments then began as the river bottom was subsequently disturbed by high flows and boat traffic, causing resuspension and redeposition of river sediment. In general, higher concentrations of PCBs are found in the silty deposits near the banks of the river than in the center, higher velocity area of the river. These bank sediments are less subject to resuspension, therefore the PCBs tend to accumulate there.

Surveys of waters for PCBs have been going on since 1970 and, except for water from the Hudson and Mohawk Rivers (a tributary of the Hudson River), PCBs are undetectable in both ground water and surface water. PCBs are undetectable north of the General Electric facilities, but were commonly detected at other sites in the Upper Hudson. Only limited data exist on PCB concentrations in the Lower Hudson, and these are from the Poughkeepsie and Troy area. Values ranging between 0.1 and 1.1 ppb have been measured.

The source of PCBs in biota is predominantly through the detrital food chain. Bottom-feeding organisms serve to transport these compounds out of the sediment environment, resulting in their wide distribution in other aquatic life. The total amount of PCBs existing in the biota of the Hudson River is very small (about 0.1%) compared to the large quantities in sediments and land disposal sites (Table 17.2).

Although very difficult to estimate, it is calculated that the Upper Hudson Basin delivered 3 tons of PCBs to the Lower Basin in 1977. It is felt that much of this comes from certain highly contaminated areas in the Upper Hudson, especially those sedimentary deposits residing above the site of the removed dam at Fort Edward. Much of this has already moved downstream, resulting in other highly contaminated areas in the Upper Basin.

17.7. Remedial Measures

The dilemma of what to do now that the problem has been defined is of immediate concern since most remedial actions become less effective as the PCBs become more dispersed. One year has been spent in evaluating the available control technology for the PCB problem in the Hudson River (Table 17.3).

The action that New York State will probably take will be partial dredging, although total dredging of the Upper Hudson Basin has also been proposed. The cost to the environment and the taxpayer will be high and the problem may simply be moved to another place as a solid waste problem, since the dredged

Table 17.2 Distribution of PCBs in the Hudson River Basin

Site	PCBs (tons)
Upper Hudson	440
Lower Hudson	220
Landfills and dumps	530
Dredge spoils	160
River biota	0.1–1

Source: Adapted from New York State Department of Environmental Conservation Technical Paper 51, 1978.

Table 17.3   Control Technology for PCB-Contaminated Sediments

Method	Status of development
Removal	
Dredging	Common practice, but technology for disposal of the dredged spoils has only been tested on a pilot scale for 1 year
Activated carbon sorption	Laboratory tested
Bioharvesting of fish	Conceptual
Sorption by oil-soaked mats	Conceptual
Destruction in place	
Degradation by UV ozonation	Pilot scale development for closed systems
Biodegradation by microorganisms	Laboratory tested (rapid development)
Chemical treatment	Conceptual
Fixing in place	
Sorption	Laboratory tested
Erosion control of river bottom	Conceptual
Chemical fixation	Conceptual
Physical covering of sediments	Conceptual

Source: Adapted from New York State Department of Environmental Conservation Technical Paper 51, 1978.

sediments will have to be placed somewhere or disposed of in some way. The proposed method of disposal is placement on a "contained" dredge spoils site, which means that the components of the dredged sediment (PCBs, etc.) as well as the degradation products from these components must be retained at the selected site by means of liners and covers. Both the location of these sites and the method of containment are two very serious problems that have yet to be resolved before such action can be taken.

Suggested Reading

Environmental Protection Agency. Scientific and Technical Assessment Report on Polychlorinated Biphenyls. EPA-600/6-75-00X. Washington, D.C., 1975.

Environmental Protection Agency. Review of PCB Levels in the Environment. EPA-560/7-76-001, Washington, D.C., 1976.

Finklea, J. F., Preister, L.E., Creason, J.D., et al. Polychlorinated biphenyl residues in human plasma expose a major pollution problem. Am. J. Public Health 62:645, 1972.

Gustafson, C. G. PCBs—Prevalent and persistent. Environ. Sci. Technol. 4:814–819, 1970.

Hetling, L., Horn, E., Tofflemire, J. Summary of Hudson River PCB Study Results. Technical Paper 51, Albany: New York State Department of Environmental Conservation, 1978.

Jensen, S. Report of a new chemical hazard. New Sci. 32:612, 1966.

Nisbet, I. C. T. Criteria Document for PCBs. EPA 440/76-021. Washington, D.C.: Environmental Protection Agency, 1976.

Riseborough, R.W., Rieche, P., Peakall, D. B. et al. Polychlorinated biphenyls in the ecosystem. Nature 220:1098–1102, 1968.

Subcommittee on the Health Effects of PCBs and PBBs. Final report. Washington, D.C.:Department of Health, Education and Welfare, 1976.

G. M. Rand
G. T. Barthalmus

18

Case History:
Pollution of the Rhine River

18.1. Introduction

Our industrially intense society and increasing population density have created some seemingly insurmountable pollution problems in many river systems of the world. In many instances appropriate measures have been taken toward pollution abatement through conventional and advanced water treatment practices. However, in Europe one major water pollution problem that has not been readily resolved is that in the Rhine River. For hundreds of years the Rhine has been a navigation channel for commerce, a source of power, a water supply, and an international sump for wastes. Over the past 10 years the quality and condition of the Rhine River water have deteriorated in spite of extensive expenditure on treatment plants and antipollution facilities. This lack of control stems from the magnitude and complexity of the pollution problems. For example, an estimated 20×10^6 tons of waste currently enters the Rhine each year from a wide spectrum of industries and municipalities. The bulk of this waste is salts, chemicals, metals, oils, pesticides, and thermal discharges from industry and power stations.

In 1950 concern over this pollution led to the establishment of the International Commission for the Protection of the Rhine River Against Pollution. In 1963 the commission was officially ratified by its five member countries (France, Germany, Switzerland, the Netherlands, and Luxembourg). The commission has made some technical recommendations to its member governments on the abatement steps necessary to restore the quality of the river. However, the commission has no authority to direct and enforce all of these actions. To complicate matters, the member nations do not always agree on the abatement steps and on the budgeting of economic priorities for the specific objectives. The commission therefore has no real power and consequently serves as an advisory board to promulgate new research.

The prospects of a clean Rhine in the future are mixed because the solution to the problem is not only scientific but political. On the scientific level there is little systematic sampling data on either the actual state of the river or on the likely effects of abatement measures. On the other hand, the lack of success may also be attributed to an absence of enforcement powers on the part of the relevant authorities.

A discussion of all the environmental issues, their effects, and the political ramifications associated with them would fill half of this text. Therefore, only some background information and a few of the major problems and possible solutions will be considered here.

18.2. Geography

The Rhine River is the most important inland waterway in Central and Western Europe although it accounts for only 0.2% of the river water in the world. The river is over 1230 km (760 miles) in total length and on its journey to the North Sea it borders on or passes through Switzerland, Luxembourg, Austria, West Germany, France, and the Netherlands (Figure 18.1).

As a result of the influences produced by snow melt in Switzerland, the river flow remains fairly constant. Low flow is one-half the median flow and usually occurs for 2 days in an average year. However, during a dry year the low flow may continue for 80 days or more. The critical periods of low flow compound the pollution problems and occur in or around October, when the snow melt has terminated.

Figure 18.1   Rhine River Basin. (From Tinker, J. Europe's majestic sewer. This first appeared in New Scientist, London, the weekly review of science and technology. Volume 56, page 194, 1972.)

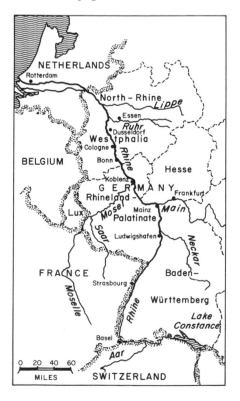

For the first 120 km of the river below Lake Constance, the area is relatively undeveloped by industry except for a few dams and hydroelectric plants; this contrasts greatly with the lower section of the Rhine. From Basel, Switzerland, to its mouth, the Rhine has heavy concentrations of industry. Below this point for the first 50 km only a small amount of water remains in the river bed because the major portion of the flow has been diverted into France to serve the Alsatian Canal.

After the river leaves the French–German border and enters Germany, it receives major augmentation from the Main, Mosel, and Ruhr Rivers. These bodies of water tend to freshen the Rhine somewhat despite the intense industrialization and dense population in the northern portion of the river basin.

18.3. Sources of Pollution

The Rhine River serves a population of over 40×10^6 people, who require its water for drinking, washing, fishing, shipping, and irrigating. The river is of equal importance to the factories located on its banks, which use the water for various industrial processes.

The river receives an influx of sewage and other domestic waste from municipalities that vary considerably in composition and strength from town to town and from country to country. The sewage is usually turbid and very dilute and contains mineral and organic matter in many forms; it consists of soap and detergent, food material, urine, fecal matter, and traces of metals in addition to living matter, especially bacteria, viruses, and protozoa. In addition, the river is a natural disposal area for industrial trade wastes whose effluents are as varied and complex as the products produced. Industrial discharges come from the iron and steel, coal mining, chemical, oil, cellulose and paper, and food industries.

The shipping on the Rhine and its tributaries constitutes another source of pollution, which consists of both human sewage and other wastes, the most important of which is oil. Finally, agriculture contributes animal wastes, pesticides, and fertilizers, which enter the waterway as runoff from the fields.

The Rhine, like other rivers, also suffers from pollution as a result of natural strains not associated with the activities of man. Pollution from this source is usually small and in the form of solid matter that drains into the river following heavy rainfall or floods. It may consist of organic, mineral, and suspended matter, and lead to problems in turbidity, color, odor, acidity, and alkalinity.

The intensity and complexity of the pollution problem dictate the need for immediate improvement or else vast stretches of water will be completely deoxygenated.

18.4. Causes and Effects of Pollution

18.4.1. Inorganic or Mineral Pollution

River waters may contain trace or larger amounts of water-soluble inorganic substances. The presence and relative abundance of these constituents in water is influenced by several factors, including surface runoff, atmospheric fallout (snow and rainfall), effluents, and biological and chemical processes in the water itself. Many of these dissolved materials are essential to the life processes of aquatic organisms.

A general term used to describe the concentration of these dissolved materials in water is total dissolved solids (salts). The total dissolved solids in natural waters and discharges may include chlorides, sulphates, nitrates, bicarbonates, phosphates, and nitrates. These anions occur in combination with such metallic cations as calcium, sodium, potassium, magnesium, and iron to form ionizable salts.

In most rivers the concentration and relative proportion of dissolved material remain low enough to support a mixed biota. However, in the Rhine River vast quantities of salt are found not only as a result of natural sources, such as erosion and atmospheric fallout, but also from artificial discharges due to mining and industry (Table 18.1). The amount from natural sources is proportional to the flow and the amount from artificial sources is constant in time. The mineral content (total dissolved solids) of river water increases with diminishing flow, as shown in Table 18.1.

The history of chloride discharges into the Rhine over the period 1885–1969 is illustrated in Figure 18.2. The periods of the first industrial revolution in the second half of the 19th century and of the second industrial revolution, which started with the second half of this century, are shown. The effects of the two world wars are apparent.

Today the artificial chloride load is over 300 kg/sec. The largest contributor (>60%) to this problem is France, from the potash mines in Alsace. The raw potash consists of 26% potassium chloride, combined with 61% sodium chloride and 13% insolubles. As a result, France discharges more than 7×10^6 tons of dissolved sodium chloride each year, the waste product of the mining of sylvinite, a compound of potassium chloride and sodium chloride.

Another 3.5×10^6 tons of salts from Western Alsace flow into the Rhine via the industries along the Moselle River. In addition, roughly 17% comes from the

Table 18.1   Mineral Loads (kg/sec) of Rhine at Dutch–German Border, 1969

Ion	Natural load at median flow	Artificial load	Global constitution and origin of artificial load
Cl^-	41	300	400 NaCl from mines (potassium and coal)
Na^+	27	170	25 NaCl from miscellaneous sources
HCO_3^-	240	—	
Ca^{2+}	110	70	70 $CaCl_2$ from soda industry
SO_4^{2-}	70	110	155 $CaSO_4$ from industry: steel, artificial silk, etc.
Total	488	650	650

Total dissolved salts
Median flow	[(488 + 650) × 1000 g/sec]/(2000 m³/sec) =	569 ppm
Low flow	[(244 + 650) × 1000 g/sec]/(1000 m³/sec) =	894 ppm
Minimum flow	[(158 + 650) × 1000 g/sec]/(650 m³/sec) =	1240 ppm
Natural state	(all flows)	= 244 ppm

Source: Biemond, C.J. J. Rhine River Pollution Studies. Reprinted from JOURNAL American Water Works Association, Volume 63, Number 1 (January, 1971) by permission. Copyright 1971, the American Water Works Association.

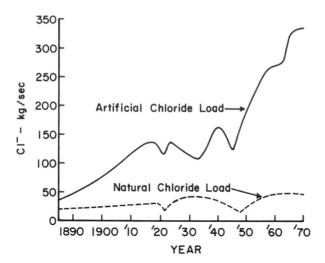

Figure 18.2   Chloride discharges into Rhine River, 1885–1969. (From Biemond, C.J. J. Rhine River Pollution Studies. Reprinted from JOURNAL American Water Works Association, Volume 63, Number 1 (January, 1971), by permission. Copyright 1971, the American Water Works Association.

German coal fields of the Ruhr district and around 20% from the soda industries in the Rhineland. The remainder may come from domestic effluents from municipalities.

These circumstances have given rise to a most crucial problem for the people in the Netherlands, where the chloride content of the Rhine has doubled since 1940. The Dutch population depends to a large extent on the Rhine for drinking water as well as for agriculture and industry. This nation uses approximately 1.5×10^9 m³ fresh water per year, and it is anticipated that the requirements will be 4×10^9 m³ by the year 2000.

The low-lying westland region of the Netherlands that extends from Rotterdam to The Hague is particularly vulnerable to this pollution. The high saline content of the ground water there, which is due to seepage from the sea, is aggravated by the salt in the river.

Some success in dealing with the salt problem was achieved at a recent (1976) Paris meeting. An agreement was made whereby the equivalent of about 50 kg/sec of chloride would be prevented from entering the river. However, 1980 is the earliest that this desired target can be achieved. It was also agreed that the salt would be stored underground, but a major problem is finding storage sites that will not present a risk of contaminating underground aquifers. The cost of this storage is also considerable. However, the Dutch have agreed to finance 30% of the estimated $12 million capital cost for the first year's storage facilities. France and West Germany will each fund 30% of the total, and Switzerland will make up the balance. Many feel the long-term solution is to take the salt by river barges or pipelines to dump it into the sea. This method, however, may also prove too expensive.

Many lawsuits have been brought against the mining industry, and it is still unclear as to how and when the salt issue will be completely resolved. The problem should not be taken lightly because the quantity and quality of dissolved solids are major factors not only in potability of water but in determining the variety and abundance of plants and animals in the river. They serve as nutrients in productivity, but in high concentrations they produce osmotic stress and direct toxicity to aquatic life. A major change in the quantity or composition of the dissolved solids may change the structure of the river system; however, the impact of such changes is difficult to predict.

The industrial wastes and mining operations also contain inorganic mineral acids and alkalies that can break down the natural buffering system of the river, alter its pH, and produce extensive damage to aquatic life. These acids and alkalies may also increase the toxicity of various components in the waters. For example, the Rhine contains significant quantities of ammonia in wastes. The addition of strong alkalies results in an increased pH and causes the formation of undissociated NH_4OH or un-ionized NH_3 in quantities that may be toxic to fish and other aquatic life. Acids and alkalies can also destroy bacteria and other microorganisms and thus inhibit or even prevent self-purification of the stream.

18.4.2. Thermal Pollution

The species composition and well-being of the aquatic community also depend on the termperature characteristics of the environment since most aquatic organisms have body temperatures that conform to the ambient water. Fish and other aquatic life can survive only within certain temperature ranges, which vary from one species to another. Tests have shown that temperature is of vital importance in controlling growth, reproduction, development, digestion, and respiration.

Temperature also affects the physical and chemical properties of the aquatic medium. For example, as the temperature increases the density and viscosity of water decrease, while the vapor pressure increases. These decreases in viscosity and density cause the settling speed of suspended particles to increase; the sediment load of the river will then settle more rapidly and possibly affect food supplies. This could be deleterious to aquatic organisms that require more food to maintain their body weights when the temperature rises.

The solubility of oxygen and other gases in water also decreases with increasing temperatures. This is of primary importance since most fish require at least 5 mg/liter for normal activities.

Higher temperatures also favor bacterial growth and increase the rates of physiological processes (two or three times for a $10°$ C change). Thus the decomposition of wastes by microbial oxidation is accelerated, increasing the BOD and the rate of oxygen depletion, and further aggravating the dissolved oxygen problem.

Most temperature changes of rivers are a result of natural diurnal and seasonal variations. However, in recent years there has been an accelerated demand for cooling waters for nuclear power stations that release large quantities of heat, causing a warming of rivers, or a rapid cooling when the artificial sources of heat are abruptly terminated. This problem is further compounded by the discharge of heated effluents from small factories and mills.

In the Rhine River thermal pollution is as big a problem as the conventional pollutants. Many power stations draw on the Rhine for cooling water, and as a result increase its temperature. A 1965 analysis showed significant thermal discharges on the Rhine and its tributaries. In 1970 between the Aar–Rhine confluence and the German–Dutch frontier there were about 19 major nuclear and conventional power stations generating between them 6100 MW of electricity. By 1976 the figure nearly tripled, and by 1985 it will have tripled again to nearly 44000 MW from almost 40 stations.

Studies by the German states have shown that at the anticipated growth of power demand in the German–Dutch frontier alone, such direct cooling at all stations would result in a peak river temperature of 35°C by 1985. This problem is further compounded because the river recovers slowly to normal temperatures after receiving thermal discharges. A 12°C increase in temperature above normal could have deleterious effects, since the dissolved oxygen content of fully aerated Rhine water drops by about 16% for each extra 1°C. When the river is low, this 12°C warm-up could cause total deoxygenation along long stretches of the river, eventually rendering the river foul and lifeless. This may also have serious effects on the Rhine vineyards, since the choice wines depend on frosts in early autumn. A warmer Rhine would also make the area more humid, cause more fog, and reduce vital sunlight during the daytime.

The Germans have agreed on three provisional measures to counteract the thermal pollution. First, all of their nuclear power stations will have cooling towers, which transfer the heat from cooling water to the atmosphere through evaporation. Second, no conventional station will heat up the river by more than 3°C. Third, the water temperatures below a power plant, after mixing, will never exceed 28°C.

Most of the plants under construction have planned for cooling towers. The Swiss Federation has also adopted the three German guidelines. However, France has a number of nuclear power plants in southern Alsace that have no cooling towers as well as more plants under construction that may raise the temperature of the Rhine by as much as 18°C.

The growing number of commercial nuclear power plants have thus far created only thermal problems, but the possibility of contamination by radioactive elements also exists. The experts say that pollution from this source is minor but this area still has to be explored.

18.4.3. Pesticides

Pesticides are categorized according to their use or intended target (eg., insecticide, herbicide, or fungicide), but their release into the environment presents an imminent danger to many nontarget species. Some degree of contamination and risk is assumed with nearly all pesticide use. The risk to aquatic ecosystems depends upon the chemical and physical properties of the pesticide, type of formulation, methods of application, and nature of the receiving system.

The pesticides of greatest concern are those that are persistent for long periods (organochlorine) and accumulate in the environment. The major sources of pesticides in water are runoff from treated lands, industrial discharges, and domestic sewage. Significant contributions may also occur in fallout from the atmosphere, drift, and precipitation. Applications to water surfaces, intentional or otherwise, will also result in rapid and extensive contamination.

The pesticide pollution in the Rhine is a result of both agricultural and industrial input. In order to monitor some of these potentially hazardous substances, in 1969 the National Institute of Public Health (Utrecht, the Netherlands) began a weekly sampling program on the river. The monitoring program analyzed organochlorine (and related substances) and organophosphate pesticides.

After almost 3 years of analysis some disturbing data began to emerge. The C_6Cl_6-compounds such as α-benzene hexachloride (α-BHC), lindane (γ-BHC), and hexachlorobenzene (HCB) were nearly always present. If one compares the concentrations of these compounds in the Rhine with other Dutch surface waters (Table 18.2), the pesticide pollution of the Rhine is quite evident. The concentration of these substances is about 10 times as high as in typically agricultural surface waters. This may mean that industry rather than agriculture is the main source of pollution. For example, the high concentration of HCB can scarcely be explained by its limited use as a fungicide. The presence of these C_6Cl_6-compounds is also important because these substances are stable, persistent, and not easily removed during processing to drinking water.

Some of the cyclodiene organochlorine pesticides (heptachlor, aldrin, dieldrin, endrin, and endosulfan) were also occasionally present but only in low concentrations. This is fortunate because many of these compounds are toxic to aquatic life. Among this group of compounds, endosulfan deserves particular attention with respect to Rhine River pollution.

In 1969 the Dutch authorities were informed of a massive fish kill in West Germany. Water samples of the Rhine were subsequently analyzed and found to contain endosulfan (α and β) at a maximum concentration of 0.70 ppb in the Netherlands. The observed quantities of endosulfan and its degradation products led to an estimation of a discharge of approximately 2000 kg near the Dutch–German border. The incident led to international publicity and concern. However, since 1970 the concentrations of endosulfan have decreased to insignificant levels.

In light of this incident a similar catastrophe should be mentioned involving the sandwich tern, a migrating sea bird. Between 1940 and 1957 the number of these birds fluctuated between 25,000 and 40,000 pairs in the Netherlands. Following an effluent discharge from a pesticide factory into the Rhine, this population fell to 650 pairs in 1965. After control measures it rose to 2000 pairs, but even so the population for Northwestern Europe has only numbered about 12,000 pairs in recent years. It is known that organochlorine pesticides have a

Table 18.2   Average Concentrations (μg/liter) of Some Pesticides and Related Substances in Dutch Surface Waters

Compound	Rhine	Maas	Other surface waters
α-BHC	0.15	0.01	0.01
γ-BHC	0.10	0.02	0.01
HCB	0.13	0.01	<0.01
Dieldrin	<0.01	0.01	0.01
Cholinesterase inhibitors (as paraoxon)	1.14	0.13	0.10

Source: Greve, P.A. Sci. Total Environ. 1:173, 1972.

detrimental effect on the growth, reproduction, and development of birds, and this fact should be carefully considered in view of the importance of these animals in the food chain.

Organophosphate insecticides (cholinesterase inhibitors) were also present in significant quantities in samples from the Rhine and its tributaries (Table 18.2). In other Dutch surface waters the concentrations were about one-tenth as high. The presence of these compounds is definitely unfavorable because they have adverse affects on the nervous systems of aquatic organisms.

18.4.4. Other Organochlorine Compounds

PCBs and terphenyls represent another class of organochlorine compounds that are widely used in industry as lubricants, heat transfer media, and insulators. These compounds have been monitored since the late 1960s for their occurrence and distribution in the Rhine River and the coastal area of the Netherlands. Both groups of compounds were found in the late 1960s in small quantities in water, fish, invertebrate organisms, and human fat. Today, however, they are found in increasing quantities; they present a potential hazard to the environment because of their persistence and biomagnification in the food chain.

18.4.5. Oil Pollution

Oil enters the aquatic environment from accidental spills, oil-carrying tankers and ships, refinery operations, and the disposal of oil waste material. Oil pollution may be in the form of floating oils, emulsified oils, or solutions of the water-soluble fraction of these oils.

The toxicity of oil is difficult to ascertain since crude oil is a mixture of many organic and inorganic components. The hydrocarbons in crude oil cover a wide range of molecular weights and include aliphatic compounds with straight and branched chains, olefins, and the aromatic ring compounds. Crude oils differ in the relative concentrations of these components.

When released into the aquatic environment these compounds react differently: some are soluble, others evaporate from the surface, form extensive oil slicks, or settle to the bottom. Although many differences exist between crude oils and their refined products, they all have deleterious effects on fish and other aquatic life, including birds. In fish, they interfere with respiration, whereas in birds they penetrate the feathers, affecting insulation and buoyancy.

As a result of the considerable amount of shipping on the Rhine, oil pollution is particularly severe, and even today, in spite of national and international regulations, the problem persists. Approximately 18,000 ships use the Rhine and the canals linked with it.

The sinking of fuel and cargo ships in the Rhine following collisions and other accidents accounts for an overwhelming degree of pollution. A more continual problem is the fact that part of a tanker cargo is discharged after it arrives at a port. The tanks are then filled up with fresh water to act as a ballast, and before the tanker docks again, the ballast, contaminated with residues of oil, is discharged into the water. Ordinary vessels that use oil for fuel can also produce oil slicks when the waste oil is dumped from their fuel tanks. Over 8000 Rhine barges normally release approximately 10×10^6 tons of oily water from their bilges each year.

In 1974 the Testing and Research Institute of the Netherlands Waterworks determined the oil content at various points along the Rhine River and Maas River (Table 18.3). Weekly samples were taken and analyzed either by spectrometry or gas chromatography. The highest concentrations of oil were measured at places where the Rhine enters the Netherlands, after which they decreased steadily. These high concentrations may be due in part to the intensive shipping near the frontiers.

There is, however, one success story to report. The Germans have formed the Bilge Drainage Association, which directs the collection of bilge oil and renders it harmless at no charge. The bilge oil collected grew from 530 tons in 1962 to over 7000 tons in 1972. The service is financed partly by the sale of oil that is removed and partly by the German and Dutch governments. This is an example of cooperation that should be followed by other countries using the Rhine as a shipping route.

18.4.6. Heavy Metals

Metals reach the aquatic environment through natural weathering as well as municipal and industrial discharges. In solution, heavy metals may constitute a very serious form of pollution because they are stable compounds not easily removed by oxidation, precipitation, and other natural processes. A characteristic feature of heavy metal pollution is its persistence and bioaccumulation through the food chain.

Along the Rhine many of the chemical industries use metals as additions to oil, gasoline, plastics, resins, soaps, and cosmetics. The metals found in solution form only a part of the total discharge from industry. The majority of the metals are bound by adsorption and found in sediment or suspended matter. Under the proper climatic conditions, the sediments on their way to the sea can undergo changes in their metal composition by mobilization of these elements as soluble metal–organic complexes. This process leads to less contaminated sediments in the lower course of the Rhine.

Table 18.3   Average Oil Concentration (mg/liter) in the Rhine River and Maas River Per Quarter, 1974

Location	Quarter, 1974				Average for year
Rhine Lobith	0.93	0.95	0.09	0.35	0.58
Waal Ochten	0.36	0.45	0.13	0.19	0.28
Waal Brakel	0.13	0.25	0.21	0.19	0.20
Lek Bergambacht	0.11	0.14	0.19	0.18	0.16
Ijssel lake Andijk	0.16	0.11	0.09	0.04	0.10
Maas Maastricht	1.45	0.97	0.57	1.42	0.90
Maas Berg	0.58	0.22	0.58	1.04	0.59
Maas Belfeld	0.36	0.32	0.27	0.29	0.30
Maas Grave	0.29	0.17	0.27	0.46	0.30
Maas Heusden	0.08	0.16	0.13	0.33	0.18
Maas Drimmelen	0.28	0.25	0.24	0.21	0.25
Amer Kerksloot	0.15	0.16	0.23	0.24	0.20

Source: Meijers, A.P., Vander Lee, R.C. The occurrence of organic micropollutants in the river Rhine and the river Maas in 1974. Reprinted with permission from Water Research 10:597. Copyright 1976, Pergamon Press, Ltd.

The National Institute of Public Health (the Netherlands) periodically analyzes samples from the Rhine River for heavy metals. Combined data on water samples and sediments in the 1970s show the presence of large amounts of arsenic, chromium, copper, mercury, lead, and zinc. These metals were found in concentrations of 20–50% of the World Health Organization limits in river water.

Eventually many of these metals may accumulate in agricultural land and have effects on plant growth and animal nutrition. For example, mercury samples in river sediments have reached concentrations as high as 23 ppm. During high flows such sediments are deposited in areas used as pastures. Fortunately, the levels of mercury in the milk and tissues of cows and other land animals have remained low thus far. Apparently the animals have been exposed to the nontoxic inorganic form of mercury that is eliminated quickly, not the more toxic methylmercury. However, with sufficient bacterial action this metallic mercury may be converted to the more toxic organometallic compound.

Although there is a large margin of safety between actual quantities delivered in the water and safe limits, the pollution by heavy metals should be under careful scrutiny because the toxicity of these elements changes drastically with changes in water quality.

18.5. Secondary Effects of Pollution

There are many secondary effects of pollution, such as physical changes (color, turbidity), biological changes (algae, fungi, bacteria, worms, etc.), and aesthetic changes (taste, odor). In view of increasing population densities, the Rhine River must be used by many municipalities for potable water supplies. For example, by the year 2000, it has been estimated that the Dutch requirements alone for clean surface water will have quadrupled. Treatment of these quantities of water for consumption will be difficult because of the immense discharges of treated and untreated sewage and wastes. A problem that will also assume considerable importance will be the concentration of chemical compounds that impart characteristic and unpleasant tastes and odors to the water.

Odors in the river may be associated with strong-smelling compounds (phenols, chlorine, sulphides, ammonia, etc.), organic materials (oils), or algae and other decomposing and putrescent organic matter. Unpleasant odors may also be due to the presence of microorganisms, different forms of nitrogen, sulfur (H_2S), and phosphorus. Taste-producing substances in polluted rivers may include many of the above substances in addition to unsaturated hydrocarbons, salts, iron, manganese, etc.

Along the course of the Rhine from 1960 to 1969 different waterworks companies collected information on odor substances and threshold values. It was shown that part of the odorous substances originate in the sewage and waste flowing into the river. This was true for the chlorinated hydrocarbons, whose average concentration in the river water was 100 μg/liter. There was also evidence that part of the odorous substances may come from biological reactions in the river. In addition, some of the odorous substances were terpenoids, which are natural cyclic hydrocarbons produced by plants. Today, there are other industrial wastes (phenols, salts, iron, ammonia, oil, etc.) that enhance these unpleasant tastes and odors.

Usually the less volatile and more polar substances contribute very little to the odor problem. The more volatile and more polar substances and the less volatile and less polar substances have the highest odor threshold concentrations.

Many of these substances can be removed by purification processes, but these less readily oxidizable substances give rise to problems. They cannot be oxidized by ozone or permanganate and are difficult to flocculate. Therefore, activated carbon has to be used for their elimination, which has the additional advantage of removing wastes. In many German waterworks, threshold odor values are reduced through bank filtration, subsequent ozone oxidation, and activated carbon treatment.

The solution to many of the secondary effects of pollution exists. However, some countries have not as yet taken advantage of the appropriate technology to remedy their situations.

18.6. Conclusions

After a decade of conferences among the Rhine Basin countries, it is obvious that results cannot and will not be achieved if these countries do not engage themselves to an equal extent in cleanup measures.

In recent years some of the authorities have increased their demands for effluent purification. Comprehensive plans and expenditures on abatement facilities are quite impressive, but the magnitude is still inadequate. Germany, for example, is taking the problem very seriously, and it should, because West Germany has the longest Rhine border of any country sharing the waterway. The large West German industries, particularly the chemical companies, have spent millions of dollars to reverse the pollution trend. Bayer, BASF, and Hoechst are three large international companies that have invested in antipollution facilities to treat their liquid effluents. Although these procedures only amount to mechanical (primary) treatment, and in some cases biological (secondary) treatment, they are a step in the right direction. On the other hand, some of the Rhine Basin countries continue to discharge untreated sewage and wastes.

In general, effluents can no longer be treated by only mechanical methods because they are not efficient in removing certain substances such as nitrogen, phosphorus, and dissolved minerals. If biological treatment is combined with mechanical treatment, the removal efficiency is better for nitrogen and phosphorus, but it does little to reduce concentrations of dissolved minerals, heavy metals, drugs, and some exotic chemicals. Because the Rhine has serious problems with many of these substances, the more advanced (tertiary) treatment processes should be used. These procedures can improve on the waste water quality to the point at which it can be reused. This is very important in view of the scarcity of drinking water for the 40×10^6 inhabitants of the Rhine Basin.

Although the thermal and salt problems are far from being settled, the environmental ministers have agreed to measures to control the discharge of certain dangerous chemicals. These chemicals are divided into two lists, each of which categorizes groups of materials according to their respective level of danger. Those in list I (or the ''black list'') include not only such nonbiodegradable toxic substances as mercury and cadmium and their derivatives, but also organohalogens, phosphorus and tin compounds, mineral oils, hydrocarbons of petroleum origin, and persistent synthetic substances. Their release into the river will be strictly limited according to a uniform community-wide system of emission standards. This will require that all emissions meet uniform requirements concerning the composition of waste water independent of the quality of the drainage channels in question. Ideally, the aim is to eliminate these chemicals completely. List II (or the "gray list") includes a range of metals and biocides not included in the black list and chemicals that affect the taste and odor of the water.

It could take almost 3 years, however, to devise such emission standards and to work out the necessary programs to safeguard the Rhine against substances on list I. The water quality objectives regarding the release of substances on list II still have to be defined. Nevertheless, this agreement is a definite breakthrough in achieving a lasting improvement in the quality of the Rhine. It provides a starting point for the Europeanization of water protection and serves to harmonize the obligations of the participating countries.

The existing International Rhine Pollution Commission must be given power to enforce its recommendations because so far negotiations between the countries have not solved enough of the complex problems that have existed for decades. If this is not the solution, then maybe a strong international pollution control authority will be required.

Suggested Reading

Duinker, J. C., Nolting, R. F. Distribution model for particulate trace metals in the Rhine estuary, Southern Bight and Dutch Wadden Sea. Neth. J. Sea Res. 10:71, 1976.

Gaessler, W. The importance of the Rhine as a water source. Effluent Water Treat. J. 11: 659, 1971.

Goldbach, R. W., Van Genderen, H., Leeuwangh, P. Hexachlorobutadiene residues in aquatic fauna from surface waters fed by the river Rhine. Sci. Total Environ. 6:31, 1976.

Greve, P. A. Potentially hazardous substances in surface waters. Sci. Total Environ. 1: 173, 1972.

Greve, P. A., Wit, S. L. Endosulfan in the Rhine River. J. Water Pollut. Control Fed., 43: 2338, 1971.

Koeman, J. H., Ten Noever De Brauw, M. C., De Vos, R. H. Chlorinated biphenyls in fish, mussels, and birds from the river Rhine and the Netherlands coastal area. Nature 221: 1126, 1969.

Meijers, A. P., Van Der Leer, R. C. The occurrence of organic micropollutants in the river Rhine and the river Maas in 1974. Water Res. 10: 597, 1976.

Montgomery, A. H., Merklein, H. Protection of the Rhine River against pollution. J. Am. Water Works Assoc. 64: 108, 1972.

Rolle, W., Koppe, P., Sontheimer, H. Taste and odor problems with river Rhine. Water Treat. Exam. 19: 120, 1970.

Tinker, J. Europe's majestic sewer. New Sci. 56: 194, 1972.

Neal E. Armstrong

19

Case History:
Galveston Bay

19.1. Introduction

The history of pollution in Galveston Bay, Texas, is closely tied to the development of urban areas, primarily the City of Houston and her associated industries, and other cities and industries on the Bay's periphery. Water quality problems from biodegradable organic wastes reached their peak in the early 1970s but have since decreased following substantial reductions in these wastes through waste treatment. The exact status of toxic materials in the bay is still unknown, however, for there have been few definitive studies to delineate toxicant concentrations and the problems they present.

The information presented below describes the Galveston Bay system, the history of urban development around the bay, particular discharges of toxic wastes, and the studies that have delineated the presence and effects of toxic materials to date.

19.2. Physical and Hydrological Characteristics

Galveston Bay, with an area of 1.35×10^5 m² and an average depth of about 2.4 m, is the largest inland bay on the Texas coast (Figure 19.1). The bay lies in the humid zone of Texas and rainfall ranges between 1067 and 1270 mm/year. The annual mean temperature is about 20.6°C.

Galveston Bay consists of four contiguous bodies of water identified on charts and maps as Galveston Bay, Trinity Bay, East Bay, and West Bay. The four-bay system is separated from the Gulf of Mexico by Galveston Island and the Bolivar Peninsula. Bolivar Roads and San Luis Pass are the passes through which bay water exchanges with the gulf. West Bay lies between Galveston Island and the mainland; East Bay lies between the Bolivar Peninsula and the mainland. Trinity Bay is the northeastern body of water in the system and receives the inflow of the Trinity River.

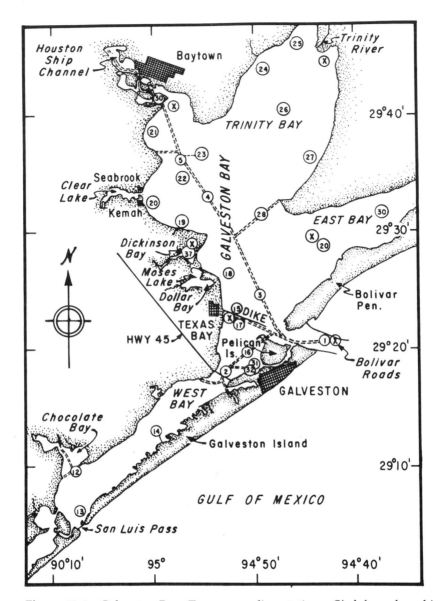

Figure 19.1 Galveston Bay, Texas, sampling stations. *Circled numbers:* biota sampling stations. *Circled X's:* sampling stations for toxicity and nutrient enrichment studies. (Adapted from Copeland, B.J., Fruh, E.G. Ecological Studies of Galveston Bay, 1969. Report to the Texas Water Quality Board by the University of Texas, Austin, 1970.)

Galveston Bay receives fresh-water inflow from several sources. It is fed by the San Jacinto River, Cedar Bayou, Clear Creek, Dickinson Bayou, and Trinity River. East Bay is fed by Oyster and East Bay Bayous and other small creeks. West Bay receives its fresh-water flow from Chocolate and Halls Bayous, which empty into Chocolate Bay.

The quantity and quality of surface water runoff in the area are changing as a result of urbanization and the control and channelization of the tributary system.

The flat coastal topography is susceptible to extensive flooding from storm water overflow of waterways and on occasion from hurricane tides and wave action.

19.3. Economic Development

The inland port of Houston, linked to both the Gulf of Mexico and the Gulf Intracoastal Waterway, is a leading oil and petrochemical center, the focal point for networks of oil and natural gas pipelines, and an aerospace research and development center. The rise of the region as a major population and industrial center has been a fairly recent development. An uninhabited swamp as late as 1836, most of its growth has taken place in the past 50 years. Much of the phenomenal growth and development of the Houston area is attributed to the construction of the Houston Ship Channel. Built along the natural course of Buffalo Bayou, the Ship Channel opened up the area to ship traffic and facilitated its growth and development from a community of a little over 50,000 in 1915, the year the Ship Channel was opened, to a metropolis of over 2×10^6 people at the present time.

The discovery of oil in the region, the concurrent development of the internal combustion engine, and the resource requirements of World War I combined to produce a heavy demand for products from this region. By 1927, 83% of the ocean-going tonnage from the Port of Houston was in the form of oil and related chemicals. In the 1930s, refineries were well developed along the channel, and Texas led all states in refining of petroleum, with Harris County leading all other counties. During and after World War II, new major industries were established, including a primary steel producer and a major ordinance plant. Construction of countless miles of pipelines, accompanied by continued development of chemical and petrochemical industries, further established the channel area as a major production and distribution center. At the same time, Texas City in Galveston County developed into the largest single concentrated point of heavy industry in the state.

As a result of this economic development, over 300 major industries are located around the bay, many on the banks of the Houston Ship Channel. The sewage from the over 2×10^6 people and waste from industries are collected and find their way to over 700 discharge points into the bay; because of the types of industries involved, substantial amounts of toxic materials are discharged with these wastes.

In addition to these point sources of toxic wastes, runoff from irrigated and nonirrigated agricultural areas sprayed with pesticides and areas sprayed for mosquito control contribute to the toxic material load to the bay. The Dallas and Fort Worth urban areas also discharge toxic wastes that may reach the bay via the Trinity River.

19.4. Toxic Material Discharges

In an attempt to define the sources of toxic wastes released into Galveston Bay, information from several sources was used to calculate the mass discharge of toxic materials to Galveston Bay from point and nonpoint sources in 1974. Information from the Corps of Engineers, which was obtained from industrial discharges as a prelude to preparing permits for discharges under the 1899

Refuse Act, was used to calculate the mass discharges. In the Houston Ship Channel, the major discharger of toxic materials was the Gulf Coast Waste Disposal Authority, and the location of heavy metal concentrations in the channel waters and sediments tended to verify this conclusion. The Trinity River was also a major source of toxins. Based on an analysis of U.S. Geological Survey data, the Trinity River mass emission rates for cadmium, copper, mercury, and zinc made up 61%, 79%, 85%, and 81%, respectively, of the total mass emission rate of each compound to Galveston Bay.

Further studies on the discharge of toxic material in Galveston Bay were carried out in 1977. In these studies, more definitive relationships between observed toxicity and the presence of specific toxicants were developed, and the presence of relative toxicity, measured as toxic units, was calculated in the Houston Ship Channel and the bay proper. In general, the geographical distribution of relative toxicity corresponded to the observed growth depression values obtained in the algal assays. Furthermore, it was shown that the levels of relative toxicity in the bay exceeded the 0.05 toxic unit receiving water standards which had been set in California coastal waters by the State of California Department of Water Resources and considered as a standard by the Texas Water Quality Board in 1976.

19.5. Toxic Material Concentrations

The presence of toxic materials in Galveston Bay was detected through the measurement of specific toxicants and through algal bioassays. The results of these tests are discussed below.

19.5.1. Specific Toxin Concentrations

Samples taken in 1968 and analyzed for heavy metals and pesticides indicated high concentrations of some metals and certain persistent pesticides. However, the results were uncertain due to unreliable analytical techniques and the small number of samples. Sampling of heavy metals on a regular basis by the U.S. Geological Survey began in 1970 in the bay and continued into 1972. Stations were sampled at various times during this period and several combinations of heavy metals were measured each time. Several laboratories with varying degrees of detection capability were involved in the analyses, thus it is somewhat hazardous to attempt an analysis of even these data.

Concentrations of each heavy metal measured were compared to the 1973 EPA Maximum Acceptable Concentrations for receiving waters at each station sampled. The number of times a measured concentration exceeded the EPA criterion was determined and converted to a percentage of total measurements; these values are tabulated in Table 19.1. Entries were made only if more than two samples were taken at a station over the period of record, and the segments listed are Department of Water Resources segments.

Except for arsenic, all heavy metals were found in Galveston Bay in concentrations greater than EPA criteria. High zinc concentrations were found in the Houston Ship Channel and in the lower portions of the bay. Lead concentrations above the EPA criteria were found with low frequency throughout the bay with no apparent gradients. Mercury concentrations were frequently above the EPA

Table 19.1   Frequency of Exceeding EPA Receiving Water Maximum Acceptable Concentrations for Heavy Metals in Galveston Bay in 1977

Segment	Station	Zinc	Lead	Mercury	Cadmium	Copper	Arsenic	Nickel
1006	9	0	0	60	43	75	0	40
1007	11	50	20	0	50	75	0	40
2421	18	20	20	60				
	22	37	14	37				
	23	0	20	60				
	28	0	20	80				
	31	0	20	80				
	33	0	20	75	0	80	0	50
	41	0	20	100				
2422	26	25	14	25				
	38	0	40	80				
	39	0	20	60				
	42	0	20	100				
2423	29	37	14	25				
2424	14	37	14	25				
2437	17	37	14	57				
2501	1	29	29	71				

Note: All values are percentages of total samples that exceed criteria.

criteria in the Ship Channel, as were copper and nickel. The importance of these data is not only that the EPA criteria were being exceeded frequently, but that these concentrations were considered hazardous to the organisms in the bay according to the National Academy of Sciences criteria.

These high concentrations of heavy metals are the result of discharges in excess of both the EPA and Texas Department of Water Resources effluent standards, of nonpoint discharges such as runoff, and of river inflows carrying toxic materials from discharges upstream.

19.5.2. Algal Assay for Detecting Toxic Materials

Researchers at the University of Texas used an algal assay technique to detect the presence of growth suppressant materials in fresh-water and waste-water inputs to Galveston Bay and in Galveston Bay waters. A blue-green algae (*Coccochloris elebans*) was maintained in pure cultures to which pasteurized water samples collected in Galveston Bay were added and the resulting growth was followed colorimetrically. The effect of toxicity was found to be a depression of the growth rate K from the optimal rate of 2.0 (or 6.6 generations per 24 hr). The results of these studies showed that significant amounts of growth suppressant materials originated in the Houston Ship Channel and in the Trinity River. Toxicity in the Houston Ship Channel was not unexpected because a very large number of industries discharge waste waters into that channel.

These studies also showed that industrial waste discharges did indeed contain materials that suppressed the growth of the blue-green algae used as the assay organisms, as did water from the Trinity River. In fact, growth suppressant materials were detected in the Trinity River up to Lake Livingston Dam and above Lake Livingston. They were not detected, however, in water samples from the lake proper nor from Lake Travis on the Colorado River in Texas.

19.5.3. Algal Toxicity Modeling

Two-dimensional mathematical models were used in the Galveston Bay Study to predict the distribution of the growth rate K through the bay system. In this experimental model, it was assumed that the experimental K value obtained from the Houston Ship Channel data had the same growth inhibitory effect as the experimental K value from other stations such as the Trinity River input. (It is possible that the effects from the toxic materials in the Houston Ship Channel on the ecosystem will be different from those from the materials from the Trinity River). Based on this hypothesis, it was further assumed that the input K values from the Houston Ship Channel, Trinity River, and Bolivar Roads were additive.

It was determined from inflow records and chlorinity measurements that the period August–October represented a sustained low inflow period and probably approximated an equilibrium condition. Thus, the distribution of the growth rate K through the bay system was made assuming a steady-state condition. K was assumed to be a conservative parameter transported by advection and diffusion through the bay with the important boundaries being Trinity River, Houston Ship Channel at Morgan Point, and Bolivar Roads. To eliminate the effect of experimental fluctuations, the data were averaged for the period July–October, and the averaged values for the boundary points were taken to be constants in the simulation runs.

Model results along with observed K's are presented in Table 19.2. These assumptions were verified by comparing the predicted model value to the actual observed K rate at Hannah's Reef, Dickinson Bay, and Texas City Dike.

19.5.4. Correlation Between K Value and Ecological Structure

The K values of various stations generated from the preliminary computer models were compared with the phytoplankton diversity indices as shown in Figure 19.2. As the toxicity of the waste increased (decreasing K), the phytoplankton diversity index decreased.

Table 19.2 Average Simulated (Tracor 1969) and Experimental K (Growth Rates) Values for Estuarine Stations in Galveston Bay

Averaging period, 1977	Dickinson Bay	Hannah's Reef	Texas City Dike
March–Oct.			
Predicted	1.33	1.20	1.65
Observed	1.51	1.40	1.59
July–Oct.			
Predicted	1.33	1.20	1.65
Observed	1.35	1.47	1.61
Aug.–Oct.			
Predicted	1.34	1.21	1.66
Observed	1.45	1.35	1.70

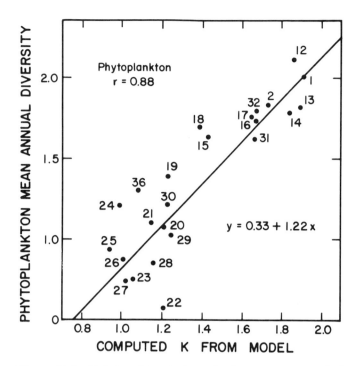

Figure 19.2 Relationship of phytoplankton mean annual diversity to computed toxicity at various stations in Galveston Bay. (Adapted from Copeland, B.J., Fruh, E.G. Ecological Studies of Galveston Bay, 1969. Report to the Texas Water Quality Board by the University of Texas, Austin, 1970.)

The correlation is highly significant in view of the limitations associated with the data. The stations in the stratified Ship Channel were not modeled because of the limitations of the steady-state model utilized. The stations in West Bay were also not part of the modeling package at that time. In addition, approximately one-half of the stations utilized were along the shoreline, where local inputs (wastewater, urban runoff, agriculture runoff, etc.) could be more significant than the inputs from the Houston Ship Channel, Trinity River, and Bolivar Roads. Furthermore, the effect of natural stresses could not be separated from what appears to be the overwhelming effect of the toxic materials.

The algal species present in the samples from the various estuarine areas substantiated this general correlation between the toxicity parameter and the diversity index. The hardier Cyanophyceae (blue-green algae) were dominant in Upper Galveston Bay and Trinity Bay, while the diatoms were the most abundant in Lower Galveston Bay, East Bay, and West Bay.

Additional indirect evidence for the above correlation was available from nutrient enrichment studies. Addition of a medium containing all nutrients stimulated the least growth in the Trinity River sample. The addition of Houston Ship Channel and Trinity River waters to those of Bolivar Roads, Hannah's Reef, Dickinson Bay, and Texas City Dike generally depressed growth below that of the control (the sample to which no other water was added) for a significant time (15 days).

If there are certain areas or inputs containing materials that are inhibitory to phytoplankton, then the water in question might affect higher organisms as well. Certainly this would appear to be the case for "harsh" pollutants such as industrial wastes and insecticides. However, the pollutant material might be limited to inhibition of only phytoplankton. Thus, the species diversity index of the fish, nekton, zooplankton, and benthos obtained from the 28 sampling stations during four seasons were compared with the K values computed from each station in the preliminary model. For all types of organisms, there was an obvious trend toward high diversity indices with an increase in K (decrease in toxicity). The most severely stressed subsystem was evidently Trinity Bay, where no correlation was evident for the zooplankton and the benthos. In fact, only in Trinity Bay, the diversity index of these particular organisms apparently varied inversely with increasing K values.

19.6. Summary

In summary, the information available to date for the Galveston Bay area indicates that some specific toxicants are present in concentrations that are believed to affect organisms in the bay. Second, toxic materials are present that suppress the growth of an algal assay organism, and this could be extremely significant for primary productivity levels in the bay. Third, the nature of this growth suppressant compound is not known at the present time but is present in the Houston Ship Channel, in the Trinity River both above and below Lake Livingston, and in Galveston Bay.

Suggested Reading

Beale, J.J. Galveston Bay Project—Summary Report. Texas Water Quality Board, Austin, Texas, 1975.

Copeland, B.J., Fruh, E.G. (1970). Ecological Studies of Galveston Bay, 1969. Report to the Texas Water Quality Board by the University of Texas, Austin, Texas, 1970.

Marine Science Institute. Toxicity Studies of Galveston Bay Project, September 1, 1971 to December 1, 1972. Report to the Texas Water Quality Board by the University of Texas Marine Science Institute, Port Aransas, Texas, 1973.

Smith, J. N. Decline of Galveston Bay. Washington, D.C.: The Conservation Federation, 1972.

Robert J. Reimold

20

Case History:
Point Source Effluents in
the Georgia Coastal Zone

20.1. Introduction

Water quality criteria protect an important resource of our nation. These criteria are designed to ensure water quality that permits the propogation of wildlife and fish and does not endanger the health of humans. Acceptable levels of toxic materials in the water are based on environmental and organismal interactions. Concern for water quality is reflected by recent requirements for environmental impact statements for projects that may cause environmental perturbations. The EPA based criteria for water quality on the effects on the most sensitive important species of fauna and/or flora. The EPA has suggested a desirable degree of regional or local variation in water quality standards to reflect local conditions. According to the EPA definition, an "important species" is one that (a) is commercially or recreationally valuable, (b) is rare or endangered, (c) affects the well-being of some species within (a) or (b), or (d) is critical to the structure and function of ecological systems.

Research on pollutants has generally been based on bioassay methodology. These bioassays have been considered to be effective and accurate methods of predicting and assessing potential dangers to specific organisms. The synergistic effects of certain combinations of pollutants, however, result in very different effects than simple additive combinations of the effects. Laboratory bioassays must explain the field results reasonably well before the laboratory test can be considered adequate.

A recent report from the National Academy of Sciences reviews the importance of community structures and diversity studies. The report recommends that changes in community diversity measured by diversity indices be used to evaluate the effects of pollution on aquatic life. A number of scientific investigators have utilized the species diversity concepts in recent years in working with estuarine communities. The relationships between the number of species and importance values (numbers, dominance, redundancy, similarity, etc.) of individuals are collectively referred to as ecological community indices.

20.2. Study Design

In order to utilize the modern techniques of community ecological studies to assess pollution abatement programs, a study was undertaken in August 1970 to assess changes in community structure reflecting pollution from a toxaphene[1] manufacturing plant in coastal Georgia. This community ecological study contrasted the nekton in the estuary adjacent to the toxaphene manufacturing plant with a nearby undisturbed pristine estuary designated by the U.S. Department of Commerce, Office of Coastal Zone Management, as one of its national estuarine sanctuaries. The study is utilized here to provide a case history on the effects of industrial point source effluents in the coastal zone.

The study areas represented estuaries adjacent to Brunswick, Georgia, and Sapelo Island, Georgia. The estuarine collection site near Brunswick was selected because of the potential contamination from a nearby toxaphene manufacturing plant and its point source effluent discharged into the estuary. The Duplin Estuarine Sanctuary near Sapelo Island was studied as a control. The Duplin Estuarine Sanctuary represented an area uninfluenced by any type of known contaminant.

Field sampling in the Duplin Estuary was conducted over a straight stretch of the estuary 1.0 km in length. Nekton samples in the Duplin Estuary were collected utilizing an otter trawl made of 32-mm mesh that was 3 m wide at the mouth of the net; two repetitive trawls were performed every 4 weeks from August 1970 through June 1976. These samples were collected between 10:00 a.m. and 12:00 noon and between 10:00 p.m. and 12:00 midnight. In addition, an 80-mm mesh otter trawl that was 16 m wide at the mouth was used to collect duplicate samples over the 1.0-km course from August 1970 through June 1972. These duplicate samples were collected both in the daytime and at night. From July 1973 through June 1976, samples were taken in the Duplin Estuary with the smaller net at 8-week intervals.

In the Brunswick Estuary, seven subsamples were collected at 4-week intervals from August 1970 through June 1975. From July 1975 through June 1976 the samples were taken at 8-week intervals. Equal numbers of samples were collected against and with the tide. Each of the seven substations in the Brunswick area was 0.14 km long. One of the seven substations was Terry Creek, the location of the toxaphene point source discharge from the manufacturing plant.

Other data collected associated with the trawls included the date, cloud cover, salinity, water temperature, and air temperature. All nekton collected were sorted, identified, measured (total length for finfish), and weighed. Wet weight biomass was measured to the nearest 0.1 g using a Mettler Model Pll balance; total length was reported to the nearest 1.0 mm for each fish. Measurement of the community indices included several diversity indices:

1. Shannon-Weaver index, $\bar{H} = - P_i \log P_i$, where P_i is the proportion of the number of individuals in the ith species to the total number of individuals.

---

[1]Toxaphene is a chlorinated hydrocarbon insecticide prepared by chlorinating camphene to 67%. It has been the most heavily used insecticide in the southeast cotton belt since about 1950.

2. Evenness index, $J. = \bar{H}/\log S$, where S is the maximum possible value of $\bar{H}$, and $\bar{H}$ is the Shannon-Weaver Index.
3. Number of moves index, $NM = N(S + 1)/2 - R_i N_i$, where N is the total number of individuals, N_i is the number of individuals of the ith species, S is the total number of species, and R_i is the rank of species i.
4. Species richness index, $d = S - 1/\log N$, where S is the number of species and N is the total number of individuals.

Computations were also made of the percent importance, the percent similarity, the number of individuals in size classes on a geometric class basis, dominance, Euclidean distance, and the Coefficient of Community for Relative Abundance. Significant differences of the $\bar{H}$ index were computed. All indices reported are on a July 1 through June 31 fiscal year basis.

20.3. Results

Figure 20.1. compares the changes in diversity measured by the $\bar{H}$ index based on the number of individuals, for all collection sites for the 5-year study period. Although there was a great disparity in $\bar{H}$ for the first 2 years of the study, the last 3 years showed less change in the index. The diversity as expressed by the J index, based on the number of individuals, for all collection sites revealed a great

Figure 20.1 $\bar{H}$ diversity index (based on the number of individuals) for all collection sites, 1970–1975.

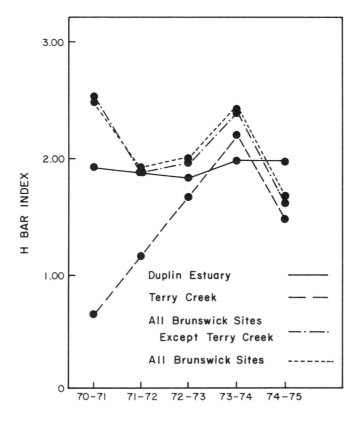

similarity of diversity at all collection locations. The NM index, based on the number of individuals, for all the collection sites revealed a great similarity of diversity during 1972–1973 and 1974–1975. A similar pattern in the d index based on the number of individuals was also found.

Comparisons of diversity indices of the community were also made based on the wet weight biomass of the organisms. Similarities in the $\bar{H}$ index based on biomass, for all collection sites, were found for 1972–1973, 1973–1974, and 1974–1975. The J index based on biomass, for all collection sites was also similar for the last 3 years of the 5-year period (Figure 20.2). The NM index based on biomass showed more dramatic annual variation. Figure 20.3 reveals changes in the d index based on biomass.

Figure 20.4 shows the diversity of the Duplin Estuary based on the number of individuals and the number of species during the study period. In this undisturbed, natural estuary, the number of species and individuals decreased during the 5-year study period; these results were used as an example of the changes in a natural system free from pollution. In 1974–1975 the diversity in the number of species and number of individuals had changed significantly from the species and individuals collected in 1970–1971. The number of species at the Brunswick Estuary collection sites remained almost constant over the 5 years, whereas the number of individuals declined; if the data from the Terry Creek collection site are excluded, the number of individuals and the number of species demonstrate a similar pattern of change.

In the Duplin Estuary collection sites there was an annual decrease in the number of species and the biomass of each species (Figure 20.5), but during 1972–1973 there was a peak in the Terry Creek collection area, the Brunswick collection sites combined, and the Brunswick collection sites with the exception of the Terry Creek collection area.

In order to assess the changes in the diversity index based on the pollution abatement procedures instituted at the toxaphene manufacturing plant, a comparison of the changes in the apparent toxaphene concentrations in the

Figure 20.2 J diversity index (based on biomass) for all collection sites, 1970–1975.

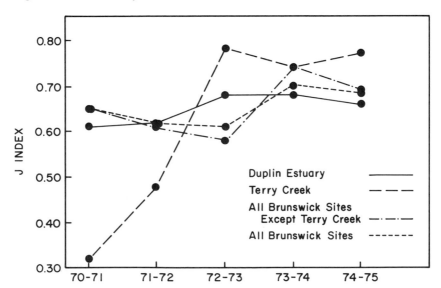

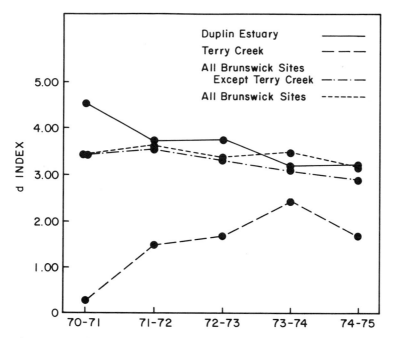

Figure 20.3 *d* diversity index (based on biomass) for all collection sites, 1970–1975.

Figure 20.4 Diversity expressed as the number of species and number of individuals in the Duplin Estuary, 1970–1975 (1970–1973, 12 collections per year; 1973–1975, 6 collections per year).

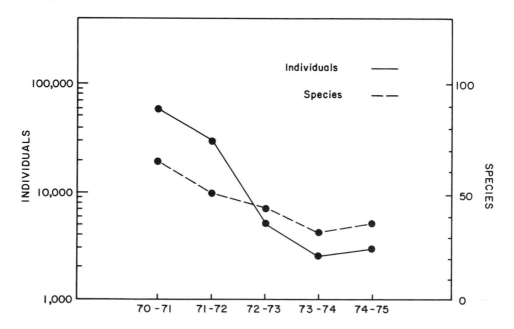

262

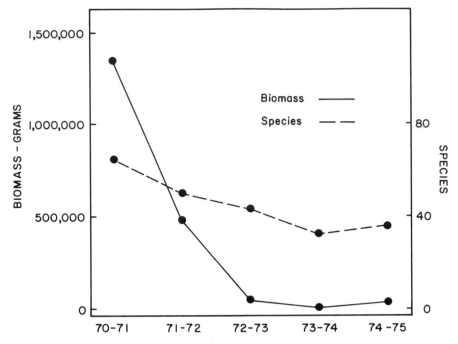

Figure 20.5 Diversity expressed as the number of species and the amount of biomass in the Duplin Estuary, 1970–1975 (1970–1973, 12 collections per year; 1973–1975, 6 collections per year).

Figure 20.6 Monthly average apparent toxaphene concentrations in manufacturing plant effluent, 1970–1975. (Data courtesy of Hercules, Inc., Wilmington, Delaware.)

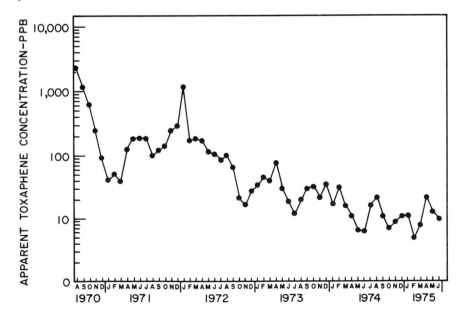

plant effluent was deemed necessary. Hourly samples collected from the effluent stream and analyzed for apparent toxaphene concentration were averaged on a monthly basis. This information, provided by the toxaphene manufacturing plant, is summarized for the 5-year period in Figure 20.6. The apparent toxaphene concentration decreased from greater than 2000 ppb in 1970 to 5 ppb in 1975.

In order to compare the actual biological make-up of the estuarine communities sampled, the species composition, number of individuals, and biomass of the estuarine community were compared. The organisms, numbers of individuals, and biomass for the Duplin Estuary for the 1970–1975 sampling period are given in Table 20.1; the same information for the Brunswick Estuary sites is given in Table 20.2.

Figure 20.7 depicts the percent importance of the six most abundant species from each area for each of four years. The most abundant organisms at all locations were the white shrimp, bay anchovy, and star drum. Similar information exists for all trawls weighted to equal distance. The percent similarity weighted for the observations made with the small net only reveals close groupings of similarities within areas compared, i.e., Duplin Estuary versus Terry Creek, etc. This close grouping of the percent similarity demonstrates the similarity between the two areas being compared.

The number of individuals in a size class (geometric size class 3) is contrasted with the number of species at all locations in Figure 20.8. The similarity in frequency of abundance between the control area (Duplin Sanctuary) and the experimental area (Brunswick Estuary and Terry Creek) can be seen. A log-normal distribution of species abundance for 1973, 1974, and 1975 also documented the similarity of the species sequence.

Dominance, percent similarity, and Euclidean distance for relative abundance per trawl were computed in order to compare the areas. These comparisons were based on equal numbers of trawls at each location. Table 20.3 summarizes the comparisons with all trawl lengths weighted to equal 1.0 km. Comparisons were also made for all trawl lengths weighted to equal 2.0 km. A final comparison involved computation of the coefficient of the community based on relative abundance.

20.4. Discussion

Communities in stable environments often have greater species diversity than those subjected to seasonal or periodic stress. Estuarine communities are naturally subject to numerous physical and chemical stresses. The various ecological community analyses that were performed reveal that over the 5-year study period there were significant variations in the natural, undisturbed Duplin Estuary ecosystem. Since diversity tends to be higher in mature, more ecologically healthy communities, the significant increases in species diversity in Terry Creek (the body of water receiving the effluent from the toxaphene manufacturing plant) indicated an increase in the stability and health of the ecosystem. This 5-year improvement in diversity was inversely related to the significant decrease in the apparent toxaphene content of the manufacturing plant effluent. During the third, fourth, and fifth years, diversity became statistically similar in all the areas considered.

Table 20.1 Number of Individuals and Biomass of Species in Trawl Collections from the Duplin Estuary, 1970–1975

Species	Common name	1970–1971	
		No.	Biomass (g)
Acipenser oxyrhynchus	Atlantic sturgeon	1	758
Alpheus normani	Snapping shrimp	19	96
Aluterus schoepfi	Orange filefish	7	26
Anchoa mitchilli	Bay anchovy	4,071	10,375
Ancylopsetta quadrocellata	Ocellated flounder	19	283
Archosargus probatocephalus	Sheepshead	2	2,331
Arius felis	Sea catfish	851	31,091
Astroscopus y-graecum	Southern stargazer	26	970
Bagre marinus	Gafftopsail catfish	38	856
Bairdiella chrysura	Silver perch	2,528	68,213
Brevoortia tyrannus	Atlantic menhaden	3,972	340,328
Callinectes sapidus	Blue crab	1,334	63,580
Caranx latus	Horse-eye jack	5	214
Carcharhinus limbatus	Blacktip shark	1	2,239
Centropristis philadelphica	Rock sea bass	1	40
Chaetodipterus faber	Atlantic spadefish	207	1,714
Chilomycterus schoepfi	Striped burrfish	23	430
Chloroscombrus chrysurus	Atlantic bumper	109	855
Clupea harengus	Atlantic herring	0	0
Cynoscion regalis	Weakfish	2,332	69,132
Dasyatis americana	Southern stingray	32	63,119
Dorosoma cepedianum	Gizzard shad	716	7,180
Elops saurus	Ladyfish	9	412
Etropus crossotus	Fringed flounder	53	349
Eucinostomus gula	Silver jenny	1	15
Fundulus heteroclitus	Mummichog	0	0
Gobiosoma bosci	Naked goby	3	3
Gymnura micrurc	Smooth butterfly ray	2	41,314
Harengula pensacolae	Scaled sardine	217	1,606
Hypsoblennius hentzi	Feather blenny	127	614
Ictalurus catus	White catfish	0	0
Ictalurus punctatus	Channel catfish	1	182
Lagocephalus laevigatus	Smooth puffer	10	204
Lagodon rhomboides	Pinfish	0	0
Larimus fasciatus	Banded drum	76	193
Leiostomus xanthurus	Spot	3,116	122,240
Lepisosteus osseus	Longnose gar	82	179,125
Lobotes surinamensis	Tripletail	1	399
Loligo brevirostrum	Squid	1,373	17,149
Lutjanus griseus	Gray snapper	0	0
Menidia menidia	Atlantic silverside	0	0
Menticirrhus americanus	Southern kingfish	200	9,736
Micropogon undulatus	Atlantic croaker	783	20,215
Mugil cephalus	Striped mullet	55	1,118
Oligoplites saurus	Leatherjacket	2	24
Opsanus tau	Oyster toadfish	28	1,194
Orthopristis chrysoptera	Pigfish	10	262
Palaemonetes pugio	Grass shrimp	0	0
Paralichthys dentatus	Summer flounder	170	0
Penaeus aztecus	Brown shrimp	718	5,147

1971–1972		1972–1973		1973–1974		1974–1975	
No.	Biomass (g)	No.	Biomass (g)	No.	Biomass (g)	No.	Biomass (g)
0	0	0	0	0	0	0	0
0	0	0	0	0	0	1	4
6	28	1	15	0	0	1	1
1,476	2,254	325	630	274	448	146	270
0	0	0	0	0	0	0	0
0	0	0	0	0	0	0	0
408	28,535	38	1,936	19	676	91	2,833
14	437	4	18	1	2	1	2
78	1,155	70	736	9	56	12	101
1,158	18,785	235	3,992	54	310	264	5,167
416	35,786	0	0	25	710	13	475
555	44,136	115	7,025	134	4,393	63	6,897
41	362	0	0	0	0	0	0
0	0	0	0	0	0	0	0
8	316	1	49	0	0	0	0
677	6,778	17	266	61	275	10	50
24	505	3	158	2	93	1	13
149	828	10	113	32	77	34	100
1	24	3	30	0	0	1	1
1,569	31,646	65	1,449	50	271	63	1,197
5	11,188	9	8,240	1	524	3	15,533
24	131	0	0	2	84	1	11
0	0	0	0	0	0	0	0
81	513	4	54	3	18	14	122
1	5	1	7	1	12	0	0
96	375	0	0	0	0	0	0
0	0	0	0	1	1	0	0
0	0	0	0	0	0	0	0
0	0	0	0	0	0	0	0
0	0	2	30	2	10	0	0
0	0	1	154	2	14	0	0
0	0	0	0	0	0	0	0
8	47	0	0	0	0	0	0
0	0	1	32	0	0	0	0
8	14	0	0	0	0	0	0
956	50,668	118	3,066	50	1,041	53	2,435
3	4,736	2	4,202	1	1,004	1	2,247
0	0	0	0	0	0	0	0
477	5,659	209	2,273	40	212	61	476
2	16	0	0	0	0	0	0
10	73	5	18	0	0	0	0
229	5,672	25	847	9	276	23	1,149
752	20,568	133	3,227	113	1,136	124	1,640
34	536	0	0	0	0	1	15
0	0	0	0	0	0	0	0
6	209	10	359	0	0	5	309
28	408	2	84	0	0	0	0
0	0	0	0	0	0	2	1
45	0	11	0	4	206	2	311
592	6,732	50	615	22	214	64	607

(Continued)

Table 20.1 Number of Individuals and Biomass of Species in Trawl Collections from the Duplin Estuary, 1970–1975 *(continued)*

		1970–1971	
Species	Common name	No.	Biomass (g)
Penaeus duorarum	Pink shrimp	55	662
Penaeus setiferus	White shrimp	33,342	205,257
Peprilus alepidotus	Harvestfish	149	6,991
Peprilus triacanthus	Butterfish	0	0
Pogonias cromis	Black drum	1	6,079
Pomatomus saltatrix	Bluefish	32	2,499
Prionotus tribulus	Bighead searobin	111	578
Rhinoptera bonasus	Cownose ray	2	17,444
Rissola marginata	Striped cusk-eel	5	49
Sciaenops ocellata	Red drum	0	0
Scomberomorus maculatus	Spanish mackerel	108	4,480
Scophthalmus aquosus	Windowpane	16	80
Selene vomer	Lookdown	175	2,217
Sphoerides maculatus	Northern puffer	16	77
Sphyrna zygaena	Smooth hammerhead shark	2	2,622
Squilla empusa	Mantis shrimp	43	316
Stellifer lanceolatus	Stardrum	911	6,050
Symphurus plagiusa	Blackcheek tonguefish	616	13,103
Syngnathus floridae	Dusky pipefish	4	31
Synodus foetens	Inshore lizardfish	3	115
Trichiurus lepturus	Atlantic cutlassfish	50	1,232
Trinectes maculatus	Hogchoker	50	1,496
Urophycis floridanus	Southern hake	78	2,045

1971–1972		1972–1973		1973–1974		1974–1975	
No.	Biomass (g)	No.	Biomass (g)	No.	Biomass (g)	No.	Biomass (g)
48	410	21	136	2	25	1	3
17,522	156,163	2,895	19,258	698	6,920	1,366	8,245
84	1,409	0	0	0	0	0	0
1	34	0	0	0	0	0	0
0	0	0	0	0	0	0	0
10	424	0	0	0	0	1	70
60	211	5	26	2	77	3	17
0	0	0	0	0	0	0	0
7	146	1	38	0	0	0	0
0	0	2	10	0	0	1	2
21	502	0	0	0	0	0	0
0	0	0	0	0	0	0	0
38	179	6	70	0	0	2	17
0	0	3	12	0	0	0	0
0	0	0	0	0	0	0	0
22	110	7	129	1	12	0	0
2,058	21,538	653	7,296	974	2,860	688	3,946
411	8,436	162	3,468	64	1,374	83	1,843
3	23	0	0	0	0	0	0
10	811	0	0	0	0	0	0
5	78	1	10	0	10	0	0
37	1,241	6	233	3	103	1	22
0	0	15	0	0	0	0	0

Table 20.2 Number of Individuals and Biomass of Species in Trawl Collections from all Brunswick Estuary Collection Sites, 1970–1975

Species	Common name	1970–1971 No.	1970–1971 Biomass (g)
Alpheus normani	Snapping shrimp	10	20
Aluterus schoepfi	Orange filefish	0	0
Anchoa mitchilli	Bay anchovy	355	597
Anguilla rostrata	American eel	1	311
Archosargus probatocephalus	Sheepshead	0	0
Arius felis	Sea catfish	85	794
Bagre marinus	Gafftopsail catfish	0	0
Bairdiella chrysura	Silver perch	18	436
Brevoortia tyrannus	Atlantic menhaden	199	11,118
Callinectes sapidus	Blue crab	63	5,679
Caranx latus	Horse-eye jack	0	0
Centropristis philadelphica	Rock sea bass	0	0
Chaetodipterus faber	Atlantic spadefish	0	0
Chilomycterus schoepfi	Striped burrfish	0	0
Chloroscombrus chrysurus	Atlantic bumper	0	0
Cynoscion regalis	Weakfish	29	1,309
Dasyatis americana	Southern stingray	0	0
Dorosoma cepedianum	Gizzard shad	0	0
Elops saurus	Ladyfish	0	0
Etropus crossotus	Fringed flounder	15	235
Eucinostomus gula	Silver jenny	0	0
Fundulus heteroclitus	Mummichog	230	3,181
Gobiosoma bosci	Naked goby	14	30
Hypsoblennius hentzi	Feather blenny	1	2
Ictalurus catus	White catfish	0	0
Ictalurus punctatus	Channel catfish	1	202
Lagodon rhomboides	Pinfish	0	0
Larimus fasciatus	Banded drum	8	47
Leiostomus xanthurus	Spot	126	4,736
Lepisosteus osseus	Longnose gar	0	0
Loligo brevirostrum	Squid	4	57
Lutjanus griseus	Gray snapper	0	0
Menticirrhus americanus	Southern kingfish	1	2
Micropogon undulatus	Atlantic croaker	17	144
Mugil cephalus	Striped mullet	0	0
Opsanus tau	Oyster toadfish	0	0
Palaemonetes pugio	Grass shrimp	9	4
Paralichthys dentatus	Summer flounder	7	545
Penaeus aztecus	Brown shrimp	22	201
Penaeus duorarum	Pink shrimp	13	57
Penaeus setiferus	White shrimp	386	4,185
Peprilus alepidotus	Harvestfish	0	0
Pogonias cromis	Black drum	0	0
Pomatomus saltatrix	Bluefish	0	0
Prionotus tribulus	Bighead searobin	2	7
Sciaenops ocellata	Red drum	1	2
Scophthalmus aquosus	Windowpane	1	44
Selene vomer	Lookdown	0	0
Squilla empusa	Mantis shrimp	3	13
Stellifer lanceolatus	Star drum	146	1,247
Symphurus plagiusa	Blackcheek tonguefish	31	704
Syngnathus floridae	Dusky pipefish	0	0
Synodus foetens	Inshore lizardfish	0	0
Trichiurus lepturus	Atlantic cutlassfish	1	13
Trinectes maculatus	Hogchoker	7	39

| 1971–1972 | | 1972–1973 | | 1973–1974 | | 1974–1975 | |
No.	Biomass (g)	No.	Biomass (g)	No.	Biomass (g)	No.	Biomass (g)
4	9	1	3	0	0	2	1
1	1	0	0	0	0	0	0
1,577	2,019	585	828	266	480	135	226
4	803	6	1,847	2	577	0	0
1	8	0	0	0	0	1	18
3	491	31	823	9	698	10	726
5	33	3	58	1	11	1	2
156	2,637	237	4,665	160	1,621	140	2,034
13	905	7	285	1	151	4	476
180	9,131	175	9,517	109	4,513	25	3,528
2	5	0	0	0	0	0	0
0	0	1	24	1	9	0	0
4	51	7	22	9	30	1	13
1	2	0	0	3	32	0	0
1	16	0	0	1	1	0	0
8	514	74	3,620	54	621	29	1,299
0	0	0	0	1	557	1	10
1	2	11	155	3	11	1	8
0	0	4	53	0	0	0	0
5	17	3	23	1	3	3	11
5	74	0	0	6	46	0	0
224	2,084	7	423	13	120	1	8
1	0	0	0	0	0	0	0
0	0	1	10	0	0	0	0
1	261	12	3,588	0	0	0	0
0	0	0	0	0	0	0	0
0	0	1	13	0	0	0	0
0	0	1	129	0	0	0	0
167	10,360	348	24,318	40	2,436	56	2,366
0	0	0	0	1	512	1	855
18	64	54	199	53	205	14	82
0	0	0	0	0	0	1	22
4	12	0	0	1	2	3	143
70	1,171	168	2,968	51	753	117	1,166
4	451	9	456	1	143	14	1,534
1	451	0	456	1	143	2	1,534
38	17	6	2	2	3	1	< 1
3	377	5	410	8	761	2	137
49	437	90	755	76	892	53	265
9	31	32	248	2	26	4	27
1,301	10,625	2,073	14,920	239	1,771	1,029	6,958
0	0	1	266	0	0	0	0
0	0	1	158	0	0	0	181
0	0	1	3	0	0	0	0
9	12	1	9	0	0	1	3
0	0	0	0	0	0	0	0
0	0	0	0	0	0	0	0
5	15	1	1	3	19	1	8
8	52	5	64	11	43	0	0
489	2,745	585	7,590	187	754	320	1,264
67	1,190	55	1,059	10	234	20	452
1	1	0	0	0	0	0	0
0	0	0	0	0	0	1	38
1	17	2	269	1	0	0	0
11	115	6	82	5	112	0	0

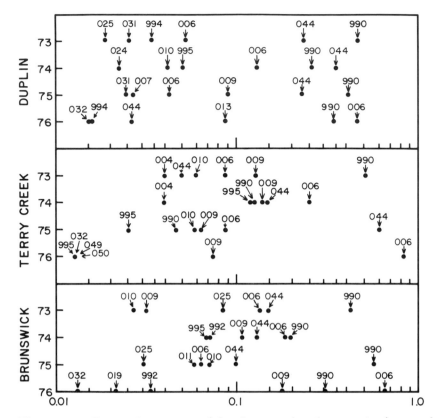

Figure 20.7 Percent importance of the six most abundant species from each area based on the number of individuals using all the data from all trawls from the Duplin, Terry Creek, and Brunswick Estuaries during study years 1972–1973 (73), 1973–1974 (74), 1974–1975 (75), and 1975–1976 (76). Species identification: *004*, mummichog; *006*, bay anchovy; *007*, sea catfish; *009*, silver perch; *010*, Atlantic croaker; *011*, gafftopsail catfish; *013*, bumper; *019*, Atlantic menhaden; *024*, spadefish; *025*, spot; *031*, blackcheek tonguefish; *032*, weakfish; *044*, star drum; *049*, Atlantic herring; *050*, threadfin herring; *990*, white shrimp; *992*, brown shrimp; *994*, squid; *995*, blue crab.

Species diversity indices are considered to be one of the best means of evaluating pollution. Diversity tends to be low in physically or chemically stressed or controlled systems and high in biologically controlled ecosystems. The 5-year study described here appears to be one of the longest continous assessments of diversity indices of nekton in a natural undisturbed estuarine ecosystem contrasted simultaneously with the changes in an estuary receiving effluent from a toxaphene manufacturing plant. The improvement in the ecological community parameters in the estuary receiving the toxaphene man-ufacturing plant effluent was associated with pollution abatement procedures at the plant.

In another study, apparent toxaphene concentration was found to be decreas-ing in fauna, flora, and substrate collected from the Brunswick Estuary. In that study, toxaphene analyses of the biota were conducted at 4-week intervals, simultaneously with the species diversity collections associated with the other study. The decreases in toxaphene content of the biota were correlated with the

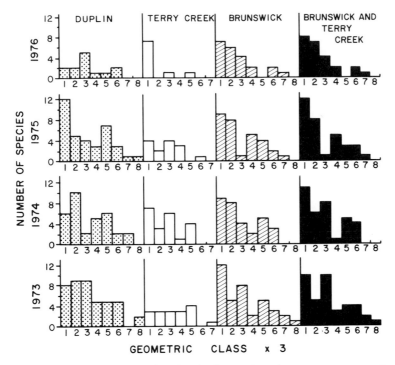

Figure 20.8 Number of individuals in size classes versus number of species at all locations, based on all data from all trawls (geometric scale). Geometric classes *1*, 1 individual; *2*, 2–4 individuals; *3*, 5–13 individuals; *4*, 14–40 individuals; *5*, 41–121 individuals; *6*, 122–364 individuals; *7*, 365–1093 individuals; *8*, 1094–3280 individuals.

Table 20.3 Comparisons of Dominance, Percent Similarity, and Euclidean Distance for Relative Abundance per Trawl Weighted for (0.1-km) Trawl Length (D = Duplin; TC = Terry Creek; BR = Brunswick)

	Dominance			
Year	D	TC	BR	B + TC
1973	0.310786	0.280419	0.217244	0.234030
1974	0.289662	0.136049	0.126337	0.130415
1975	0.266978	0.362737	0.342039	0.292099
1976	0.507333	0.804841	0.418089	0.431444

	Percent similarity					
Year	D–T	D–B	D–(B+TC)	T–B	T–(B+TC)	B–(B+TC)
1973	0.71171	0.73796	0.77165	0.67938	0.73777	0.94161
1974	0.52852	0.59524	0.58920	0.76867	0.81133	0.95734
1975	0.49931	0.74195	0.79802	0.45780	0.52307	0.93473
1976	0.56055	0.78876	0.77510	0.69725	0.71413	0.98311

	Euclidean distance					
Year	D–T	D–B	D–(B+TC)	T–B	T–(B+TC)	B–(B+TC)
1973	0.16185	0.13015	0.12236	0.13843	0.11294	0.02983
1974	0.26438	0.24215	0.24276	0.10300	0.08441	0.02213
1975	0.35667	0.15572	0.10412	0.49219	0.43223	0.05997
1976	0.30619	0.18169	0.19033	0.27091	0.25554	0.01547

dramatic increases in diversity of the estuarine nekton. However, during the EPA National Estuarine Monitoring Program, toxaphene was never found in biota from any collection sites in Georgia or South Carolina.

Several factors that may regulate diversity include niche size and overlap, natural environmental stress, man-induced environmental stress (pollutants), productivity, competition, trophic structure of the community, and space. In reviewing the changes in diversity as expressed by the various indices, it becomes evident that any assessment of pollution stress must include several indices of diversity to reflect both the number of individuals and the biomass of the community.

Suggested Reading

Boesch, D. F. Species diversity of marine macrobenthos in the Virginia area. Chesapeake Sci. 13:206–212, 1972.

Copeland, B. J., Bechtel, T. J. Species diversity and water quality in Galveston Bay, Texas. Water, Air, Soil Pollut. 1:89–105, 1971.

Environmental Protection Agency. Proposed Criteria for Water Quality, Vol. 1. Washington, D. C., 1973.

Hutcheson, K. A test for comparing diversities based on the Shannon formula. J. Theor. Biol. 29:151–154, 1970.

Livingston, R. J. Impact of kraft pulp-mill effluents on estuarine and coastal fishes in Apalachee Bay, Florida, U.S.A. Marine Biol. 32:19–48, 1973.

Margalef, D. R. Information theory in ecology. General Systems 3:21–36, 1958.

National Academy of Sciences and National Academy of Engineering Water Quality Criteria, 1972. EPA-R3-73-033. Washington, D. C.: Environmental Protection Agency, 1972. third edition.

Odum, E.P. Fundamentals of Ecology, Philadelphia: Saunders, 1971, pp. 140–161.

Pielou, E. C. The measurement of diversity in different types of biological collections. J. Theor. Biol. 13:131–144, 1966.

Wilhm, J.L. Comparison of some diversity indices applied to populations of benthic macroinvertebrates in a stream receiving organic wastes. J. Water Pollut. Control. Fed. 39:1673–1683, 1967.

E. D. Ermenc

21

Case History:
Air Pollution Control in Cincinnati

21.1. History and Demography

Cincinnati is a city of 420,000 inhabitants located on the Ohio River in the southwest corner of the State of Ohio. The city covers an area of 78 square miles but is a part of an air pollution control region covering four counties in Ohio, two counties in Indiana, and three counties in Kentucky. The City of Cincinnati, Division of Air Pollution Control has jurisdiction over those four counties in Ohio: Hamilton, Butler, Clermont, and Warren Counties. This area covers 1700 square miles and services 1,300,000 inhabitants.

Many people think air pollution control is of relatively recent vintage; however, the first action on smoke abatement in Cincinnati was taken in 1886. The first smoke ordinance to reduce emissions was passed in 1903, and an engineer was appointed to be Chief Smoke Inspector in 1914.

Minor modifications were made to the city ordinances over the years until 1947, when low-volatile coal (maximum 26% volatiles) was prescribed for residential heating and industrial restrictions on fly ash emissions (0.85 lb/1000 lb gases) were instituted; installation permits were required plus specifications on boiler construction. By 1969 the emphasis changed from a mechanically oriented to a chemically oriented program, and the City of Cincinnati passed an ordinance restricting smoke plume to 40% maximum opacity, particulate matter emissions on boilers to 0.3 lb solids/1000 lb gases for new facilities and 0.5 lb solids/1000 lb for existing facilities; coal sulfur content was restricted to 1.25%. In addition to the emissions standards, ambient air standards were established for sulfur oxides (0.02 ppm maximum annual average) and total suspended particulate matter (TSP; 100 μg/m^3 maximum annual average).

After the Clean Air Act of 1970 was passed by Congress and the State of Ohio established emissions and ambient air standards, the City of Cincinnati established more stringent standards in 1972 as promulgated by the State of Ohio. The ambient air standards are shown in Table 21.1, and the Kentucky and Indiana standards are given as well.

Table 21.1   Ambient Air Quality Standards for Ohio, Kentucky, and Indiana

Pollutant	Ohio	Ky.	Ind.
Sulfur oxides (μg/m^3)			
Annual arithmetic mean	60	80	80
24-hr conc.	260	365	365
Particulate matter (μg/m^3)			
Annual geometric mean	60	75	75
24-hr conc.	150	260	260
Carbon monoxide (mg/m^3)			
8-hr conc.	10	10	10
1-hr conc.	—	40	40
Photochemical oxidants (μg/m^3)			
24-hr conc.	40	—	—
4-hr conc.	79	—	—
1-hr conc.	119[a]	160	160
Hydrocarbons (μg/m^3)			
3-hr conc. (6 a.m.–9 a.m.)	126	160	160
Nitrogen dioxide (μg/m^3)			
Annual arithmetic mean	100	100	100

[a]Not to be exceeded.

21.2. Legislation and Resultant Action

The Federal Air Quality Act of 1967 started the new era of chemically oriented air pollution control, but insufficient monies were appropriated to move the program along. It wasn't until passage of the Clean Air Act of 1970 that sufficient funds were allocated by Congress to provide the necessary impetus to local and state agency programs. The Clean Air Act of 1970 also established the new EPA, which took over the reins from the Department of Health, Education and Welfare.

The State of Ohio provided an implementation plan, as required under the Clean Air Act of 1970, and both ambient air and emission standards were set up. Citizen input at public hearings held around the state resulted in more stringent ambient air standards in Ohio than in Kentucky and Indiana (Table 21.1).

The City of Cincinnati had instituted an Intercommunity Program in the middle 1950s, and seven suburban communities (Lockland, Wyoming, Glendale, St. Bernard, Arlington Heights, Elmwood Place, and Reading) for a nominal fee, joined in it, setting and regulating air pollution control standards; by 1970 two additional cities (Evendale and Sharonville) had been added for a total of nine. As a result of the increasing emphasis on air pollution control, the State of Ohio requested the Cincinnati agency to consider extending air pollution control to the counties of Hamilton, Butler, Clermont, and Warren. Seed money of $57,500 was proffered by the State if the four counties could be signed up to accept air pollution control. By 1972 Hamilton, Butler, and Warren Counties had agreed to join with the State in air pollution control under the aegis of the City of Cincinnati. As a result, the EPA granted $115,000 to further add to the program's effectiveness.

The Clean Air Act of 1970 required that standards be met by July 1, 1975; this date was extended to April 15, 1977, when standards were not met. The problem of noncompliance required the immediate attention of Congress, but several years passed before the Clean Air Act Amendments of 1977 were passed. These amendments required the following:

1. Present stationary facilities emitting sulfur oxides and TSP must be in compliance by July 1, 1979.
2. Stationary facilities emitting ozone-oriented pollutants and carbon monoxide were required to be in compliance by no later than July 1, 1982.
3. Mobile sources (automobiles) required evaluation of strategies to meet ozone standards by July 1, 1982.
4. Based upon good faith efforts, the deadline in item 3 could be extended to July 1, 1987.

Two controversial concepts were confirmed by the Clean Air Act Amendments of 1977: one requires industry to "offset" emissions in noncompliance areas where new plants are to be built; the second, Prevention of Significant Deterioration (PSD), requires a 1-year period of monitoring a specific site in a compliance area before any construction can begin (see Section 21.5). Up to 2.5 years could elapse before a construction permit is granted.

21.3. Monitor Systems

It would be impossible to conduct an air pollution control program without knowing the concentrations of the various pollutants in the atmosphere; hence a well-planned monitoring system must be provided. Figure 21.1 shows the extent

Figure 21.1 Monitoring sites in Cincinnati in 1969. There were no sites in the four-county area of southwestern Ohio.

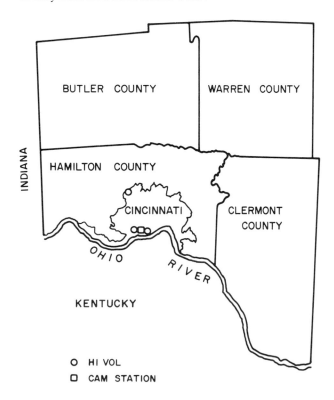

of monitoring for the City of Cincinnati in 1969—1 continuous automatic monitor (CAM) station and 3 Hi-Vol stations. By 1978, 6 CAM, 39 Hi-Vol, and 10 bubbler stations were on line. Figure 21.2 shows the improvement in the monitoring system as of 1978. Simply put, a Hi-Vol is a glorified vacuum cleaner in which a paper filter catches the atmospheric dirt over a period of 24 hr. The concentration is easily determined from knowledge of the volume of air handled. The system was designed to provide a systematic measure of concentrations of pollutants in the area.

The greater number of meters are located in the areas where the industrial concentration is the greatest, the Cincinnati area (Figure 21.2). As the rural areas are reached, the number of measuring instruments is decreased due to the lower concentrations of contaminants present. The variables measured and types of continuous measuring instruments are shown in Table 21.2.

21.4. Pollutants

The two primary pollutants, sulfur oxides and suspended particulate matter, result from the use of coal by many utilities and industries. Chemical processes are other major contributors of sulfur oxides and suspended particulate matter. Table 21.1 shows the standards adopted by Kentucky and Indiana, and the more

Figure 21.2   Expansion of monitoring sites in the four-county area of southwestern Ohio from 1969 to 1978 as a result of the Clean Air Act of 1970.

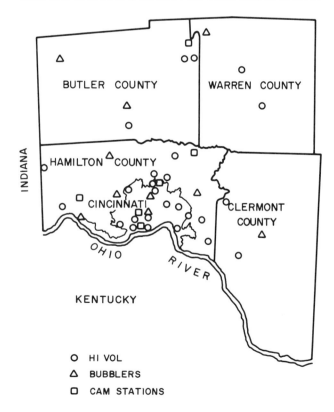

Table 21.2 Parameters Measured and Instrument Types Used at Continuous Automatic Monitor Sites in Southwestern Ohio, 1976

Site	SO₂ (ppm)	Part. COHS	NO (ppm)	NO₂ (ppm)	O₃ (ppm)	CO (ppm)	Total hydrocarbons (ppm)	Methane (ppm)	Wind speed (mph)	Wind direction	Ambient air temp.	Dew point	Source of funds to purchase	Source of funds to operate
Drake	ML 8100 (colorimetric)	RAC 5000 (light transmission)	ML 8100 (colorimetric)	ML 8100 (colorimetric)	Beckman 950 (chem.)	Intertech URAS-2 NDIR	MSA PN455874 FID	MSA PN455874 FID	Climet 011-1	Climet 012-10	Yellow Springs 700	Yellow Springs 91	City	City
Univ. Cam	ML 8100	RAC 5000	ML 8100	ML 8100	ML 8400 (chem.)	Intertech URAS-2	Beckman 400 FID	Beckman 400	Climet 011-1	Climet 012-10	Yellow Springs 700	Yellow Springs 91	City	City
Sycamore Cam	ML 8100		McMillan 1200 (chem.)	McMillan 1200 (chem.)	ML 8400	Beckman 865-17 NDIR	Beckman 400	Beckman 400	Climet 011-1	Climet 012-10	Climet 015-3	Climet 015-12	Hamilton County	Hamilton County
Middletown Cam	Beckman 906A (coulometric)				Beckman 950	MSA Lira 202 NDIR							Federal and state	Federal and state
Gest St. Lab.	Beckman 906A		Bendix 5513802 (chem.)	Bendix 5513802 (chem.)	Beckman 950	Beckman 865-17-7-3							City	City
Batavia	Beckman 906A				Beckman 950								Clermont County	Federal and state
Lebanon					Beckman 950								Federal and state	Federal and state

Note: COHS, coefficient of haze; ML, Monitor Laboratories; RAC, Research Appliance Corp.; MSA, Mine Safety Appliance; NDIR, nondispersive infrared; FID, flame ionization detector.

stringent standards adopted by Ohio. Since the City of Cincinnati, by law, could only adopt standards no less stringent than those of the State of Ohio, those regulations were adopted.

The secondary pollutants are primarily from automobile emissions: carbon monoxide, hydrocarbons, nitrogen oxides, and photochemical oxidants. The standards are given in Table 21.1. Considerable discussion has been generated in 1977–1978 regarding the loosening of standards for several pollutants and changes may be made in the future.

Four other pollutants have been formally adopted for control: asbestos, beryllium, lead, and mercury. Most areas have to contend with asbestos and lead; beryllium and mercury are distributed less generously.

21.4.1. Suspended Particulate Matter

As an example of how the Hi-Vol data are handled, an isopleth is shown in Figure 21.3. Thus, it is possible to detect areas of low or high pollution immediately without going through the time-consuming process of reading individual values.

The major sources of suspended particulate matter are the utilities burning coal. Pulverized coal is utilized, resulting in heavy emissions of fly ash unless

Figure 21.3 Isopleths of suspended particulate matter in the four-county area of southwestern Ohio, 1976.

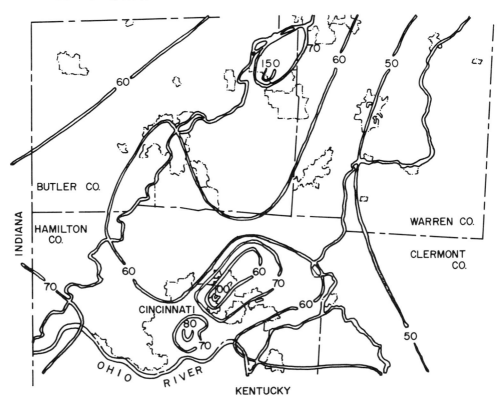

controlled by suitable pollution control devices such as multiclones, electrostatic precipitators, bag houses, etc.

Every control officer is particularly concerned about the improvement of air quality over a period of years. Due to the effect of weather on pollutant concentrations, it is not pertinent to compare any single year's value with another, and only a 5–10-year comparison can be significant. The values from the central core of the City of Cincinnati over the past 15 years have been plotted in Figure 21.4; the continuing trend downward is very significant, indicating that the control program is working.

21.4.2. Sulfur Oxides

The history of sulfur oxides concentrations in Cincinnati shows a marked improvement over the years, as seen in Figure 21.5. The values shown were recorded in the heart of the city and reflect the shift from the usage of coal to natural gas. An ordinance was passed in 1970 that the sulfur content of coal could not exceed 1.25% in the City of Cincinnati area. This standard was changed to 1.0% in 1972 to conform with the new State standard of 1.6 lb $SO_2/10^6$ Btu.

In the period of time reflected in Figure 21.5, the utilization of coal in the Cincinnati area dropped from over 1,000,000 tons/year to approximately 350,000 tons/year, with natural gas substituted for coal. Thus the drop in coal usage was fundamental in reducing concentrations of sulfur oxides in the ambient air. This

Figure 21.4 Improvement in suspended particulate matter concentrations in ambient air in Cincinnati, 1960–1976.

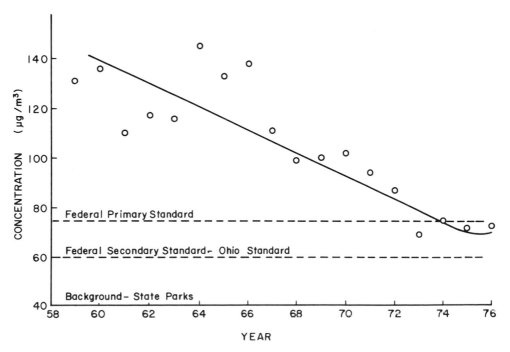

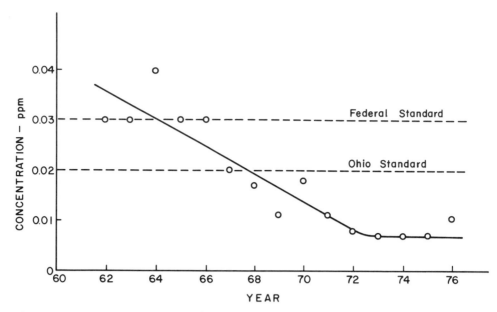

Figure 21.5   Improvement in sulfur concentrations in ambient air in Cincinnati, 1962–1976.

reduction in coal usage also had a marked effect on the suspended particulate matter concentrations in the city.

A specific major factor in the reduction of sulfur oxides in the Cincinnati area was a fuel change in the Front Street Station of the Cincinnati Gas and Electric Company located on the Ohio River in the central part of the city. In 1967, natural gas was substituted for pulverized coal, resulting in a marked drop in ambient air concentrations of sulfur oxides as well as suspended particulate matter.

21.4.3. Carbon Monoxide

Generally, carbon monoxide values are on the high side when measured within 70 ft of either side of the major throughways of any city. Only one of these stations in the City of Cincinnati has occasionally shown values exceeding the carbon monoxide ambient air standard, and this station is within 100 ft of a major artery.

21.4.4. Ozone (Hydrocarbons and Nitrogen Oxides)

Smog is composed of ozone and photochemical oxidants. Ozone (O_3) is the allotropic form of oxygen (O_2). Photochemical oxidants are generally peroxidized hydrocarbons, which are formed as very fine particles in the atmosphere and thus reduce visibility. PAN is one form of photochemical oxidants. In the low concentrations that are present in the atmosphere, ozone is a colorless gas; hence a high-ozone day with low photochemical oxidants can still be a clear day. Generally, ozone values comprise 90–95% of the total oxidants, and therefore the dry analytical method provides for determination of ozone alone.

The emissions of unburned gasoline vapor and nitrogen oxides combine in the atmosphere under the proper weather conditions to form ozone and photochemical oxidants. The following weather conditions are favorable to the formation of these compounds:

sunshine (UV)

low cloud cover (less than 50%)

temperatures above 70° F

low wind velocities (less than 5 mph)

stable weather conditions (little change over the previous 24–48 hr)

lack of rain over previous 3–7 days.

It is interesting to note that one of the control points for prediction of ozone values is high nitric oxide concentrations in the morning, which generally presage high ozone values in the afternoon. As morning traffic increases in the summertime, the nitric oxide concentration increases, followed by oxidation of the nitric oxide to nitrogen dioxide and then formation of ozone by early afternoon. Usually, by 6:00 p.m. to 10:00 p.m., ozone values decrease markedly and then reach zero. The chemical cycle can be simply put as follows:

$$N_2 + O_2 \longrightarrow 2\,NO$$
$$2NO + O_2 \longrightarrow 2\,NO_2$$
$$NO_2 \xrightarrow{\text{UV}} NO + (O)$$
$$O_2 + (O) \longrightarrow O_3$$

Ozone can participate in oxidation reactions with hydrocarbons to produce various peroxy-type compounds. Table 21.3 shows the history of ozone concentrations between 1973 and 1977 in Cincinnati, and Figure 21.6 shows a plot of maximum hourly concentration versus years.

21.4.5. Other Pollutants

In 1977 only three other pollutants had been placed under control: asbestos, beryllium, and mercury. Lead should also be placed on the control list in the near future with other heavy metals to follow.

Table 21.3 Days of Ozone Levels over the Federal Standard and the Alert Level, Including the Highest Concentration in Any One Hour, 1973–1977

Year	No. of days over 0.08 ppm federal standard	No. of days over 0.10 ppm alert level	1-hr high (ppm)
1973	56	22	0.187
1974	34	16	0.196
1975	36	19	0.154
1976	77	38	0.172
1977	90	59	0.208

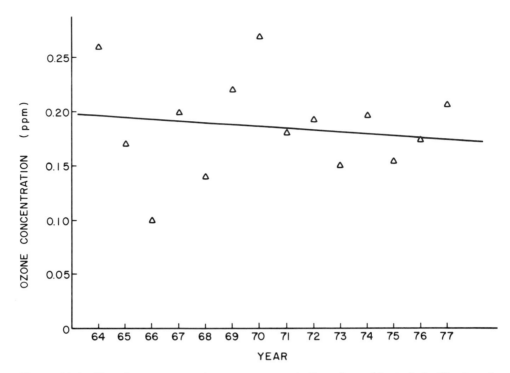

Figure 21.6 Slow improvement in ozone concentrations in ambient air in Cincinnati, 1964–1977. Triangles represent highest values in each year.

Beryllium and mercury were of little concern in Cincinnati since there were no industries using these metals. Most of the problems with mercury have been due to losses from mercury cells producing chlorine and caustic, such as found in the Detroit and other areas. Beryllium problem areas were primarily in the Cleveland and Chicago areas.

Asbestos is a complex magnesium silicate compound and most areas have some exposure to this very useful material. The two primary groups of asbestos are serpentine and amphibole. Serpentine is primarily the white variety known as chrysotile, largely obtained from Quebec, Canada. Of the amphiboles, crocidolite (blue asbestos) and amosite (brown asbestos) are the two commercially available varieties; these two are found in large quantities in South Africa. There are other asbestos crocidolite types but they are of minor commercial importance.

There is evidence that asbestos is a carcinogenic agent over the long term. It is particularly of concern to cigarette smokers who are exposed; it has been indicated that cigarette smokers are 10 times more likely to contract asbestosis or malignant tumors. Those individuals who saw cut asbestos-containing materials such as insulation, millboard, or asbestos–cement materials are the most highly exposed.

Table 21.4 indicates the regulations for asbestos, beryllium, and mercury. Cincinnati enforces the regulations for asbestos, particularly for demolition of old buildings in the area. Old buildings generally contain asbestos-containing insulation and inspectors check out such sites. Samples are removed for

Table 21.4   Regulation Summary for Asbestos, Beryllium, and Mercury

Material	Regulation
Asbestos	Asbestos spray products prohibited Demolition of buildings containing asbestos: permit required; wet down asbestos debris; place asbestos debris in plastic bags; bury debris in landfill not to be disturbed Baghouse for processing asbestos and products
Beryllium	10 g/24 hr maximum
Mercury	2300 g/24 hr maximum for mercury ore processing for mercury cells 3200 g/24 hr maximum for incineration of waste-water treatment plant sludges

examination by experts in the Division of Air Pollution Control and a permit is issued if asbestos is found. The permit provides for surveillance of the site to be sure procedures are followed.

21.5. Standards

The ambient air quality standards for Ohio and the neighboring States of Kentucky and Indiana are shown in Table 21.1. Ohio is in process of changing its standards to those of Kentucky and Indiana, which in turn are replicas of the national standards.

The Clean Air Act Amendments of 1977 provide for different regulations governing compliance and noncompliance areas. A noncompliance area is an area in which ambient air standards are not being met and new industry must provide for an "offset" of the pollutants emitted. In other words, an industry proposing to emit 200 tons/year of hydrocarbons must provide a reduction of at least 200 tons/year from some other source in the area. In addition, the people in the area must provide a reduction in the vehicle miles traveled through various strategies such as car pooling, use of public transportation, reduction in parking places in the congested areas, emission testing of automobiles, etc.

The compliance area is one that meets ambient air standards, and a PSD policy is applied. Thus if ambient air measurements for suspended particulate matter are 50 μg/m³ and the standards are 75 μg/m³, room is available for a new industry to enter the area so long as the standard is not exceeded. It is possible that as long as 2.5 years could be required for an installation permit to be issued to the prospective new industry.

In addition to ambient air standards, emission standards have been promulgated that are theoretically geared to meeting the ambient air standards. These emission standards must be met before an operating permit is granted. Emission standards tables are quite lengthy since many industries are individually covered. However, as an example of a general emission standard, the density of issuing fumes from stacks is an excellent control. Black smoke emitted from boilers is observed for the degree of opacity, which is measured by the inspector's eye by what is known as a Ringelmann number. The Ringelmann number ranges from 0 to 5:0 indicates a clean stack and 5 indicates completely black smoke. White fumes issuing from a stack are also measured by the degree of opacity, but on a different scale. Zero opacity indicates a clean stack and 100% opacity indicates that no light is passing through the plume.

21.6. Air Quality Index System

A new index system as a measure of pollution levels has been proposed by the EPA for national use. Up to this time there has been little uniformity in index systems across the United States. Hence there was no good way for the lay person to evaluate pollution conditions from city to city or state to state other than by concentrations of each pollutant; this type of reporting is too complex for comprehension by the average citizen. An index system with one number representing the air quality is the easiest to understand. Table 21.5 shows the index system correlated with the concentration of pollutants.

The index system ranges from 0 as the indicator of no pollution to 500 as a level of significant harm. Now, how does it work in practice? Hydrocarbons and nitrogen oxides are not shown since ozone is the resultant of the reaction of those compounds in the atmosphere. Generally, in Cincinnati, the summertime index almost always reflects the ozone value. In the winter, the index most often reflects the concentration of suspended particulate matter. Thus, in the summer an index value of 100 would indicate that the ozone standard had been reached; a value of 200 would show alert conditions based on ozone, an unhealthy condition, and industries emitting hydrocarbons would be required to cut back operations. For those persons with lung disabilities (emphysema, bronchitis, etc.), a health alert would be called at an index of 117 (0.10 ppm) to warn them to cut down on physical activity.

Table 21.5 National Index Levels Correlated with Descriptors and Concentrations of Ozone, Suspended Particulates, Sulfur Dioxide, and Carbon Monoxide

Index	Descriptor	O_3 ($\mu g/m^3$)	TSP ($\mu g/m^3$)	SO_2 ($\mu g/m^3$)	CO (mg/m^3)
0		0	0	0	0
100	Standard	160 (0.08)	260	365 (0.140)	10 (9.0)
200	Alert	400 (0.20)	375	800 (0.30)	17 (15.0)
300	Warning	800 (0.40)	625	1600 (0.60)	34 (30.0)
400	Emergency	1000 (0.50)	875	2100 (0.80)	46 (40.0)
500	Significant harm	1200 (0.60)	1000	2620 (1.00)	57.5 (50.0)
Measurement time (hr)		1	24	24	8

Note: Values in parentheses are in parts per million.

21.7. Enforcement

21.7.1. Inspection

The inspection group is the enforcement arm of the Division of Air Pollution Control and consists of two groups, the City Section and the County Section. The City Section covers an area of 78 square miles, and each inspector is assigned a section of approximately 10 square miles to patrol; the County Section covers around 1600 square miles, and sectors per inspector range from 150 square miles to 400 square miles.

Inspectors are the sensory organs of an operating agency and make sure that all facilities are in compliance. Inspectors are required to have a background as an operating engineer (in other words, experience in operating boilers) or experience in process industries. With that type of background the inspectors are better able to understand problems that occur and can recommend improvements to prevent recurrences of violations.

Before citing anyone to court, inspectors will first issue a warning to the violator; should two warnings occur within a 4-month period, a notice to appear (NTA) is issued. The violator is summoned to appear at the Superintendent's office to determine the reasons for the violation and what is to be done to correct the problem. If satisfactory actions are to be taken by the violator to prevent future violations, no further action is taken. Should additional violations occur without satisfactory explanations, the violator can be summoned to appear in court for action by the judiciary.

Inspectors also conduct annual inspections of at least the major industries, defined as those industries emitting over 100 tons/year of pollutants from any source in the facility. Significant sources are those emitting over 25 tons/year and are to be inspected annually as the inspector is able.

21.7.2. Engineering

The engineering group handles all permits covering installations and operations of facilities as well as inspection of more complex facilities where an engineering background is necessary. All plans are reviewed by that group, and emission levels are determined dependent upon the type of control equipment used.

Emissions from all facilities in the area are inventoried annually to determine the reduction in levels from each facility from year to year. The emission inventory is a valuable adjunct to the ambient air levels measured by the monitor system as a means of determining the effectiveness of control measures.

21.8. Transportation Control Program

The prime problem in Cincinnati is high levels of ozone, which run well over the federal standard of 0.08 ppm. As a result the EPA mandated that the City of Cincinnati and Hamilton County institute emission testing of automobiles. The City instituted its program on January 1, 1975, and Hamilton County on August 1, 1975.

The programs were generally not well accepted by the citizenry and considerable criticism was evoked. It was felt that a better public relations program was required and that initially a voluntary effort would be best to introduce the

Table 21.6 Automotive Emission Standards (g/mile), 1968–1981, for Hydrocarbons (HC) Carbon Monoxide, and Nitrogen Oxides Compared with Uncontrolled Emissions for Same Period

Pollutant	Uncontrolled	1968	1973	1975	1977	1980	1981
HC	11	3.4	3.4	1.5	1.5	0.4	0.4
CO	80	39.0	39.0	15.0	15.0	7.0	3.4
NO_x	6	—	3.0	3.0	2.0	2.0	1.0

program. However, the final decision provided for rapid institution of emission testing.

The prime reasons for emission testing are to maintain high efficiency of gasoline usage, thus reducing the hydrocarbon emissions, and to make sure that automobile manufacturers are meeting the standards established by the EPA. Table 21.6 lists the automotive regulations the manufacturers must meet in contrast to the uncontrolled emissions of earlier automobiles.

The period of greatest testing was reached in 1976, when 220,000 cars were tested, about 43% of the cars in Cincinnati and Hamilton County. The year 1977 showed a reduction to about 180,000 cars tested. Once a car has gone through the test lane a windshield sticker is applied; if the car has passed, a valid sticker is applied and testing is complete until the next year. Should the car fail, a temporary sticker is applied and 30 days are granted for correction. Table 21.7 shows the Cincinnati emission regulations, based solely on an idle test.

The failure rate was initially about 30% in 1975, but was reduced to 18% in 1977. Approximately 80–85% of the failures were due to high carbon monoxide emission and about 15–18% to hydrocarbons or both carbon monoxide and hydrocarbons. The remaining failures were for miscellaneous causes, such as heavy tail pipe smoking.

To provide for full compliance with the mandated orders of the EPA, the procurement of a license plate should be tied in with a successful emission test. This action would ensure 100% enforcement of the emission testing law. It is expected that by 1982 most states will have instituted emission testing tied in with license plate procurement.

Table 21.7 Emission Standards (Maximum Allowable) Used on Cincinnati Emission Test Lanes (Idle Test) for Various Model Years of Automobiles

Model Year	Hydrocarbons (ppm)	Carbon monoxide (%)
Pre-1968	1000	6.0
1968–1969	600	5.0
1970–1974	500	4.0
1975 and later	250	1.5

21.9. Financial Aspects

It is interesting to note how the Cincinnati agency grew as a result of the passage of the Clean Air Act of 1970. This act allocated the monies to provide the necessary impetus to enable states and cities to obtain the personnel for proper air pollution control.

Table 21.8 shows the rapid increase in financing that occurred due to funds obtainable from the EPA. The peak in personnel was reached in 1974, but relatively constant funds are now being allocated by both the State of Ohio and the EPA. The fund allocations are provided by the following political entities:

Contributor	Percent of budget
City	30
County	5
State	20
Federal	45
	100

Because the funds are relatively constant, personnel attrition continues to be necessary to keep within budget bounds.

Most agencies are having similar financial difficulties, and it is hoped that corrections will be made in the near future to prevent the loss of all that has been gained in the struggle to control air pollution.

Table 21.8 Budget Growth, Budget Contributors, and Personnel History, Cincinnati Division of Air Pollution Control, 1970–1977

	1970	1971	1972	1973	1974	1975	1976	1977
Funds ($)								
City	150,000	330,000	205,000	260,000	260,000	330,000	340,000	345,000
County	—	—	50,000	50,000	60,000	50,000	50,000	50,000
State	—	60,000	60,000	110,000	258,000	258,000	253,000	253,000
Federal	50,000	170,000	435,000	565,000	581,000	528,000	541,000	541,000
Total	200,000	560,000	750,000	985,000	1,159,000	1,166,000	1,184,000	1,189,000
Personnel(No.)								
City	15	19	23	23	23	21	20	18
County	—	—	—	—	—	—	—	—
State	—	14	15	19	23	19	17	17
Federal	6	6	14	23	23	22	20	23
Total	21	39	52	65	69	62	57	58

Suggested Reading

Air Pollution Engineering Manual. EPA Publ. AP-40. Washington, D.C., 1973.

Air Quality Criteria for Carbon Monoxide. DHEW Publ. AP-62. Washington, D.C., 1970.

Air Quality Criteria for Nitrogen Oxides. DHEW Publ. AP-84. Washington, D.C., 1971.

Air Quality Criteria for Particulate Matter. DHEW Publ. AP-49. Washington, D.C., 1969.

Air Quality Criteria for Photochemical Oxidants. DHEW Publ. AP-63. Washington, D.C., 1970.

Air Quality Criteria for Sulfur Oxides. DHEW Publ. AP-50. Washington, D.C., 1969.

Control Techniques for Carbon Monoxide, Nitrogen Oxide, and Hydrocarbon Emissions from Mobile Sources. DHEW Publ. AP-66. Washington, D.C., 1970.

Control Techniques for Hydrocarbon and Organic Solvent Emissions from Stationary Sources. DHEW Publ. AP-65. Washington, D.C., 1970.

Control Techniques for Particulate Air Pollutants. DHEW Publ. AP-51. Washington, D.C. 1969.

Control Techniques for Sulfur Oxides. DHEW Publ. AP-52. Washington, D.C., 1969.

Ermenc, E. D. Controlling nitrogen oxide emissions. Chem. Eng. 77: 122–125, 1970.

Ermenc, E. D. Careers—Air pollution control. Chem. Eng. 78: 122–125, 1971.

Ermenc, E. D. Odor control by adsorption and odor control by absorption. Air Pollution Control Association Specialty Conference, Pittsburgh, 1977.

Transporation Controls to Reduce Automobile Use and Improve Air Quality in Cities. EPA Publ. 400/11-74-002, Washington, D.C., 1974.

J. R. Bradley, Jr.

22

Pesticide Effects upon the Agroecosystem

22.1. Characteristics of Pesticides

Pesticide use has increased tremendously during the past 30 years; current estimates of the total quantity applied annually in the world exceeds 4×10^9 lb. Approximately one-half of this amount is used in the quest for increased productivity of agricultural crops. This enormous figure will continue to increase with the evolution of agriculture in less developed countries. These countries are currently utilizing only about 8% of the total world pesticide production despite the fact that they include approximately 72% of the world-wide total usable land. Current annual rates of increase in pesticide use in these countries are herbicides 32%, fungicides 25%, and insecticides 21%. The acceleration in demand for chemical pest control in developing countries is due, in part, to the fact that pesticides in general, and herbicides in particular, are relatively new agricultural tools for most countries; as such, their full potential for increasing crop production remains relatively unexploited. Furthermore, it is obvious that the drastic changes in the agroecosystems of less developed countries brought about through "green revolution" technology has intensified losses to pests. Current estimates suggest that by 1985 the pesticide requirements of these countries would have to increase fivefold over 1970–1971 levels before a real impact is felt in food production through a significant reduction in preharvest and postharvest food losses (estimated to be approximately 50% at present).

In the United States, over 0.5×10^9 lb of pesticides are applied just to farm and croplands; 53% are insecticides, 36% herbicides, and 10% fungicides. However, of the nearly 900×10^6 acres of cropland in the United States, only 10% is treated with insecticides, 15% with herbicides, and 0.5% with fungicides. Within the United States, pesticides are not evenly distributed across all areas or crops. For example, nearly 50% of all insecticides used in agriculture are applied to a single crop, cotton. Cotton acreage accounts for only 1.5% of the U.S. cropland and one-half of the cotton acreage is not treated with insecticides.

(Volumes and types of pesticides produced and amounts used on specific crops are discussed in greater detail in Chapter 2.)

22.1.1. Advantages of Pesticides

Pesticides possess several unique characteristics compared to alternative pest management tactics that have led to their typically serving as man's first line of defense against agricultural pests. Among these features are the following:

1. They are highly effective—greater than 90% control of susceptible pest populations can easily be achieved.
2. Their effect upon the pest population is often immediate, so delayed use of the tactic to the point of imminent disaster is possible.
3. Pest populations over very large areas can be brought under control almost immediately, whereas most natural controls have delayed effects and often can be implemented only under specific environmental conditions.
4. They can be conventionally manufactured, transported, stored, and employed as needed.
5. They can be used in much less sophisticated systems with far less understanding of the complexity of interactions occurring within the agroecosystem than can many alternative control methods.

22.1.2. Disadvantages of Pesticides

Pesticides have been associated with increased agricultural productivity, quality, efficiency, and stability since World War II, but serious drawbacks to sole reliance on chemicals for pest control have developed. The most frequently encountered drawbacks have been the following: (a) target pest resurgence following chemical application; (b) destruction of beneficial species, i.e., parasites, predators, pollinators, and alternative hosts; (c) release of secondary pests from the constraints of natural enemies; (d) phytotoxicity and alteration of host plant phenology; (e) selection of resistant strains of pests or species population shifts; (f) residues, hazards, and legal problems; and (g) expense of pesticides in programs characterized by repeated applications.

22.1.2. a. Resurgence of Pest Populations

Croplands are subject to invasion pressure from many actual and/or potential pest species throughout the growing season, and each species has a characteristic population pattern (e.g., multivoltine species may exhibit population peaks corresponding to each generation). Due to this consistent (though not constant) invasion pressure, a pest species may be temporarily eliminated from a field only to become reestablished as soon as conditions become suitable (e.g., after dissipation of toxic insecticidal residues). In some cases, conditions following temporary suppression of a pest may be more favorable for its rapid population growth than beforehand. The reestablishment and rapid growth of a pest population after temporary suppression (as with a pesticide), known as resurgence, is due to a complex of factors differing to some extent in each situation. For a crop growing optimally and with few herbivores present, food and space are not limiting and the stage is set for an invading pest species to realize much of its biotic potential without the constraints of intraspecific or interspecific competition (at least initially). In addition, temporary suppression tactics often remove the natural enemies of pests and these species reinvade and reestablish more slowly than their pest hosts. Consequently, resurging populations experience an initial period of lower than normal natural enemy mortality. The resurgence phenomenon has been observed to be particularly pronounced when insecticides have been applied against certain multivoltine insects. The rapid population rebound after one application often necessitates another application, setting in motion the classical "pesticidal treadmill."

22.1.2.b. Effects on Beneficial Species and Secondary Pests

Pesticides usually have a broad spectrum of activity and are toxic to a wide range of organisms. Repeated applications have a destructive effect upon beneficial species, often resulting in crop fields or orchards becoming "biological deserts" characterized by uniform stands of a single plant species. The consequences of the decimation of parasitic and predaceous organisms may be the eruption of secondary pests formerly held below damaging population levels by natural enemies as well as pest resurgence discussed above. Natural control can also be upset indirectly by disruption of food chains, resulting in the same effect on pest populations. For example, if prey (e.g., aphids or thrips) of omnivorous insect predators such as coccinellids, nabids, geocorids, and chrysopids are eliminated by early season chemical treatments that are harmless to the predators directly, the predator populations would still decline due to starvation or emigration in search of food. A late season invasion of such an area by a mobile pest would result in much more rapid pest population build-up in the absence of predator attack.

Destruction of insect pollinators is often a very serious adverse effect of using insecticides and perhaps arsenical herbicides on crops. The annual value of bee-pollinated crops exceeds $1 billion in the United States. The honeybee is estimated to pollinate 80% of the deciduous fruits, vegetables, legumes, and oil seed crops in addition to annually producing honey and beeswax valued at $50 million. There are countless documented cases of crop pollination problems resulting from insecticide application that caused far greater crop yield reduction than would have been expected from damage by the uncontrolled pest population. A restructuring of the agroecosystem has occurred in areas where frequent insecticide applications to one crop prevented pollination of an adjacent crop, resulting in the latter crop having to be withdrawn from the area. Structural changes of this type are partially responsible for the continued trend toward monoculture in crop production.

22.1.2.c. Effects of Pesticides on the Crop Plant

Many pesticides may and often do affect phenological development of crop plants. Herbicides, for example, must be applied at precise rates dependent upon soil type and other local environmental factors or stunting of the crop species may develop to the ultimate benefit of weed competitors. The organophosphate insecticides, particularly methyl parathion, are known to delay maturity of cotton to the extent that protection from late season insect pests must be prolonged. Some pesticides may cause direct phytotoxicity to the crop plant under certain environmental conditions, rates of use, and timing of applications (some stages of the crop plant are more susceptible than others). Even a moderate phytotoxic response may reduce leaf area, resulting in increased susceptibility to insect herbivores.

22.1.2.d. Pesticide Resistance

The phenomenon of pesticide resistance is a simple matter of genetic selection. Within almost any pest population, there are individuals that are more proficient at detoxifying pesticides or escaping toxic action through behavioral modifications than the remainder of the population. As selection pressure increases through repeated applications, an increasing proportion of the population becomes resistant to the pesticide. The speed at which this process occurs depends upon the pesticide and its use pattern, the genetic make-up of the organisms, and the extent to which the entire population is exposed to the selection pressure. Resistance is certainly one of the major contributors to increased insecticide use in agriculture. This problem now has developed into a frantic race by entomologists to develop new insecticides in order to keep one step ahead of genetic selection in pest populations. In cotton alone there are 33 known species of arthropod pests resistant to one or more insecticides. Resistant strains of plant parasitic fungi are also developing at an alarming rate in response to increased pressure of continuous applications of fungicides.

Resistant strains of formerly susceptible weed species have been slow to develop, but weed species population shifts in response to increased selection pressure by herbicides are well documented. In cotton fields, for example, annual grass weed species (e.g., crabgrass) are declining in importance and far fewer species of annual broadleaf weeds now occur, as specific broadleaf weeds (e.g., velvetleaf, cocklebur, prickly sida) less susceptible to currently used herbicides are becoming predominant.

22.1.2.e. Residues, Hazards, and Legal Problems

Residues, hazards, and legal problems are all functions of the overall pesticide load placed on the agroecosystem. The significance of these problems is at best poorly understood on a world-wide basis because developing countries do not have the technological systems necessary to monitor pesticide distribution and degradation in the environment. (This subject is presented in detail in Chapter 23.)

22.1.2.f. Cost of Pesticide Programs

The production, formulation, packaging, delivery, and application of pesticides require significant quantities of energy. It is estimated that in the United States alone, 500×10^6 gal of fossil fuel equivalents are used annually to produce and apply our pesticides. This is a financial burden on society and the farmer, in addition to a further drain on limited fossil fuel supplies. There is a positive side to increased cost of pesticides, and that is the likelihood that farmers and others responsible for agroecosystem structure will be forced by spiraling costs to develop more energy-efficient systems. Production systems less dependent upon pesticides must be developed immediately for some crops because pest control costs are causing decreased plantings and production shifts to other crops. For example, the increased cost of pest control has resulted in a 50% reduction of cotton acreage in the southeastern United States over the past 5 years and the bulk of that land is now planted to soybeans. These trends magnify the presently serious problem of agroecosystem instability.

22.2. Characteristics of Agroecosystems

The agroecosystems that are subjected to these pesticides are man-altered systems characterized by their simplicity (as compared to natural systems) and sensitivity to disruptive factors. They usually include a group of associated agricultural fields of one to several crop types, adjacent uncultivated areas, the overall conditioning environment, and the total complex of organisms living within the area. In parts of the world, agroecosystems are distinct units spatially separated by geological barriers (e.g., mountain ranges or deserts) or by large expanses of native vegetation (e.g., forest, jungle, or swampland); whereas in other areas, particularly in developed countries, agroecosystems are continuous over rather large land masses (e.g., coastal plains of the southeastern United States and the Mississippi River valley) and are virtually indistinguishable except for changes in host crop complexes and associated organisms. After 30 years of intensive use of pesticides, man is beginning to understand and appreciate the extent and significance of the effects of these chemicals upon agroecosystems.

22.2.1. Causes of Pest Problems in the Agroecosystem

Despite the intensive use of pesticides (especially insecticides), we are currently losing as much of our potential crop yields to pests as we did 30 years ago. For example, the overall percentage of crop losses to diseases and insects has increased even though use of pesticides to control these organisms has increased 10-fold over the same period. One of the excuses most frequently offered for this seeming lack of progress in pest control is that success in pest control has been documented by increased agricultural productivity. While it is obvious that production of food and fiber could not have reached current levels without chemical pesticides, the rationale for continued dependency upon this pest control strategy needs examination. Philip S. Corbet proposed that today's crop pest problems owe their genesis primarily to four separate developments in man's history:

1. The development of agriculture, involving conversion of ecosystems from natural to artificial productivity and the provision of a rich, uniform food substrate for man and pests.
2. The development of economics, involving the use of food as a medium for trade.
3. The development of preventive medicine, involving a reduction in human mortality (without a compensating reduction in natality).
4. The application of high-energy technology to agriculture and its supporting activities, which involves a short-term increase in productivity based on subsidies from fossil fuels and mineral ores.

It seems logical that all crop pest problems owe their creation to the existence of agriculture. Furthermore, the major causes for accelerated pesticide use accompanied by increased crop loss to pests are changes in agroecosystems (in quest of greater productivity of selected crops) that have favored pest population increases as well as pest control strategies of independently operating pest control disciplines that interact in a counterproductive fashion. Paradoxically, the protective cover provided by pesticides is responsible for the following changes in agroecosystems that have produced pest problems which require increased pesticide inputs.

22.2.1.a. Production of Susceptible Crops in High-Risk Areas

In most cases the decision as to whether to produce a crop in an area is determined by suitability of climate and soils with little concern as to the probability of pest attack. The (erroneous) assumption has been that pest problems could be alleviated through pesticides with little regard for economic and environmental considerations. The continued effort to produce sweet corn in the coastal plains of the southern United States provides an excellent example of this problem. Farmers often make as many as 25 insecticide applications in that area to meet fresh-market demands that the produce be free of damage by lepidopterous larvae, whereas in low-risk areas fewer than 5 insecticide applications usually suffice.

22.2.1.b. Increased Susceptibility of Improved Varieties to Pests

Newly developed crop cultivars designed for quality and high yields are usually more susceptible to insects, pathogens, and weeds. Prior to the pesticide era, farmers saved their own planting seed from plants that survived best under the local cultural conditions and produced the highest yield. These genotypes naturally possessed alleles resistant to insects and pathogens as well as competitive to weeds in response to the forces of coevolution. However, crop breeders today usually conduct their genetic selections under a protective blanket of pesticides that excludes development of resistance to pests.

22.2.1.c. Planting Genetically Uniform Crop Cultivars

An objective of modern agriculture has been maximum production, and to meet this goal agroecosystems have been characterized by continuous monocultures of uniform crop stands over wide areas. This practice aims at providing the maximum possible yield of a uniform food substrate for man but inadvertently does the same for pest species. The much publicized southern corn leaf blight epidemic of 1970 that destroyed 25% of the crop in the United States corn belt is an example of the consequences of a narrow germ plasm base within a crop. Prior to 1970 southern corn leaf blight was considered to be a minor disease, largely restricted to the southern United States. However, the 1970 epidemic was caused by the new race, T, of the fungus, which attacked not only the leaves, but also stalk, ears, and other plant parts. Furthermore, race T has a lower optimum temperature, so it was not restricted to the warmer southern corn production region. The new race was designated T because the corn hybrids produced by using the "Texas type" of cytoplasmic male sterility were most susceptible. Unfortunately, at least 80% of the 1970 corn crop consisted of hybrids produced by using the Texas type of cytoplasmic male sterility. The product of that genetically uniform corn crop and environmental conditions favorable to development of the southern corn leaf blight fungus was a crop failure. Such a catastrophe might easily occur with other crops and pests if sound crop production and management strategies are not utilized.

22.2.1.d. Multiple or Successive Cropping

Continuous production of a single plant species on the same land area over successive years or the production of more than one crop during the same year has increased pest outbreaks profoundly. With few exceptions, the second planting of a crop in a specific field (whether it is during the same year or in successive years) can be productive only under a strict pesticide regimen. For example, in North Carolina the insecticide requirements for protection of the first annual planting of silage corn are minimal; however, the second crop can be produced only through repeated insecticide applications for control of fall armyworm and European corn borer. The grape colaspis is one of several pest species that develops damaging populations in soybeans only when rotation is not practiced. Crop rotation is one of man's most powerful tools with which to combat pest populations, but it is often ignored in favor of pesticides if there is a strong economic incentive to produce one crop continuously.

22.2.1.e. Increased Use of Fertilizers and Irrigation

The increased use of chemical fertilizers has drastically altered phenological development and productivity of crop plants. In so doing, pest populations have been presented favorable substrates upon which to develop for longer time periods, often permitting additional annual generations. Fertilizers also may change the plant nutrient ratios in favor of pest reproduction. Increased water availability to crop plants has had a similar effect, especially in arid areas. However, the major effect of irrigation has been the development of large-scale, highly intensive agricultural systems in areas of historically marginal production. The ultimate effect of both fertilizers and irrigation has been increased crop yields, more severe pest problems, and added pesticide load on the agroecosystem.

22.2.1.f. Agroecosystem Structure

Selection of crops produced and ratios of mixed crop systems have a profound effect on crop-associated organisms, beneficial or pest, but seldom are these organisms given consideration during the agroecosystem structuring process. Crop production specialists mold agroecosystems to meet production goals with little regard to whether the systems favor pest or beneficial species. The cropping system may favor pest outbreak through providing food and other requisites for successive generations of mobile, multivoltine species. For example, the corn earworm has essentially changed from a secondary or occasional pest to a key pest in the southeastern United States in response to increased corn acreage, decreased cotton acreage, and a later maturing cotton crop caused by increased use of fertilizers and pesticides. The corn earworm prefers corn to cotton as a host when both are in attractive phenological stages. As recent as 15 years ago, corn and cotton matured essentially at the same time, and the corn earworm rarely developed to damaging levels on cotton. However, a late maturing cotton crop now provides an ideal site for development of the F_3 corn earworm generation well after maturity of corn. The late maturing cotton has bridged the gap from the F_2 to the overwintering population and may be partially responsible for the increased pest status of the corn earworm.

22.2.2. Interactions Between Pest Control Disciplines

Interactions between pest control disciplines often result in a situation in which a control tactic (usually chemical) used in one discipline is counterproductive to the pest management efforts of a second discipline. The most obvious interactions are those involving pesticides since their effects upon segments of the agroecosystem are readily visible. The result of interactions of this type is usually an increased pesticide burden to an already loaded agricultural environment. The extent and severity of interactions between pest control disciplines is poorly understood, and this lack of knowledge frustrates efforts to integrate pest management strategies into programs compatible with the goal of more stable agricultural ecosystems.

22.2.2.a. Interactions Between Weed and Insect Management

Clean culture as associated with chemical weed control severely reduces or eliminates reservoirs and alternative hosts for arthropod natural enemies of key insect pests. The maintenance of pure stands of a single crop plant through use of herbicides is thought to have been responsible for the shift in preference of certain insect species from weed hosts to crop hosts. For example, a cerambycid beetle, *Dectes texanus texanus* (LeConte), is thought to have expanded its host range to include soybean in response to the reduced occurrence of native hosts (e.g., ragweed) brought about through increased herbicide usage.

Herbicides not only affect weed species, but under certain environmental conditions they may alter crop plant growth and development. The effect is often stunted plants that are more susceptible to certain phytophagous insects, resulting in damage thresholds being met or exceeded at much lower population levels. Reduced root system development often follows herbicide application and causes plants to be more susceptible to insects as well as nematodes that feed upon crop roots.

Arsenical herbicides applied as broadcast sprays to cotton fields may interfere with natural control of *Heliothis* species through toxicity to hemipterous predators.

Insecticides applied to protect crop plants from phytophagous insect pests also affect phytophagous insects that feed upon weed roots, stems, leaves, or seeds. The extent to which this interference affects the biological control of weed species is unknown.

22.2.2.b. Interactions Between Disease and Insect Management

The control of parasitic fungi on crop plants is rapidly increasing but not without serious interactions with insect pest management systems. Fungicides used to control plant parasitic fungi may cause a significant reduction in fungal parasites of insect pests and spider mite pests (e.g., *Entomophora*) thereby releasing these pests from the constraints of natural controls, necessitating pesticide applications to relieve another pesticide-induced problem.

Nematicides are known to indirectly affect insect pest populations through disruption of natural controls. Certain nematicides (e.g., aldicarb and carbofuran) are very broad-spectrum biocides, which, when applied to the soil, not only protect the crop root system, but may be transported throughout the plant by its vascular system. These chemicals may reduce beneficial arthropods (e.g., parasites or predators) by direct toxic action or through food chain alterations that cause parasites and predators to emigrate in search of acceptable hosts. The net result of reduced natural enemy populations is usually increased population levels of phytophagous pests. This phenomenon has been documented in soybeans when aldicarb used for nematode control reduced hemipterous predators of the corn earworm, resulting in a fivefold increase in numbers of that pest.

Nematicides also affect seasonal longevity of crop plants by maintaining a functional root system free of nematode damage. Oftentimes this ensures sufficient food supplies for insect pests developing in late season that contribute to the overwintering population. It has been observed that control of nematode pest populations on tobacco with nematicides or resistant tobacco varieties may increase late season tobacco plant biomass and tobacco hornworm larval populations severalfold.

The product of interactions between nematode and insect management tactics is invariably an increased use of pesticides.

22.3. Conclusions

Pesticides have served mankind well over the past three decades despite the continued misuse of these tactical weapons through a heavy-handed approach to pest management. Pesticides have often been used as a club rather than a tool—as an expendable commodity rather than a resource.

The use of pesticides without regard to the complexities of agroecosystems, especially the fundamental aspects of the population dynamics of the species involved, has been one of the major causes for serious ecological perturbations that have characterized agricultural areas. Furthermore, improvements in crop protection from pests continue to be offset by changes in crop production technology that were designed for the singular purpose of maximizing yields with little consideration for the environmental consequences. These crop production goals must change and the pest management specialist must cooperate with other agricultural specialists as architects of future agroecosystems.

Pesticides will continue to be basic tools in pest management since there are many pest situations for which there are no known alternative management methods, and pesticides must serve as "fail-safe" mechanisms in the event that alternative management tactics do fail. The increased acceptance of the "treat when necessary" philosophy advocated by proponents of integrated pest management is dependent upon highly effective pesticides that can rapidly be employed against pest populations that reach economic threshold levels. Nonetheless, future pesticides must be more selective and their fate in the environment more predictable, or the ecological consequences of their use may dictate acceptance of greater crop loss in lieu of higher chemical inputs into agroecosystems.

Suggested Reading

Corbet, P. S. Pest management in ecological perspective. In Apple, J. L., Smith, R. F. (Eds.). Integrated Pest Management. New York: Plenum Press, 1976, pp. 51–56.

Glass, E. H. Pest management: Principles and philosophy. In Apple, J. L., Smith, R. F. (Eds.). Integrated Pest Management. New York: Plenum Press, 1976, pp. 39–49.

Metcalf, R. L. Insecticides in pest management. In Metcalf, R. L., Luckmann, W. (Eds.). Introduction to Insect Pest Management. New York: Wiley, 1975, pp. 235–273.

National Academy of Sciences. Pest Control: An Assessment of Present and Alternative Technologies. Vol. 3., Cotton Pest Control. Washington, D.C., 1976.

Pimentel, D. World food crisis: Energy and pests. Bull. Entomol. Soc. Am. 22:20–26, 1976.

Reynolds, H. T., Adkisson, P. L., Smith, R. F. Cotton insect pest management. In Metcalf, R. L., Luckmann, W. (Eds.). Introduction to Insect Pest Management. New York: Wiley, 1975, pp. 379–443.

Smith, R. F., Reynolds, H. T. Effects of manipulations of cotton agroecosystems on insect pest populations. In Farvar, M. T., Milton, J. P. (Eds.). The Careless Technology—Ecology and International Development. Garden City, N.Y.: Natural History Press, 1972, pp. 373–406.

Frank E. Guthrie

23

Pesticides and Humans

23.1. Introduction

The very fact that millions of pounds of toxic chemicals are applied directly for control of noxious organisms, some of which have physiological and biochemical features not unlike those of humans, is sufficient reason for concern among health authorities over possible acute and chronic effects of pesticides. The recent trend toward greatly reducing the use of persistent, fat-soluble chemicals and substituting more transient ones has caused a drastic shift in associated health problems, although sizable quantities of toxaphene and endrin are still used on agricultural crops and dieldrin-related compounds are used for termite control. As chlorinated hydrocarbon insecticides are being replaced by organophosphate and carbamate insecticides (cholinesterase inhibitors), the problems of acute toxicity have tended to increase as the problems of chronic toxicity decrease. This change in potential hazards has not received adequate comment in recent environmental texts, which report the health problems associated with chlorinated hydrocarbons as a current rather than a rapidly declining problem.

Health problems may be due to acute effects (primarily accidents) and chronic effects (long-term exposure to small quantities, with food residues the primary concern) of pesticides. One or more Poison Control Centers (associated with hospitals) in each state, EPA Community Pesticide Safety Programs (and successor programs), which are regional programs directed to research, and federal and state agricultural extension programs have been established to treat these problems.

Important legislation concerning pesticide safety has been passed by federal and state governments. These regulations will be only briefly mentioned in this chapter as they relate to specific problems. Chapter 35 is concerned with legal aspects of environmental contamination, and the interested student should also consult the appropriate reference at the end of this chapter.

23.2. Acute Health Hazards

Despite carefully written instructions on the label of every pesticide container, some 50–60 persons are fatally poisoned by pesticides each year in the United States, and there have been some poisoning episodes in other parts of the world involving hundreds, and even thousands, of persons. It is an axiom among public health pesticide safety specialists that for every reported nonfatal poisoning, there are some 10–15 not reported. Legislation may drastically reduce accidents (particularly gross ones), but total avoidance seems impossible.

A very large segment of the population has access to potentially dangerous chemicals for pest control even though recent legislation has imposed a number of important restrictions on availability, especially in household situations.

The toxicities of pesticides vary tremendously; the LD_{50} varies from a few milligrams per kilogram to several grams per kilogram (Table 23.1). The compounds that have been of most concern are a relatively small group of organophosphate and carbamate insecticides, although pesticides in use before 1945 also contribute substantially to acute accidents. Some rather gross accidents have resulted from the misuse of certain metal-containing fungicides. Most deaths caused by herbicides (much less common than deaths caused by insecticides) have resulted from accidental ingestion of paraquat or arsenic-containing compounds (Table 23.2). Misuse of insecticides is the major cause of

Table 23.1 Relative Acute Toxicities of Pesticides by Category of Use

Pesticide category	Total No.	Percent of compounds with oral LD_{50} (mg/kg) for rat in the range			
		0–50	51–250	251–1250	>1250
Herbicides	70	4	7	34	55
Organophosphates	56	52	23	23	2
Other insecticides	49	24	18	24	34
Fungicides	22	5	9	50	36

Source: Edson, E. F., et al. World Rev. Pest Control 4:36, 1965.

Table 23.2 Pesticide Poisonings by Major Category

Pesticide category	No. of Poisonings
Pesticide combinations	33
Insecticides	3035
Rodenticides	1535
Fungicides	119
Herbicides	267
Animal repellents	198
Insect repellents	236

Source: Data from National Clearinghouse for Poisons Control Centers Bulletin, Sept.–Oct., 1972.

Note: Nearly 70% of poisonings reported occurred in children under 5 years of age.

pesticide poisoning, and rodenticide poisonings, not surprisingly, run a close second.

The hazards from acute toxicity of pesticides differ greatly among the occupational and nonoccupational groups exposed. The occupational hazards today primarily are related to the use of organophosphate insecticides. In the nonoccupational groups, accidental exposure, usually ingestion, is unrelated to use, and the other chemical classes are also of importance.

23.2.1. Industrial Workers

As the manufacture of pesticides is controlled by large industries, the protection of workers is normally carefully monitored by industrial hygienists as regulated by the Occupational Safety and Health Act (OSHA). A number of studies of workers heavily exposed to several groups of insecticides (DDT, dieldrin type, and organophosphates) have failed to reveal any problems during the relatively short (15 years) time period of those studies. Synthetic processes are carefully controlled, and routine safety and health surveillance guards against appreciable direct contact with pesticides. Prompt detection of potential problems is ensured, especially those of an acute nature. In the rare instances in which workers in controlled situations showed adverse effects, there was usually an element of carelessness by a worker who had received adequate instructions.

There have been some rather dramatic, although rare, exceptions to this record in recent years. A well-authenticated case of nearly 50 worker poisonings in a poorly supervised factory preparing a moderately toxic insecticide, chlordecone (Kepone), and a less well-documented episode (15 workers) of a more sophisticated plant operation involving the manufacture of leptophos (not permitted for sale in the United States) have been reported. In both cases, severe neurological symptoms occurred among workers, but no deaths were reported. Despite these atypical episodes, one would have to judge the record of safe manufacture of pesticides as very good in regard to acute toxicity, especially in light of the potential hazards and the tonnage of chemical product.

The problem of chronic toxicity is not so well understood, although several studies on the long-term health effects on persons exposed to both persistent and nonpersistent insecticides have typically reported negative results. However, the number of subjects in the studies and the length of direct pesticide-associated work activity among these workers may not be sufficient to draw long-term conclusions. The mobility of the work force involved, at least in the United States, probably precludes an adequate examination of this potential chronic hazard and assessment of this problem will probably rely most heavily on laboratory animal studies.

23.2.2. Formulators

Although there were a large number of small formulating plants preparing finished formulations during the period 1950–1965, the majority of all finished pesticide concoctions are now produced by a few large formulating industries. During the early period, there were relatively few safety precautions in evidence, and in some cases these workers were subjected to appreciable exposures. The possible chronic effects from exposure to the now defunct chlorinated hydrocarbons by that highly exposed, casually monitored worker class must be viewed with some concern. A few accidents in formulating plants were reported each year throughout the United States during this improperly supervised era, but the total numbers were surprisingly low when one recalls the often complete disregard for toxicity of these compounds during formulation. The amount of DDT components in body fat of high-exposure groups was determined to be 35–600 ppm (1100 ppm in one individual) in contrast to 12 ppm found in the general population during that period. In more recent years, in the more carefully regulated large formulating plants (subject to OSHA regulations), the risk to workers has been reduced by a considerable degree.

23.2.3. Applicators

It is in this group of 5×10^6 plus individuals that the greatest acute hazards exist, and the problem is primarily that of dermal toxicity. The education and training of the members of this group—housewives, farmers, commercial applicators, regulatory workers, scientists, etc.—differ enormously. Recent EPA regulation has attempted to ban the more dangerous pesticides (category I pesticides) from availability to some members of the group (particularly house-wives and home owners), but there has been no workable solution to the potential hazards manifest in applications of highly toxic compounds by many poorly educated farm workers, even though they may be "certified applicators." In order to permit the farm workers to use the pesticides necessary to their business enterprise, some method of registration was necessary, and, as many of these persons have minimal formal education, certification procedures were greatly simplified in many instances. A combination of extensive educational programs and availability of less hazardous formulations is expected to reduce accidents in the coming years, but the potential is evident. A recent study has shown that nearly 3000 farmers and agricultural workers are hospitalized from pesticide poisoning each year, primarily due to organophosphate insecticides. The study further showed that the incidence of hospitalized pesticide poisonings in this group increased from 6.7/100,000 in 1971, to 9.3 in 1972, and to 11.4 in 1973, probably a reflection of the shift from chlorinated hydrocarbon to or-ganophosphate insecticides.

The majority of agricultural lands are treated by aerial applicators, whose level of education and training should make them a less accident-prone group. Studies in past years showed that an alarming number of aerial applicators have reduced cholinesterase levels (from exposure to organophosphate and carba-mate insecticides) that might preclude normal functioning during flying. Strenuous legislation, especially by state governments, has reduced this poten-tial problem. The workers loading the planes are exposed to high concentrations of some very toxic insecticides (particularly with low-volume applications), and accidents are not infrequent among this group.

One large group of applicators that has been closely monitored over the past 30 years is the World Health Organization (WHO) crews involved in spraying insecticides to reduce the incidence of insect-borne disease. Through careful cholinesterase monitoring procedures, large-scale studies have distinguished those compounds that can be safely applied and those that have tended to reduce enzyme levels; the latter are no longer used. During their earlier use of chlorinated hydrocarbons this group also received careful supervision; it was the most closely monitored large applicator group in high contact with these compounds with questionable chronic effects. Thus, through a large-scale program supervised by adequate technology, this international group of applicators experienced minimal deleterious effects from the use of insecticides.

Studies with these high-exposure groups are especially important in detecting any adverse effects, as they would first be found in such groups. Using this as a "sensor" population, possible adverse effects on the total population should be quickly detected. Experience with this highly exposed group is a major reason the official WHO policy has not favored the ban of chlorinated hydrocarbon insecticides.

23.2.4. Nonapplicator Agricultural Workers

Much concern has been expressed in recent years regarding worker exposure to previously treated foliage during crop harvest or other work activities not directly related to application per se. As a result of certain well-publicized accidents on the west coast of the United States, the establishment of reentry periods has been offered as a solution to the problem. Following application, a minimum number of days must pass before workers are permitted to enter fields to harvest and perform other activities. Federal standards were established at 48 hr as the minimum period for the most toxic insecticides, and less dangerous compounds have a 24-hr reentry interval. However, in California (where over 90% of the accidents have been reported) the reentry periods are much longer, over 3 weeks in some instances. Worker activities that are most suspect when pesticides are applied during critical cropping periods include citrus fruit, grape, tobacco, and sweet corn harvesting, peach thinning, and professional scouting in pest management programs. Although over 500 poisoning cases have been reported in the United States since 1960, only 1 death has been reported. In this case, reentry periods for parathion were ignored, and a grower permitted tobacco harvesters to enter a field treated less than 24 hr before. The reentry restrictions have been directed to cholinesterase-inhibiting insecticides only; worker activity in the chlorinated hydrocarbon era was never regulated by such standards, although several monitoring studies were conducted (see Section 23.3.3.).

23.2.5. Accidental Poisonings

In a complex society, a number of poisons may become available to individuals and groups who themselves are not actually involved in using the chemical. Pesticide poisoning accidents are somewhat more common than food poisonings in the United States. These accidents range from accidental ingestion, spillage, suicide attempts, and a variety of other exposure situations. Although suicide attempts in the United States represent less than 10% of fatal poisonings (primarily in Florida), world wide there were 500 suicides involving parathion annually during 1955–1960: this rate is now much reduced due to stringent legislation. The number of poisonings with pesticides world wide was recently estimated to be 500,000/year, and slightly over 1% were believed to be fatal. This estimate is not derived from verified records in most countries and can only be considered tentative. Although U.S. records of pesticide poisonings are better than those of most countries, it is not mandatory to report poisonings in most states (California's excellent reporting system is an exception), and estimates are primarily based on reports to Poison Control Centers. Although the number varies each year, there are approximately 6,000–10,000 reported pesticide poisonings each year. The yearly mortality rate has decreased markedly over the past 10 years—from over 150 to 50 or less. (The ratio of nonfatal to fatal cases is slightly less than 100:1). The U.S. mortality rate from pesticide poisonings is about $0.25/m \times 10^6$, which is 100–400 times less than that in underdeveloped countries but slightly higher than that in Europe.

Nearly one-half of the pesticide poisonings in the United States involve children under 5 years of age. Although many such accidents involve careless storage of synthetic insecticides, a number of accidents are attributable to exposure to inorganic insecticides (materials available before 1945). In ghetto areas especially, a frequent method of pest control involves arsenical baits, which are at least as attractive to infants as they are to the pests. In the past 5 years the fatal accident rate has dropped significantly due to greater restrictions on the purchase of pesticides and their application. Recently there has been a trend toward decreased accidental poisoning in large cities (reflecting inaccessibility of most dangerous insecticides in urban areas) and an increased incidence of poisoning in cities of less than 2500 (where conventional channels are in more common use).

Many episodes of poisoning have occurred in areas outside the United States where pesticides were accidentally incorporated into foods (Table 23.3). In Mexico,16 persons were killed and more than 500 made ill when parathion was mistaken for flour, and similar accidents have been reported with endrin (690 ill in Qatar) and other pesticides. The widespread poisoning episode (450 killed and at least 6500 made ill) resulting from the use of mercury-contaminated seed grains in Iraq illustrates the attributes of such episodes. After the seeds of wheat

Table 23.3   Ten Major Epidemics of Accidental Poisonings by Pesticides, 1940–1975

Compound	Pesticide class	Cause	Total poisonings	Deaths	Location and year
Methylmercury	Fungicide	Mixed with food[a]	6530	459	Iraq, 1973
Endrin	Insecticide	Mixed with food	691	24	Qatar, 1970
Parathion	Insecticide	Mixed with food	600	88	Colombia, 1967
Parathion	Insecticide	Uncertain	559	16	Mexico, 1968
Parathion	Insecticide	Uncertain	360	102	India, 1958
Ethylmercury	Fungicide	Mixed with food	321	35	Iraq, 1961
Sodium fluoride	Insecticide	Eating formulation	260	47	U.S.A., 1943
Parathion	Insecticide	Mixed with food	200	8	Egypt, 1958
Endrin	Insecticide	Mixed with food	183	2	Saudi Arabia, 1967
Endrin	Insecticide	Mixed with food[b]	159	0	Wales, 1956

Source: Data from Hayes, W. J. Toxicology of Pesticides. © 1975, The Williams & Wilkins Co., Baltimore. Used with permission.

[a]Seed grain (labeled "POISON") sold for consumption.

[b]Flour shipped in railroad cars contaminated 2 months earlier by insecticide spill.

were treated with an organic mercury fungicide for control of soil diseases of newly planted grain, they were sent to Mexico. The bags were clearly marked as unfit for human consumption and bore the familiar skull and crossbones poison designation. A number of bags entered international trade and were eventually sold for human consumption in Iraq. The final purchaser was unable to read the warning labels, and the skull and crossbones were not a warning signal in that culture.

It is predicted that pesticide use will increase appreciably with attempts to feed a burgeoning world population. This increase will undoubtedly result in increased accidents, especially where populations are relatively ignorant of the hazard. There are areas of the world, Central America among the most studied recently, where wealthy planters apply large quantities of toxic insecticides within the immediate vicinity of native premises. Thus, the problem appears to be both ignorance on the part of the applicators and peasants, and apathy on the part of those who should act more responsibly. For example, well-authenticated statistics show that in El Salvador (a country of 4×10^6 people) the rate of poisoning (Table 23.4) is over five times that in the United States, and organophosphate insecticides are the primary offenders.

23.3. Chronic Health Hazards

After application, a pesticide may remain in or on a surface for varying lengths of time depending upon the opportunity for metabolism, photochemical degradation, weathering, or substrate binding. These residues present a possible chronic (rarely acute) hazard to animals consuming treated parts, to invertebrates and vertebrates living in treated areas, or, in the case of certain residual herbicides, to sensitive plants introduced into the soil many months after treatment. Other chapters are devoted to the effects on insects, birds, fish, and mammals; this discussion is limited to the effects on humans. We must recognize that overuse of chlorinated hydrocarbon insecticides has resulted in a residue problem of such magnitude that essentially every living creature on the planet has detectable quantities of DDT or other chlorinated products, even in areas several thousands of miles from sites of application. Detectable amounts of such residues are expected to remain in humans for one or more decades.

Legislation directed to controlling the problem of synthetic pesticide residues on food was enacted in the United States and many other countries early in the

Table 23.4   Pesticide-Caused Poisonings in El Salvador

Year	Nonfatal cases	Fatal cases
1963	1104	11
1964	965	2
1968	938	1
1969	583	7
1970	474	7
1971	586	10
1972	2787	5

Source: Davies, J. Proceedings of the 10th Inter-American Meeting on Foot and Mouth Diseases and Zymoses Control. Pan American Health Organization, Sci. Publ. 358, pp. 79–86, 1978.

1900s and has been quite rigorous since 1960. The major international organizations, FAO and WHO, have also been active in circumventing a possible pesticide residue problem by providing guidelines and expertise to underdeveloped countries.

Although a sizable number of people are exposed to pesticides by virtue of their work activity, the vast majority of the population will not be exposed to appreciable quantities of pesticides unless they consume treated food (Table 23.5). It is very important to ensure that residues in food are in quantities known to be safe. This discussion will be concerned with U.S. legislation, which is similar to that of other developed countries. However, it must be recognized that at least 50% (and more likely 75%) of the world population is not protected by such legal regulation. It is fortunate that many of these countries use little insecticide but unfortunate that some do use sizable quantitites of insecticides without adequate governmental supervision.

23.3.1. Pesticide Residue Tolerances

In the United States, several federal agencies cooperate in establishing pesticide residue tolerances on food (the EPA has final authority). Establishment of these tolerances is a very time-consuming and expensive task; specific details are available in the literature listed at the end of the chapter. Simply stated, the government permits a residue estimated to be safe, based on scientific experiments, for consumption over a lifetime. Most residue tolerances contain a 100-fold (or greater) safety factor to account for individual and animal differences. Contrary to the belief held by several well-meaning, but sometimes emotional, environmental groups, the steps leading to the granting of a tolerance are very carefully controlled and require at least 5 years of background data. Tolerances are translated for the farmer, who reads on the pesticide label that he must wait a certain number of days before harvest. Thus, the potentially toxic residue must dissipate after application to nontoxic levels by the time of harvest, as illustrated by the residue disappearance curve (Figure 23.1).

The FDA enforces this legislation by periodically sampling a portion of food shipped in interstate commerce. Although most states also have residue laws,

Table 23.5 Sources of DDT Intake in North America

Source	DDT intake (mg/year)
Food	30
Miscellaneous (house dust, cosmetics, etc.)	5
Air	0.03
Water	0.01
Total	35
Acceptable yearly intake (FAO/WHO) for 70-kg man	255

Source: Kraybill, H.F. Significance of pesticide residues in foods in relation to total environmental stress. Originally published in Can. Med. Assoc. J. 100:204, January 25, 1969.

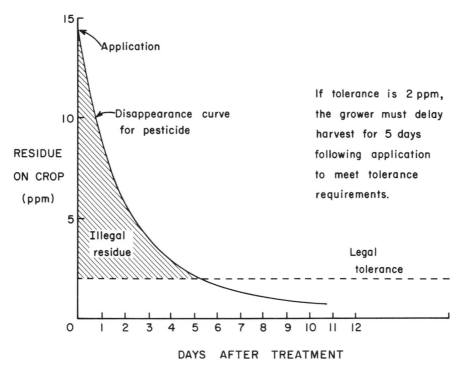

Figure 23.1 Translation of pesticide disappearance curve to harvest waiting period to permit growers to comply with federal pesticide residue tolerances.

they are not as rigorously enforced, and food in intrastate commerce is less well monitored.

23.3.2. Monitoring Programs

There are a number of monitoring programs in the United States directed toward detecting pesticide residues in nonhuman populations (especially fish, birds, and certain mammals), in water and air (these programs have shown that current pesticide levels do not present a health hazard), in food, and in humans. The most important human studies have been concerned with monitoring residues in the food, the fat, and the serum of the human population. Several heavily populated countries in other parts of the world have similar programs.

In the United States, two food sampling procedures are primarily used. In the market basket method, a typical family's weekly supply of food is analyzed for pesticide content. In the second method, a meal purchased at a restaurant is analyzed. Table 23.6 presents some of the data and includes typical intakes and amounts designated acceptable daily intakes by FAO/WHO.

The conclusion one must draw is that nearly all food consumed in the United States was contaminated with one or more chlorinated hydrocarbons before the drastic curtailment of their use. However, the vast majority of the pesticide residues in food were well within the acceptable limits established by FAO/WHO. It should be noted, however, that some food residues (dieldrin, for

Table 23.6 Comparison of Daily Intake of Selected Pesticides in the United States with FAO/WHO Acceptable Intakes

Pesticide	Intake (mg/man/day)						FAO/WHO acceptable intake (mg/70-kg man/day)
	1965	1966	1967	1968	1969	1970	
Arsenic	0.069	0.005	0.03	0.14	0.075	0.057	ND[a]
Bromides	27	15	20	28	17	16	70
Lindane	0.004	0.004	0.005	0.003	0.00	0.001	0.88
DDT and DDE	0.049	0.069	0.043	0.034	0.027	0.025	0.35
Dieldrin	0.005	0.007	0.004	0.004	0.005	0.005	0.007
Carbaryl	0.150	0.026	0.007	—	0.003	—	0.7
Diazinon	—	0.001	<0.001	<0.001	<0.001	0.001	0.14
Malathion	—	0.009	0.010	0.003	0.012	0.013	1.40
Parathion	—	<0.001	0.001	<0.001	<0.001	0.001	0.35
2,4-D	0.005	0.002	0.001	0.001	<0.001	<0.001	ND
Dithiocarbamates	0.026	—	0.005	0.003	—	<0.001	1.75

Source: Hayes, W. J. Toxicology of Pesticides. © 1975, The Williams & Wilkins Co., Baltimore. Used with permission.

[a]ND: not determined.

example) were uncomfortably close to accepted standards. Since the use of chlorinated hydrocarbons has been greatly restricted, the residue levels in food have dramatically decreased. The residues of insecticides that have replaced the chlorinated hydrocarbons (organophosphates and carbamates) have been consistently low—at least an order of magnitude below acceptable daily intakes. In many cases they are below detectable levels.

A second major area of study has been the quantities of insecticides found in fat samples procured from selected populations. The results presented in Figure 23.2 for DDT components in body fat of the U.S. population and in Table 23.7 for levels of other chlorinated hydrocarbons in human body fat in many countries show that these levels did not reach alarming proportions. As would be expected, residues of organophosphates and carbamates have not been detected in fat tissue. This is a reflection of the rapid dissipation and lack of propensity for fat storage of the heavily used organophosphate and carbamate insecticides. Potentially "tissue storable" pesticides containing lead, mercury, and other elements have not been found in significant amounts because they are not applied to crops in direct consumption.

It is interesting to note that average levels in the U.S. population had reached approximately 12.5 ppm DDT components (and smaller amounts of other chlorinated hydrocarbon insecticides) in the 1960s, but levels have declined in recent years. Highly exposed groups had about three times the average level of DDT in their fat, and one apparently healthy formulator had over 1100 ppm. As these fat-soluble, persistent compounds are not readily subject to metabolism, it is expected that DDT components will not decline to levels lower than 0.5 ppm until 1985 (Figure 23.2).

The data for DDT components can be somewhat misleading without an explanation of the contribution by DDE. This compound represents about 75% of the DDT components in human fat. It arises primarily as a contaminant in technical DDT, thus its most important route of entry is consumption of DDT-contaminated food. It is also a minor component of DDT metabolism.

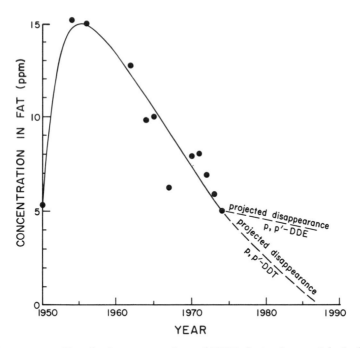

Figure 23.2 Trend of concentration of DDT-derived materials in body fat of general population of the United States and projected disappearance of DDT and DDE at no intake level.

Although most DDT would be eliminated in 1–2 decades if dietary intake were eliminated, elimination of DDE would probably require over 50 years.

23.3.3. Epidemiological Studies

Studies on sizable populations living in areas of great pesticide use have been conducted to obtain evidence to support, or deny, the existence of long-term health effects of pesticides. Perhaps the best known study concerns the so-called Mississippi Delta population. In that very large study area, 20 or more pesticide applications per year (first the chlorinated hydrocarbons and now their substitutes) are commonplace on agricultural land, much of which is in close proximity to residences and populated areas. Studies of segments of this population have included medical examinations, employment records, leave absences, school records, and a battery of questions directed to subtle actions that may have been caused by pesticides. The studies have thus far concluded that the health of the population has not been affected.

In a different type of study, a group of nearly 4600 persons in an agricultural area of California was studied to determine if enzyme levels in farm families (potential direct exposure) differed from those in nonfarm families (potential indirect exposure). A very small, but significant difference in cholinesterase levels was noted; this difference would probably be considered unimportant by the majority of informed scientists. Nonetheless, the enzyme decline in the farm family group was significant, which suggests that the physiology of the group was altered despite the fact that only casual exposure was manifest. The

Table 23.7 Representative Concentrations of Chlorinated Hydrocarbons in Body Fat of General Populations of Various Countries

Country	Year	Level in body fat (ppm)		
		BHC isomers	Dieldrin	Heptachlor epoxide
North America				
Canada	1966	0.07	0.22	0.14
U.S.A.	1962	0.57	0.11	—
	1964	0.60	0.29	0.24
	1967	—	0.21	—
	1970	0.10	0.18	0.08
South America				
Argentina	1967	2.44	0.38	0.19
Venezuela	1964	0.16	0.60	—
Europe				
Denmark	1965	—	0.20	—
England	1964	0.02	0.21	0.01
	1969	0.29	0.16	0.03
France	1961	1.19	—	—
West Germany	1970	0.45	—	—
Italy	1966	0.08	0.68	0.23
Netherlands	1967	0.11	0.20	0.01
Middle East				
Israel	1968	0.47	0.12	<0.0001
Asia				
India	1964	1.43	0.04	—
Japan	1972	0.12–1.28	0.13	0.02
Oceania				
Australia	1966	0.68	0.67	0.02
New Zealand	1966	—	0.35	—

Source: Hayes, W. J. Toxicology of Pesticides.© 1975, The Williams & Wilkins Co., Baltimore. Used with permission.

significance of these small changes is controversial, but the data should not be ignored.

23.3.4. Concerns for the Future

The evidence that pesticides can have severe detrimental effects on humans is undeniable. The lack of education concerning the safe handling of pesticides, especially the lower socioeconomic group in the United States, is a major problem that must be corrected. Moreover, if sizable quantities of pesticides are to be manufactured or purchased by underveloped countries, the necessary educational programs must be instituted before widespread application of toxic materials is undertaken. Even in developed countries, an attitude persists among too many individuals that one can take some risks. Thus, it seems debatable whether governmental regulation in the United States will enable much further reduction of the number of accidental deaths, a remarkably low number (50/year) at present (Figure 23.3). "No risk" legislation seems to be nearly impossible, but hazards that can be controlled must be.

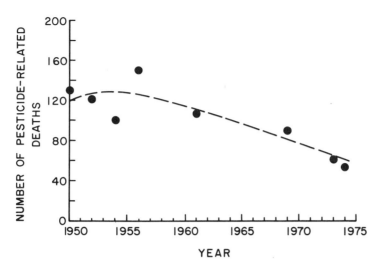

Figure 23.3 Trend of mortality due to pesticide poisoning in the United States 1950–1974.

The problem of chronic toxicity of pesticides on food would appear to have been largely circumvented by the substitution of degradable, nonpersistent compounds for those now considered to have been potentially hazardous. This does not erase the problem of a very sizable population that had extensive exposure to chlorinated pesticides for a period of 15–20 years. Latent action from these compounds, if it exists, will probably persist for another decade. A considerable body of evidence from experimental animals suggests that such actions are unlikely. A recent report of the National Cancer Institute suggests that DDT is not a carcinogen, refuting some earlier studies. The proposed increases in pesticide use as a major tool for increased food production must, and undoubtedly will, be closely monitored, and the fact that individual pesticides, or groups of pesticides, may have effects not yet detected will continue to warrant consideration by toxicologists and governments.

Although this chapter has been concerned with hazards of pesticides, the benefits from pesticides regarding human health should not be overlooked. The ability to control vector-borne diseases by pesticides (a recent development) has saved hundreds of thousands of lives and hundreds of millions of illnesses from malaria alone since 1945, and similar contributions have been made toward controlling other diseases. A significant contribution to the world population problem has resulted from this area of disease control.

Suggested Reading

Davies, J. E., Edmundson, W. F. Epidemiology of DDT. Mount Kisco, N.Y.: Futura, 1972.

Edwards, C.A. Persistent Pesticides in the Environment, second edition. Cleveland:CRC Press, 1974.

Environmental Protection Agency. Pesticides: A Legal Compilation, Vols. 1–4 plus supplements. Washington,D.C., 1973 (and other years).

Hayes, W. J. Toxicology of Pesticides. Baltimore:Williams & Wilkins, 1975.

Jager, K.W. Aldrin, Dieldrin, Endrin and Telodrin: An Epidemiological and Toxicological Study of Long-Term Exposure. Amsterdam:Elsevier, 1970.

Milby, T. H. (Ed.). Occupational Exposure to Pesticides, Report to the Federal Working Group on Pest Management from the Task Group on Occupational Exposure to Pesticides. Washington, D.C.,1974.

Morgan, D. B., Roan, C. C. The metabolism of DDT in man. Essays Toxicol. 5:39–97, 1974.

U. S. Public Health Service. Vital Statistics of the United States. Washington,D.C. (see appropriate year).

World Health Organization. Safe Use of Pesticides. 20th Report of the W.H.O. Expert Committee on Insecticides. W.H.O. Technical Report Series No. 513, Geneva, Switzerland, 1973.

World Health Organization. Information circulars on the toxicity of pesticides to man. Geneva, Switzerland (many circulars available from VBC/TOX series).

Richard B. Mailman
Judy A. Sidden

24

Food and Food Additives

24.1. Introduction

Although direct environmental effects on human health may occur after exposure to toxicants through respiratory or dermal absorption, the dependence of animals on the intake of substantial quantities of water, minerals, and preformed organic molecules is indicative of the importance of the diet as a possible vector for toxic substances. The Industrial Revolution and the subsequent birth of the chemical industry caused new problems relating to food contamination, and although the primary emphasis of this text is on the effects of human-induced alterations in the environment, it is important to realize that there are also naturally occurring toxicants. Some mechanisms by which toxicants may occur in the human food chain are surveyed in this chapter, and a framework for the evaluation of these potential hazards is offered.

24.2. Evaluation of Food Hazards

24.2.1. Historical Perspective

There are two primary protective mechanisms against the naturally occurring toxins present in the human diet. First, higher animals have a variety of biochemical systems that minimize the offensive nature of ingested toxicants. These include physiological barriers to the absorption of xenobiotics or their penetration to sensitive tissues, as well as several modes of chemical alteration that allow foreign compounds to be eliminated more readily. Second, it may be presumed that man, like lower animals, will avoid repetitive intake of foodstuffs that cause noxious responses.

In addition to essential nutrients such as proteins, lipids, carbohydrates, vitamins, and minerals, a variety of other chemical agents occur naturally in food, as manifested by their contributions to color, taste, odor, and texture. These chemicals are representative of nearly every class of organic molecule known, and thus provide a potpourri of putative physiological insults. It is not known what the toxic effects of these normal dietary constituents have been, nor how they interact with dietary constituents that result from environmental pollution or deliberate additions to foods.

24.2.2. Methodology and Philosophy

Many issues are involved in the assessment of toxic inputs through our diet. Although the most critical of these may appear to involve scientific or medical factors, the interface of these factors with philosophical, economic, and political questions (e.g., cost-effectiveness) has made this an extremely volatile issue. Some of the important questions may be summarized as follows:

1. What is the chemical identity of the "toxicant" of interest?
2. What are the biological effects of the exposure of target organisms (e.g., neonates versus adults) to different doses of the toxicant, and what methods are used to measure these effects?
3. What is the analytical sensitivity of the techniques used to detect or measure the toxicant in foodstuffs?
4. What concentrations of the toxicant occur in the food supply?
5. What is the cost–benefit relationship between the health consequences of the toxicant and the cultural or medical advantages of exposure to the toxicant?

It is unfortunate, perhaps, that the cost–benefit issue is a complicated policy decision requiring evaluation of the scientific evidence in concert with political, ethical, and/or social considerations. It should be explicitly stated that while certain scientific questions, such as the identity and concentration of a chemical in food supplies, may be answered with some degree of rigor, judgments about the resulting courses of action are political decisions that may often appear to be inconsistent with the scientific evidence on which they are based.

24.2.3. Toxicological Hazards

Historically, the primary manner in which a food-borne health hazard was detected was through epidemiological methods. Epidemiology—the study of the distribution and determinants of disease prevalence in man—is the deductive mode in which causes are elucidated retrospectively. The benefits of an epidemiological evaluation are the determination of the source and identity of a suspected toxicant and/or the evaluation of the interaction of toxicants with other physiological or environmental factors, such as drugs, dietary agents, or other environmental contaminants.

The primary deficiency of epidemiological methods is that they must, of necessity, occur ex post facto. The more easily a problem is identified, the more severe are the health implications of exposure to the particular toxicant. Furthermore, epidemiological investigations may be inhibited by the fact that sequelae of toxicant exposure may not be apparent for decades afterward, although the human health costs may ultimately be staggering. Thus, while these methods are of tremendous importance in toxicological assessments, by their very nature they are an admission of scientific or social failure. Additionally, even conclusive epidemiological data linking human disease to a specific toxicant are often dismissed because cessation of toxicant exposure would require dramatic alterations in behavior, e.g., the reaction to the Surgeon General's report on cigarette smoking. This is symptomatic of the difficulty that exists for both scientists and laymen in separating scientific decisions from those of a sociopolitical nature that are, finally, public policy decisions.

24.2.3.a. Prospective Risk Assessment

Obviously, prospective methods would be more valuable in protecting public health. If a putative toxicant has been identified and techniques have been developed for its quantification, the critical issues remaining are the doses, times of exposure, and types of toxic effects that will occur in humans. The strength of the field of toxicology has been the ability to conduct detailed pathological examinations of test animals exposed to various doses of a chemical and to detect and quantify various untoward effects. These acute toxicological studies are not, unfortunately, the defining limits of hazard; rather, epidemiological studies have indicated that effects of apparently innocuous chronic exposures may constitute the greatest health hazards. Asbestosis and reactions to radiation exposure are two examples of these long-term changes that are almost always expressed as carcinogenic or teratogenic changes. In fact, the problem of evaluating carcinogenicity has not, to date, been adequately resolved.

If doses of a chemical (at concentrations similar to those encountered in the human diet) cause cancer in several species of laboratory animals, there is little disagreement that the material is probably carcinogenic in man and should be banned from our diet. However, easily definable test results are often not obtained; for example, often only one species of animal shows a response to the agent, or an exceptionally high dose of the compound is needed to cause an effect. The resulting problems may be exemplified by the hypothetical dose–response curve shown in Figure 24.1. One unknown not directly amenable to further experimentation is the effect of toxicant exposure at lower concentrations than those that were found to elicit a response in the test of interest. For example, if one makes a linear extrapolation to zero effect ("0%" on the ordinate axis), the intercept on the abscissa is a dose that should cause no detectable response (the "threshold dose"). This prediction is consistent with the existence of protective mechanisms that allow the target organism to detoxify the chemical or physiologically repair or compensate for low frequencies of biological injury. Advocates of a "threshold model" would assert that limited exposures to low levels of many carcinogens are essentially risk free. However, an alternative method of interpreting this data is to assume that the dose–response curve in the extrapolated region is actually concave upward (Figure 24.1). This idea predicts a finite hazard from every toxicant exposure, although the hazard would not be statistically evident until a sufficiently large sample was examined.

These interpretations are necessary because of the practical problems inherent in toxicity testing. There are several limiting factors for any test, the obvious one being the number of animals that can be tested for any one compound. Since the cost of an experiment using desirable numbers of animals (e.g., 100,000–1,000,000) is prohibitive, the best available compromise is to use apparently excessive doses of the chemical being tested in smaller numbers of animals. Thus, for there to be statistical significance in a carcinogenicity study, it is

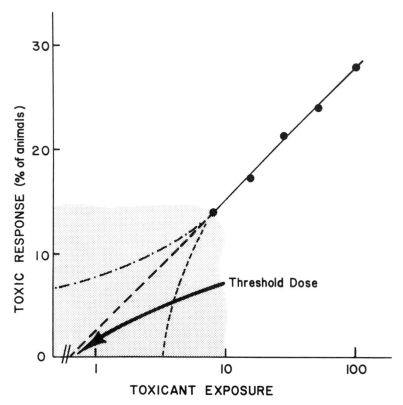

Figure 24.1 Hypothetical dose–response curve from toxicological study. The toxicant exposure (abscissa) may be a combination of dose–time interactions. In this hypothetical study, insufficient numbers of animals are tested (about 100) to evaluate the effects of very low doses of the toxicant. Three of many possible extrapolations are indicated: — · — · concave upward extrapolation, implying that there may not be a "no-effect" dose; —— linear extrapolation, implying a linear log–dose–response and a "threshold dose"; — — — — concave downward extrapolation, implying repair or other protective mechanisms that cause decreased effects at lower doses.

generally required to demonstrate an induced tumor incidence of 5%. In a study conducted with 100 animals fed a food constituent at a level of 1% of the diet, the failure to find any tumors would lead to the assumption (at the 99% confidence level) that the actual incidence of tumors was less than 4.5%. If the data suggest, for example, that human exposure would occur at 10 ppm, then the risk in rats (<5%) would be, simplistically, equivalent to a risk of less than 0.005% in humans. This negative toxicity test would therefore be indicative of potential risk to a substantial number of affected individuals (in this example, more than 10,000 for the population of the United States) if the actual risk were just below that detectable in this experiment. This is one reason an arbitrary safety factor (often 100) is chosen to help ensure safety. There are several ways to increase the precision of these determinations, the most obvious being to conduct the toxicological tests on larger numbers of animals. For example, the test described above would be 10 times more sensitive if 1000 rather than 100 animals were used. However, the ideal design utilizing low doses of toxicant in large numbers of animals is limited by excessive costs of "mega-mouse" or "mega-rat" experiments.

Finally, the theoretical framework in which these types of experiments are evaluated can dramatically alter the interpretation of the obtained data. Figure 24.1 illustrates how three different models yield very different predictions of toxicity; it is for this reason that the use of alternative analyses such as probit or Mantel-Bryan extrapolations will affect the interpretation of data. Further research may specify better criteria that would increase the validity of experimental analyses.

Another approach to toxicity testing has resulted from fundamental experiments in bacterial genetics. The Ames test (a product of the research of Bruce Ames and his co-workers) measures the mutagenicity of chemicals by their ability to cause back mutations in strains of the bacteria *Salmonella typhimurium* selected for their inability to grow without the addition of a particular amino acid. Mutagenic agents cause these bacteria to "revert" to their wild type pattern of not needing the specific amino acid, and mutagens that involve different mechanisms can be detected using several mutant strains of bacteria. Since all known carcinogens have ultimately been shown to be mutagens (though the converse is not true), and since there is a good correlation between their mutagenic and carcinogenic potencies, this test has developed into the simplest and potentially most usable prospective method to evaluate carcinogenic materials. Further research has demonstrated that in vitro metabolism of the agents being tested by liver microsomal extracts, or in vivo metabolism followed by urinary recovery of metabolites, increased the correlation with the induction of animal cancers. Further development and validation of this test may help answer many of the questions discussed in this chapter. Additional test systems may also be developed that will more sensitively evaluate mutagenic–carcinogenic materials. Other models utilizing lower animals having unusual metamorphogenic stages may eventually provide even more sensitive test systems.

24.2.3.b. Delaney Clause

The public policy resolution of many of these perplexing scientific issues was codified in the Food, Drug and Cosmetic Act of 1938. In 1958, as a result of hearings in the House of Representatives chaired by James J. Delaney, this act was amended to include several measures. The first was publication of a list of substances that were "generally recognized as safe" (the GRAS list), and the second was the so-called Delaney Clause. The latter provides that "no additive shall be deemed to be safe if it is found to induce cancer when ingested by man or animal, or if it is found, after tests which are appropriate for the evaluation of the safety of food additives, to induce cancer in man or animal." The consequences of this wording are that any compound that is shown to be carcinogenic in man or in any species of laboratory animal, at any dose, shall be banned from foods, although this apparently simple definition of safety is complicated by several pragmatic factors.

Although the intent of the Delaney Clause to protect the consumer from exposure to food-borne carcinogens is a generally accepted goal, the application of this legislation has been controversial. First, the proposal of a new food additive for approval requires a significant financial investment (and profit motivation), which, under adverse circumstances, may generate less than conservative attitudes toward toxicity evaluation. This negative attitude is caused, in part, by the expense and practical difficulties of testing a proposed additive, and is further influenced by the lack of an accepted theory of risk assessment (Section 24.2.3.a.). The concept of making dose–response extrapolations after testing of doses of toxicant several orders of magnitude larger than would be generally consumed by man has also been criticized. It is questioned whether feeding test animals diets containing several percent of a xenobiotic may result in metabolic or other physiological imbalances that do not reasonably reflect the hazard of the compound when it is consumed at trace doses. Conversely, it has been argued that one should assume that humans are the most sensitive species and are also subject to toxic insults from a variety of sources, possibly amplifying the hazards of exposure to apparently safe levels of one chemical. Finally, the FDA has been criticized for both its laxity and severity in interpreting food and drug laws. These difficulties are accentuated by the fact that food constituents may interact with each other by direct chemical reactions as well as by one chemical altering the physiological impact of another. These interactions, discussed in more detail in Section 24.5, contribute to problems of interpretation inherent in toxicology.

24.3. Unintentional Food Adulterants

The effects of environmental alterations on the human food supply have been well publicized, but it is important to realize that industrial or agricultural chemicals are not the only toxicants that may appear in our diets. Many food adulterants are "natural" or "organic" constituents that either are integral constituents of the food or may be present if carelessness in harvesting or processing occurs. In this section not only the by-products of industrial processes are considered, but also toxicants resulting from these other factors. One major source of contamination, for example, is microbial contamination, which may occur by several routes.

24.3.1. Bacterial Infections and Toxins

The most direct route of food adulteration is contamination by bacteria that can cause human infection directly. For example, *Salmonella* species are found widely in nature, often residing in the intestinal tract of poultry. Ingestion of sufficient quantities of the bacteria may cause an infection resulting in severe gastroenteritis, although this is usually not fatal in healthy individuals. Salmonellosis is a concern primarily when nonacid foods are left unrefrigerated prior to consumption for periods of time that permit the bacteria to multiply to levels sufficient to cause infection. Gross negligence in handling may also result in sufficient concentrations of *Salmonella* to present a hazard. Fortunately, the nature of the infection limits salmonellosis to isolated incidents requiring consumption of the contaminated food. Other food-borne infections, such as cholera or typhoid, are problems primarily in countries where sanitation is poorly controlled.

Food-borne toxins are a more important problem than direct bacterial infections because the toxins may persist after the source organism is no longer present. Staphylococcal enterotoxin, for example, is a protein resulting from *Staphylococcus* growth due to carelessness in food preparation and handling. The bacteria grow under aerobic conditions in nonrefrigerated contaminated foods, and the enterotoxin they produce causes severe gastroenteritis, which may be fatal to weakened individuals. The conditions necessary for toxin production usually limit staphylococcal food poisoning, like salmonellosis, to localized outbreaks.

Probably the most serious problem, however, results from the exotoxins produced by strains of the bacteria *Clostridium botulinum*. Except, possibly, for certain infants, the growth of this anaerobe in humans presents no health hazard; however, in culture these bacteria produce a series of proteinaceous neurotoxins that are generally considered to be the most toxic materials known, with an LD_{50} for man of approximately 1 μg. The growth of this bacteria requires a nonacid, oxygen-free environment with little or no competition from other organisms. Modern food distribution has resulted in two situations where this may commonly occur—in canned foods, and in vacuum packed meats or fish. Contamination of the former is the most prevalent, usually resulting from either insufficient heat treatment of the cans (permitting survival of *C. botulinum* spores), or can leakage that allows inoculation with the spores followed by sealing of the leak with food particles. In either case, spore germination and bacterial growth result in toxin production in the food. With canned foods, the growth of the bacteria may result in sufficient gas production to cause noticeable can deformation, although this may be overlooked. The botulinum toxins, like most proteins, are denatured by heating; however, this cannot be relied on as a protective measure because the required heating may cause undesirable changes in food quality and thus may not be carried out for sufficient periods of time. Botulism usually results from home canning, although commercial processors can present a more important public health hazard because of the widespread distribution of the commercial products. To minimize these risks, processing times are based on heat treatments needed to kill botulinum spores located in the most resistant location of the can. Although botulinum antitoxins are available, damage to both the central and peripheral nervous systems may be sufficiently severe when symptoms are observed to preclude the possibility of complete recovery.

24.3.2. Mycotoxins

The oldest documented episodes of mycotoxosis were epidemics that resulted from the production of ergot alkaloids as a result of the growth of the fungus *Claviceps purpurea*. This fungus, found particularly on grains such as rye, found its way into the food supply in bread. There has been speculation that several incidents of populations "going mad" (possibly including the Salem witch trials) were the result of ergotism. Awareness of this problem and better storage conditions for grains have minimized the incidence of ergotism; the last documented outbreak of any consequence occurred in France in 1951.

A more prevalent problem is contamination by aflatoxins, the fungal alkaloids produced by the *Aspergillus flavus* molds. First identified only 2 decades ago, aflatoxin contamination has been shown to be a widespread problem of tremendous health significance. In certain areas of the world where the incidence of liver cancer is high (such as Africa and Southeast Asia), aflatoxins are believed to play a significant role in its etiology. These results are consonant with animal studies demonstrating the highly carcinogenic nature of these materials. The entry of aflatoxins into the human food chain occurs by two pathways. First, animals in the human food chain may ingest fungus-contaminated feed. Although residual aflatoxin in flesh may be important, a more critical problem is the secretion of an aflatoxin metabolite into cows' milk, the resulting material (aflatoxin M) being nearly as potent a carcinogen as the original toxin. Second, many vegetable crops may be contaminated by *A. flavus*, especially if they are allowed to become moldy during harvesting or processing. The widespread occurrence of mold on certain foods (such as peanuts) has made the presence of aflatoxins an important and persistent problem.

Other mycotoxins are also known to create health problems, including products of *Penicillium* species (islandotoxin and patulin are carcinogens; cyclopiazonic acid is a neurotoxin; and luteoskyrin is a hepatotoxin) and *Fusarium* species (diacetoxyscirpenol and zearalenone), as well as other *Aspergillus* by-products (ochratoxin A is a hepatotoxin). It is apparent that measures to minimize the growth of these molds on foodstuffs or removal or inactivation of the toxicants will be important to protect the consumer.

24.3.3. Plant Alkaloids

Although only a small percentage of plants contain materials that are highly toxic, because all of the human food supply ultimately results from the plant kingdom, these materials pose the primary problem in contamination of the food chain. There are periodic instances of contamination of foodstuffs with highly toxic plant materials—for example, the contamination of lima beans by nightshade berries. Generally, this route is not one of major toxicological concern since these toxicants are either avoided or eliminated during processing. Poisoning (with primarily acute consequences) has also resulted from consumption of food fish contaminated by ingestion of dinoflagellate plankton ("red tide") that produce powerful neurotoxins, such as saxitoxin.

A more interesting question concerns trace food constituents whose toxicity has not been well studied. For example, hepatotoxic alkaloids from the tansy ragwort have been reported to occur in honey produced from nectar of that species. These compounds are carcinogenic, but fortunately they are distinguished by a bitter off-taste when they are present in honey at concentrations sufficient to cause acute poisoning. However, it is not known whether consumption of smaller quantities, not detectable by taste alterations, would have long-term effects. Similarly, quercetin and similar flavenoids are commonly found in vascular plants that are used for foods. These compounds have been found to be mutagenic by the Ames test, although at higher levels than carcinogens such as aflatoxin B_1. These results reiterate the problems of evaluating the health hazards of compounds of low, but detectable, carcinogenicity.

24.3.4. Poisons of Animal Origin

Whereas the edible tissues of terrestrial animals are remarkably free of toxic compounds of natural origin, many fish contain toxic xenobiotics. Many factors influence the occurrence of these toxins in the fish, including water temperature, time of year, and locale of the fish—all of which add additional variability to toxicity predictions. The most well-documented poisoning occurs from ingestion of certain species of puffer fish, which emanate tetrodotoxin and related compounds from the ovaries and liver. Ingestion of these parts, or lack in care of preparation, can result in ingestion of the extremely potent neurotoxins. Generally, these types of exposure are easily controlled by dietary restriction.

24.3.5. Elemental Contaminants: Heavy Metals and Radiochemicals

Contamination of the food chain by elemental materials usually implies an obligatory role of man in altering the environment. Although several chapters of this book examine these subjects directly, several examples should be reiterated in the present content.

During the era of widespread atmospheric testing of nuclear weapons, the entry of radioactive isotopes into the food chain was a problem. The concentration and passage of ^{90}Sr into cows' milk received particular attention because of its consumption by infants and children. The limitation of atmospheric testing has minimized this contamination, but there has been a concomitant increase in the number of nuclear power plants. Although the emissions from proper plant operations do not contribute significantly detectable levels of radioactivity to the environment, the dispersal of spent fuel or power plant malfunctions may be possible sources of contamination of the food supply in the future. Because many of the isotopes have extremely long half-lives, this contamination may result in long-term problems.

Heavy metals have been a more important problem in relationship to the food supply. The outbreak of Minamata disease (discussed in Chapter 3), resulting from the accumulation of methylmercury in fish, led to increased awareness of the presence of heavy metals in foods. There are two primary routes by which foods may be contaminated: the first involves direct, accidental contact with foodstuffs; but the more difficult problem is the accumulation and biomagnification of heavy metals at one or more steps of the food chain with subsequent presence in the final food product. It should be noted that the assumption that the mercury occurring in the food chain is a direct result of industrial activities may be incorrect, since the presence of elevated mercury concentrations in preserved fish indicated that a significant portion of the residue is a result of natural processes.

24.3.6. Chemical Residues in Food

24.3.6.a. Pesticide Residues

The presence of pesticide residues in food is solely the result of the activities of man in agricultural, public health, or related activities. The permissible levels of pesticides and tolerances for the presence of these agents on foodstuffs in the United States are established by the EPA, to be enforced by the FDA. These chemicals are discussed in detail in other chapters of this book, but specific facts are of importance with regard to the food chain. Acute food toxicity from pesticides generally results from careless handling. For example, during the past decade this has resulted in contamination and subsequent destruction of thousands of chickens in Mississippi that had been exposed to high concentrations of dieldrin. One outbreak in Jamaica in 1976 from parathion-contaminated flour resulted in 17 deaths and nearly 100 illnesses. There have also been several instances in which the less persistent pesticides (e.g., the carbamates or organophosphates) were applied too soon before processing or consumption, resulting in significant residues in the foodstuff.

Another important problem is the effect of low pesticide levels in foods. Since animals may biomagnify compounds such as the organchlorine insecticides, levels found in adipose tissue may be far greater than those presumably ingested at any single time. This may present two hazards. The first may result directly from ingestion of contaminated animals or fish that had accumulated these materials. Second, these compounds may also accumulate in human adipose tissue, where they may be mobilized during extreme physiological stress. Exposure to low levels of pesticides may also involve the risk of carcinogenicity, and the use of captan as a fungicide in raisins has recently been questioned for this reason.

Finally, pesticides may interact with other compounds in the food or other components of the diet. The fruit and vegetable fungicide ethylene thiourea was found to form a carcinogenic product after cooking, although the native molecule was itself not a major hazard. For this reason, its use on foods was eliminated. The use of more degradable pesticides, such as carbamates or organophosphates, as replacements for the more persistent organochlorine compounds may possibly result in new interactions between some of their degradation products and other food constituents.

24.3.6.b. Animal Feed Residues

It is estimated that more than three-quarters of all the meat, milk, and eggs consumed in the United States comes from animals that have been treated with various drugs placed in their feed or injected directly during some or all of their life. These drugs serve a variety of functions, but their usage raises several questions with regard to contamination of the food supply.

Hormone supplements. The two major classes of growth promoters used in food production are hormones and arsenicals. For almost 3 decades, nearly all the swine and poultry produced in the United States have been fed various organic arsenic compounds. In the past several years, there have been no reports of the established safe tolerance levels (usually less than 2 ppm) being exceeded in poultry muscle, although a small but significant fraction (4%) of tested swine liver or kidney exceeded the 2-ppm tolerance. There are no known hazards associated with this level of contamination.

A more important health hazard is thought to involve the synthetic estrogen diethylstilbestrol (DES), which was used as a feed additive in cattle to promote rapid weight gain. Use of this drug had been restricted to certain species for only specific periods of their life span, with sufficient time allowed after withdrawal of the drug to permit elimination of the drug from the tissues of the animal. The use of DES as a synthetic estrogen led to reports linking it to increases in a rare genital tract tumor in young women whose mothers were given DES when pregnant. Later studies have also suggested that prenatal exposure to DES may result in reproductive tract abnormalities in male mice. These consequences of

DES administration have caused reevaluation of its use and an attempt to ban it as a feed additive, as well as raised questions about the use of other sex hormones as feed supplements.

Antibiotics and related drugs. Antibiotics, principally penicillin and tetracyclines, have also been used as growth promoters in animal feeds. Prophylactic use of these antibiotics minimizes premarket infections and has been reported to have a tremendous economic advantage for meat producers, although there may be several health problems associated with this use. First, the presence of the antibiotics may serve as an immunological challenge to sensitize susceptible individuals. These people will then not be able to use these antibiotics therapeutically because of severe allergic responses. Second, the presence of low levels of the antibiotics may serve to increase the number of drug-resistant strains of bacteria both in animals and humans via selection of plasmid-containing bacteria bearing genes conferring resistance. The awareness that more and more bacteria are becoming resistant to formerly effective antibiotics has made the FDA, and certain critics of present livestock practices, question the wisdom of using these antibiotics. However, since their use has demonstrable economic value, especially in poultry raising, this issue will not be easily resolved.

Other drugs are used less widely as supplements of animal feed, including other antimicrobial, antiprotozoal, and antihelminthic agents. The effects of chronic exposure to these agents have not yet received the scrutiny applied to the drugs discussed earlier, and further study may cause some reevaluation of the application and restriction of these agents.

24.3.6.c. Miscellaneous Manufacturing By-products as Food Contaminants

This text has emphasized mechanisms by which industrial products and by-products may be released and dispersed in the environment. The wide distribution of these materials and the ubiquitousness of the human food chain afford many opportunities for contamination of the food supply. For example, PBB, a fire retardant, contaminated cattle feed in the Midwest through mishandling. More than 30,000 cattle and thousands of other farm animals were destroyed to prevent human consumption, but it was believed that some animals with elevated PBB levels did enter the food chain. Similarly, PCBs, used in many industrial applications, have been reported to occur widely in the food chain. Destruction of poultry because of PCB contamination from heat exchangers in the processing plant has been necessary, and fish (such as Hudson River salmon) have been contaminated by industrial PCB effluents.

Minerals have also ended up as food contaminants: asbestos was found in table salt in the United States in 1975. Another suspected industrial source of contamination has been certain of the packaging materials used. Under some circumstances plasticizers or monomers may migrate from acrylonitrile or polyvinyl chloride containers into the foods they contain.

Finally, materials used as aids in food marketing or production may contaminate foods. One example with PCBs has already been cited; other contaminants may include fumigants, such as ethylene oxide or methyl bromide, which may interact with food constituents, destroying essential nutrients. Both ethylene and propylene oxide have also been reported to react with foods containing inorganic chlorides to form toxic chlorohydrins.

24.4. Deliberate Food Additives

The food additives industry has a volume approaching $1 billion annually. The widespread addition of various chemicals to our food supply, although deliberate, constitutes a major route by which toxic chemicals may be added to our food. There are several goals that producers have when they add chemicals to foods.

24.4.1. Agents That Prolong or Preserve Food Quality

The modern food industry has spurred the use of food additives for two reasons: first, because it has become more centralized and methods are needed to preserve food quality between processing and consumption; and second, a new generation of previously unknown food products (e.g., "snack" foods) has developed. A whole series of food additives are used to prevent alterations in food quality between processing and purchase, or to aid in the preparation of food of a desired quality (Table 24.1). In general, these classes of food additives have been demonstrated in animal tests to be reasonably inert physiologically and have a low order of toxicity—results that have been consistent with the lack of gross effects on humans. However, continued testing and more sensitive methods of evaluating physiological risk may change this perspective.

24.4.2. Agents That Improve or Alter Food Quality

Some chemicals are added to foods to improve the taste or color of the foods rather than aid in processing or maintaining quality. Examples of these agents and their respective functions are listed in Table 24.1. For special reasons, these chemicals have been subjected to increasing scrutiny during the past few years; the artificial sweeteners, artificial colors, and nitrites have been of special concern.

24.4.2.a. Artificial Sweeteners

The first artificial sweetener used in foods was saccharin. Discovered in 1879, saccharin began to be used by the end of the 19th century and was the sole nonnutritive sweetener used until cyclamate was discovered in 1944. The potential hazards of both of these compounds began to receive increased attention in the 1960s when animal tests indicated that cyclamate preparations caused bladder cancer in rats. In 1969, these results led to the banning of cyclamates under the Delaney Clause. More recently, additional animal tests have demonstrated that saccharin, despite its apparent safety after decades of human use, also causes bladder cancer in laboratory rats. These results were confirmed using the Ames test, which gave a new sweetener, xylitol, a clean bill of health.

Despite this evidence indicating putative hazards in saccharin usage, there has been reluctance to ban it from foods. One argument that is used is that obesity is a major health problem in the United States, and banning of the major noncaloric sweetener would aggravate this and result in increased deaths from cardiovascular illnesses, diabetes, and related causes. This argument is coun-

Table 24.1 Examples of Uses of Deliberate Food Additives

Class	Examples
Agents that prolong, preserve or aid in processing food	
Acids, alkalais, buffers	Acetic acid
	Citric acid
	Alkalai hydroxides; carbonates
Anticaking agents	Magnesium carbonate
Antioxidants	Butylated hydroxytoluene (BHT)
	Butylated hydroxyanisole (BHA)
	Propyl gallate
Bleaching and maturing agents	Benzoyl peroxide
Humectants	Propylene glycol
	Glycerol
Mycostatic agents	Sodium benzoate
	Sorbic acid
	Propionates
Preservatives	Sodium chloride
	Sodium nitrate
Sequestering agents	Ethylenediaminetetraacetate (EDTA)
	Tartaric acid
Surfactants (emulsifiers; stabilizers; texturizers)	Polyoxyethylene sorbitan fatty esters
	Mono- and diglycerides
	Vegetable gums
	Acacia (gum arabic)
	Carrageenan
Coloring agents	Synthetic colors
	Natural colors (e.g., carotene)
Flavoring agents	Synthetic flavors (mixtures of chemicals)
	Spice extracts and essential oils
Flavor enhancers	Monosodium glutamate (MSG)
Meat curing agents	Sodium nitrites
	Natural and artificial smoke
Nutrients	Vitamins and minerals
	Amino acids
	Iodide
Sweeteners	Saccharin (nonnutritive)
	Corn syrup (nutritive)
	Various sugars

tered by the lack of evidence indicating that saccharin usage by obese individuals actually prevents excess intake of carbohydrates; some have suggested that it may synergistically exacerbate the very problem for which it is used. A second argument against banning saccharin notes that the best epidemiological studies have not found that saccharin causes an increase in bladder cancers in humans. However, because a carcinogen may cause different types of cancer in different species, those studies (even if valid for the entire population) did not assess saccharin-induced cancers in other tissues. Finally, the political impact of banning a household substance on the basis of scientific evidence always involves difficulties—if the overwhelming laboratory and epidemiological evidence indicating that cigarettes or their pyrolysis products are carcinogenic can be ignored, why will the public accept less clear-cut evidence about saccharin? As a footnote, more recent studies on cyclamate have demonstrated that the native compound itself may be safer than saccharin, and a manufacturing contaminant may have been responsible for the production of the cancers in laboratory animals.

24.4.2.b. Artificial Colors

More than three dozen different chemicals had been approved for use as colors in foods. These were both certified (each batch must be tested and approved for compliance by the FDA) and noncertified (mineral pigments or natural colors with low orders of toxicity and high tinctoral power). In recent years, many of these agents have been shown to be carcinogenic and have been banned from usage. Furthermore, there has been anecdotal evidence suggesting that artificial colors may cause allergic or other untoward responses resulting, according to some sources, in hyperkinesis in susceptible children. The latter speculations have, in most cases, not as yet received experimental confirmation in well-controlled laboratory or clinical studies, but they do raise concern about the use of coloring agents that are otherwise apparently acceptable. A key argument for banning these agents is that since they do not improve food quality, shelf life, or nutritive value, there is no justifiable reason to utilize them, especially in foods that will be consumed by children (who may be the most sensitive members of the population).

24.4.2.c. Nitrites and Nitrates

Many types of muscle tissue, in both fish and land animals, have historically been treated with nitrates and nitrites. It is now known that the preservative qualities of these salts are derived from the nitrites (nitrates are converted to nitrites in vivo), which inhibit bacterial growth (especially of species such as *Clostridium botulinum*), thereby providing a safety factor against mishandling of the treated foods. Furthermore, the nitrites impart a pleasing pink color to the treated tissue, which results in the appearance that is expected in hams, sausagelike products, and certain cured fish. However, it has recently been shown that under physiological conditions, nitrites can combine with certain amines present in foods or the gut to form nitrosoamines—chemicals with defined mutagenic and carcinogenic potential. Consistent with these results, well-conducted studies in one strain of rats have indicated that nitrites are indeed carcinogenic.

However, several facts mitigate against banning this chemical. First, recent work has demonstrated that only about 20% of the nitrites entering the gut are of direct dietary origin and some of these are from natural sources; the rest are a result of conversion and secretion from the salivary glands. Nitrites are also reported to be synthesized in the gut. This raises the question of whether banning cured meats, in which nitrites serve both a cosmetic and preservative function, would make a significant difference in the total physiological load of nitrites. It is plausible that only certain types of foods, such as raw fish prevalent in Japanese diets, present a significant hazard to human health, but this issue is still unresolved.

24.5. Food Contamination Caused by the Interaction of Chemicals

In the previous discussion of nitrites it was noted that the chemical itself is not directly responsible for toxicity, but rather required the presence of another ingredient for the noxious moiety to form. The chemical complexity of our diets suggests that chemical reactions occurring in the foods themselves, during processing (including cooking), and after ingestion, may markedly alter what may be considered, a priori, nontoxic food additives or contaminants. Interactions have been demonstrated with food additives, food contaminants, and endogenous materials that can result in the formation of potentially toxic materials.

An example of a food additive that was apparently innocuous was the antimold agent, diethylpyrocarbonate. This compound was supposed to have the particular advantage of self-degrading in the food after a few days, leaving no persistent residues. However, it was found that the compound could react with ammonia, present in most foods, to form urethan, a known carcinogen. Similar to the situation with nitrites, a chemical that was apparently innocuous alone had toxic possibilities when added to foods.

Similarly, natural food constituents may interact to form new toxic "adulterants." Recent studies have determined that carcinogens may be present in cooked meats. One source of these carcinogens appeared to be polycyclic aromatic hydrocarbons, such as benzo[a]pyrene, which forms during the pyrolysis of fats in grilled meats. However, it has recently been shown that other mutagens, which are distinguishable from the polycyclic aromatic hydrocarbons, are formed when ground beef is cooked, or when beef stock is concentrated. Whether these compounds are responsible for the increase in gastrointestinal cancers reported to be associated with meat consumption has yet to be determined. Other decomposition products of natural food constituents, such as malondialdehyde (resulting from peroxidized fatty acids), have been shown to have mutagenic potential and may be responsible for some of the untoward effects of ingestion of certain unsaturated fatty acids. Finally, the formation of lysinoalanine, a renal toxicant, has been reported to occur when high-protein foods are heated under alkaline conditions. Although the levels formed under normal conditions are apparently insufficient to cause toxic effects, certain susceptible individuals, such as those with preexisting kidney disease, may be at added risk.

The interaction of dietary components is an area that has received insufficient attention; because of the trend toward the addition of food additives and the use of "artificial" foods, as well as the possibility of contamination with environmental agents, this factor may be due additional attention.

Selected Reading

Fishbein, L., Flamm, W.G. Potential environmental hazards. II. Feed additives and pesticides. Sci. Total Environ. 1:31–64, 1972.

Furia, T.E. (Ed.). Handbook of Food Additives, second edition. Cleveland: Chemical Rubber Company Press, 1972.

Halsted, B.W. Poisonous and Venomous Marine Animals of the World (3 vols.). Washington, D.C.: U.S. Government Printing Office, 1965.

Hunter, B.T. Food Additives and Federal Policy: The Mirage of Safety. New York: Scribner's, 1975.

Kingsbury, J.M. Poisonous Plants of the United States and Canada, Englewood Cliffs, N.J.: Prentice-Hall, 1964.

LeRiche, W.H. Epidemiology in food safety evaluation—Past and present, Clin. Toxicol. 9:665–690, 1976.

Lijinsky, W., Coulston, F., Wolfe, S.M., et al. News Forum: Should the Delaney clause be changed?, Chem. Eng. News pp. 24–46, June 27, 1977.

Marquardt, H., Rufino, F., Weisburger, J.H. Mutagenic activity of nitrite-treated foods: Human stomach cancer may be related to dietary factors. Science 196:1000–1001, 1977.

National Research Council, Food Protection Committee. Chemicals Used in Food Processing. Publ. 1274. Washington, D.C.: National Academy of Sciences, 1965.

National Research Council, Food Protection Committee. Toxicants Occuring Naturally in Foods, Second edition. Washington, D.C.: National Academy of Sciences, 1973.

Newberne, P.M. Diet and nutrition. Bull. N.Y. Acad. Med., 54:385–396, 1978.

Rodricks, J.V. (Ed.). Mycotoxins and Other Fungal Related Food Problems. Advances in Chemistry Series, No. 149. Washington, D.C.: American Chemical Society, 1976.

Walker, E.A., Griciute, L., Castegnaro, M., et al. (Eds.). Environmental Aspects of N-nitroso Compounds. Lyon, France: International Agency for Research on Cancer, 1978.

Lynne A. Stirling

25

Microorganisms and Environmental Pollutants

25.1. Introduction

Life on earth depends on the cyclic turnover of a number of essential elements such as carbon, nitrogen, sulfur, oxygen, and phosphorous. The earth has only a finite amount of these elements, and for continuity of life these elements have to be used and reused. Microorganisms are indispensable agents in these "life-maintaining" processes, better known as the cycles of matter. The sheer ubiquity of microorganisms and their significant contribution to the biosphere in terms of total bulk of living material (about 50% of the total biomass of the biosphere is in fact microbial) highlight their overall importance.

The carbon cycle is a process fundamental to the circulation of carbon in the biosphere. This cycle is dependent for its continuation upon the degradative ability of microorganisms in the mineralization of a wide range of organic molecules to atmospheric carbon dioxide, which can then be fixed by photosynthesis. The role of microorganisms in this cycle is outlined in Figure 25.1. Thus microorganisms maintain the carbon cycle, preventing the accumulation of vast amounts of organic matter in the biosphere, which would preclude the existence of any living forms within a relatively short period of time.

The nitrogen cycle is of prime importance in crop nutrition. Through a series of microbial reactions, organic nitrogen is transformed into nitrate, the most valuable form for crops. Figure 25.2 outlines the various steps in this cycle. The sulfur cycle (Figure 25.3) is in many respects similar to the nitrogen cycle, although different microbial species are involved in the transformations. Sulfur is available to living organisms principally in the form of soluble sulfates or reduced organic sulfur compounds.

Many bacterial species are involved at various stages of these cycles, thus microbial types and populations must remain reasonably stable over long periods to ensure that the necessary transformations can take place. These cycles do not function in isolation. The balanced maintenance of *all* these cycles of

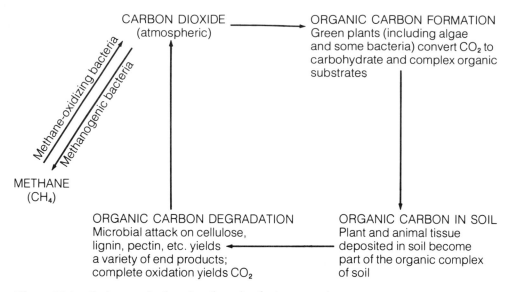

Figure 25.1 Carbon cycle showing the role of microorganisms.

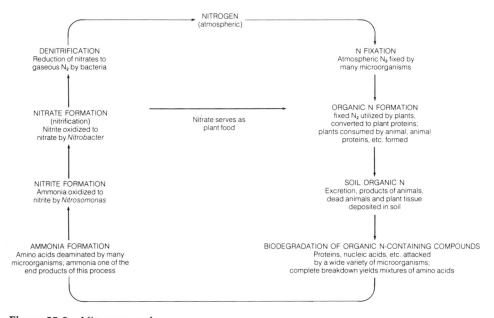

Figure 25.2 Nitrogen cycle.

matter is necessary to ensure a constant supply of those elements required by plants, whose photosynthetic abilities initially harness solar energy, making any life on earth possible. Any disruption of these major cycles would have far-reaching effects on the biosphere as a whole. For more detailed information on these cycles the reader should consult any standard microbiology textbook.

Microorganisms perhaps make their presence most felt as the causative agents in many diseases, but their role(s) in the pollution of our environment are of

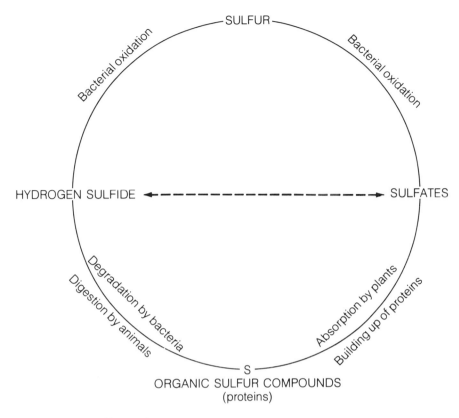

Figure 25.3   Sulfur cycle.

almost equal significance to man. Microorganisms play a dual role in pollution in that they can both generate toxicants and detoxify potentially harmful substances. In this chapter these aspects of microbial action are dealt with and the effects of a number of environmental pollutants on microbial systems themselves are discussed. Although by no means comprehensive, it is hoped that this discussion will provide the reader with the necessary stimulation to examine some of these subjects in more depth.

25.2. Effects of Toxicants on Microorganisms

Environmental pollutants can be divided into three broad categories: those occurring naturally, those either transformed or concentrated by living or nonliving systems, and those produced by man's activities. Some of these pollutants are listed in Table 25.1. One should note that "natural" is not always synonymous with "harmless," and by the same token man-made substances are not always hazardous. The crucial point to remember is that a balance has to be maintained, and when this is upset by either natural or man-made events the background levels of many compounds in the biosphere increase to such an extent that they pose a threat to many living forms. *Any* substance that is added to the environment at a rate greater than it can be removed, i.e., cycled, will

Table 25.1   Origin of Pollutants

Naturally occurring	Transformed and concentrated	Synthesized
Nitrogen oxides	Sewage	Pesticides
Nitrate	Fertilizers	Surfactants
Nitrite	Acid waste	Radionuclides
Asbestos	Fuel combustion products	Synthetic polymers
Heavy metals	Heavy metals	Petrochemicals
Radionuclides	Radionuclides	
Hydrocarbons and their derivatives	Pesticides	
Allergens	Hydrocarbons	
	Petrochemicals	

Source: With permission from Higgins, I. J., Burns, R. J. The Chemistry and Microbiology of Pollution. Copyright 1976 by Academic Press Inc. (London) Ltd.

build up. The capacity of a compound to persist for long periods of time and become a pollutant will depend on a number of its inherent physico-chemical properties and also its toxicity to all living forms.

25.2.1. Heavy Metals

A number of metals are required in minute amounts by most living organisms for normal maintenance. Some metals, particularly the heavy metals, have been found to be environmental pollutants. Lead and mercury are perhaps the most infamous, but others, such as cadmium, zinc, nickel, and chromium, when present at sufficiently high concentrations, can also pose a threat to living systems.

Lead is used in significant quantities by most industrialized nations. Electrical batteries, cable sheathing, metal piping, paint pigments, wood primers, rust inhibitors, polyvinyl chloride, plastic stabilizers, and "antiknock" agents in gasoline all use lead in their manufacture. Thus its potential for environmental contamination is enormous, and in recent years its accumulation in the environment has been the cause of much concern. Lead has no nutrient value and is, in fact, quite toxic to microorganisms. Much research has centered on this characteristic. The retardation of organic matter decay by microbes following lead treatment has been observed and is thought to be due to lead binding to selected sites on enzymes essential for microbial growth to the exclusion of other required elements such as magnesium, manganese, and iron.

The many properties of mercury, both medical and mystical, have been known for over 2000 years. Mercury is a natural component of the environment, occurring as metallic mercury and mercuric sulfide. A whole range of manufacturing industries have increased the background level of this metal. Batteries, street lamps, and circuit breakers, all of which are discarded after use, include mercury in their manufacture. Mercuric chloride catalysts are employed in the manufacture of vinyl chloride and urethane plastics. Phenylmercuric acetate is a fungicide in paints, and a number of other mercury compounds are used in agriculture. The largest contributor to environmental mercury levels is the chloralkali industry, with other minor contributions from fossil fuels, paper and pulp industries, dental preparations, antiseptics, and floor waxes.

Both elemental mercury and mercuric sulfide are volatile and are thus able to cycle, with a little help from man, between soil, water, air, plants, and animals. The effects of mercury on soil microbes, enzyme activities, and rates of carbon and nitrogen mineralization have been the subject of much investigation. The organomercurials (compounds containing both mercury and organic moieties) have been found to be more inhibitory than their inorganic counterparts. For example, methylmercuric chloride is 20 times more potent than mercuric chloride in decimating the number of soil microbes in experiments carried out under laboratory conditions. Ammonification and nitrification, necessary biotic processes for soil fertility, are retarded by relatively low concentrations of either phenylmercuric acetate or mercuric chloride, with the former more potent than the latter. Theoretically, the effects shown in the laboratory (where high concentrations of mercury are used) should not occur when a "normal" background level of mercury is present in the environment. However, if the levels of mercury in the environment are abnormally increased via industrial usage and dispersal, the inhibitory effects on essential microbiological processes could have serious consequences from an economic, ecological, and public health point of view.

25.2.2. Pesticides

Pesticides can be defined as those chemicals employed by man to destroy or inhibit life forms considered by him to be a nuisance. The survival of mankind depends upon the economical and abundant production of food. To ensure this production, pest outbreaks, whatever form they may take, must be controlled. Since the end of World War II the production and use of organic pesticides has increased enormously. It was at first assumed that microbes were infallible in their ability to degrade these compounds (after they had served their purpose) and thus could remove them from the environment. However, in the 1950s it became apparent that pesticides were persisting where they were ineffective, distributing where they were not wanted, and concentrating to levels deleterious to many living systems.

Pesticides can be divided into three broad groups: inorganic compounds, organic compounds, and organic compounds containing metal ions. Many of them have rather complex chemical structures. The structures of those mentioned in the text are given in Figure 17.1. The literature on various aspects of pesticide persistence, toxicity, and degradation is voluminous. Pesticides influence microbial populations by altering their metabolic and physiological activities. These effects are most pronounced when pesticides are applied in large amounts or at frequent intervals. Microbial carbon dioxide production, oxygen consumption, growth rates, nitrification, and legume nodulation are all used as indicators of pesticide response. If, under laboratory conditions, any of these processes is inhibited one must then seek a correlation between in vitro and in vivo and also in situ conditions. It should be borne in mind that many of the results described in this chapter were obtained under laboratory conditions and might not truly represent environmental conditions, where a host of other parameters come into play. Extensions from the laboratory to the environment are always fraught with pitfalls—liquid culture versus soil, micro- versus macroclimate, uneven distribution in situ, the need to use organic solvents in vitro, and so forth.

Pesticides appear to affect both actual numbers of microorganisms and those transformations dependent upon microorganisms. Much laboratory work has involved the use of 10–1000 times the levels normally applied to soil, which is not really that far removed from reality when one considers the uneven concentration of pesticides in many environmental niches. The influence of pesticides on total numbers of microorganisms in soil and on particular genera has merited much attention. High levels of a pesticide may radically change the total soil zoological population, destroying many highly evolved communities and, as a result, changing the comparative levels of organisms. Fungicides can destroy plant and animal fungal pathogens, altering the microbial flora to a significant extent. Different microbial species may then dominate in a particular environmental niche, altering the whole ecology of that niche.

Nitrification and nitrogen fixation are the most frequently assessed soil microbial activities in relation to effects of pesticide application. It does appear that the microorganisms most susceptible to pesticides are those that are involved in key biogeochemical cycles. Nitrification is inhibited by some pesticides at low levels, whereas others have to be present at high levels before there is any decline in nitrification rates. Herbicides apparently do not affect nitrification, whereas selected fungicides have been shown to decrease nitrification to some extent. It has been suggested that organophosphate insecticides may significantly inhibit some microbial enzymes, but again relatively high concentrations need to be applied before any major microbiological changes are induced.

25.2.3. Hydrocarbons

Hydrocarbons are compounds consisting of carbon and hydrogen only. In nature, animal, plant, and microbial activities produce a wide range of hydrocarbons which can be divided into three broad groups: the paraffins (alkanes, isoalkanes, and alkenes), the cycloparaffins (cycloalkanes and naphthenes), and the aromatics. In addition there are massive reservoirs of hydrocarbons on earth in the form of coal and crude oil. The most obvious detrimental introduction of hydrocarbons arises from large-scale release by industry or spillage in the transport of crude oil.

Low molecular weight hydrocarbons such as hexane (C_6) and heptane (C_7) are quite toxic to a variety of microorganisms. This is due to the fact that these are effective lipid solvents and can thus destroy bacterial cell membranes and cell wall lipids. Other n-alkanes can inhibit the growth of selected microbes in the laboratory, especially if they are added at high concentrations. Hydrocarbons can be utilized for growth by many bacterial types, and microbes appear to be able to cope with many of the simple hydrocarbons that occur in the environment. However, the complexity of substances such as crude oil creates problems that will not be dealt with here.

Aromatic hydrocarbons, especially polynuclear hydrocarbons, are known to be carcinogenic for many animals. The effects of these compounds on microorganisms have not been rigorously defined, but data from Russian laboratories suggest that such compounds are inhibitory to microorganisms, although the mechanistic details are still unclear. Halogenation of hydrocarbons appears to increase their toxicity to living forms. Studies with PCBs have shown that these compounds are inhibitory to marine microorganisms. The difficulties encountered in isolating organisms in the laboratory able to degrade halogenated compounds highlights their potential toxicity. This toxicity has been the basis of their inclusion in a number of pesticides.

25.2.4. Air Pollutants

Air pollutants can be conveniently divided into two groups: those arising from natural sources and those produced by man's technology. Today the major sources of air pollution include transportation, industry, power plants, heating, and refuse disposal together with those outputs from plant and microbial allergens and spray aerosols. Nature's contributions include methane and hydrogen sulfide, usually present as the result of microbial metabolism.

The types of pollutants that commonly occur in air include sulfur and nitrogen compounds, carbon monoxide, hydrocarbons, and ozone. Many gaseous hydrocarbons are effective inhibitors of spore germination. Symbiotic nitrogen-fixing organisms are adversely affected by sulfur dioxide, nitrous oxide, and aldehydes. Peroxyacetyl nitrate has been found to inhibit a number of bacterial enzymes. Ozone is lethal to bacteria in low concentrations; the site of attack is thought to be the cell membrane. Carcinogenic hydrocarbon air pollutants can also adversely affect microorganisms. Under laboratory conditions, the main target of these pollutants is microbial lipid synthesis. Air pollutants can affect the normal microbial flora of the human skin, altering the populations that are found there. The major problems associated with air pollutants are the disruption of microbial interrelationships and the introduction of these compounds into food chains. Microbes are capable of accumulating some of these pollutants, and thus they eventually enter higher animals.

It is important to remember that most of the compounds mentioned only affect microorganisms in a deleterious fashion when events cause their levels to be elevated to hypernormal proportions. Industry must be vigilant in its endeavor to ensure that its activities will not disrupt the delicate and necessary balances that exist between microorganisms and their environment.

25.3. Generation of Toxicants by Microorganisms

25.3.1. Toxic Products of Pesticide Metabolism

As well as being the victims of many environmental pollutants, microorganisms can also play the villain and generate potentially harmful compounds in a variety of ways. Pesticides are indeed toxic, but they are, or can be, transformed microbiologically to new toxicants that act on species also inhibited by the original compound. Thus, instead of the environment containing only the original pesticide, it may also contain an additional two or three toxic products. In addition, several pesticides that are active in their original forms are converted microbiologically to new inhibitors that act not only on the original species but also on a wider range of organisms; e.g., a fungicide may be converted to a human carcinogen.

An examination of the structure of chlorinated hydrocarbon insecticides, DDT, and aldrin (see Figure 17.1) illustrates clearly how new and more persistent products can be generated from an already durable parent. The widely known pesticide DDT controls a wide array of insects. It can be converted to DDD (loss of a chlorine), which is likewise insecticidal and acts on a somewhat different spectrum of insects than its precursor. A high percentage of the bacteria isolated from marine waters and raw sewage are very successful in their capacity to convert DDT to DDD.

Aldrin is subject to microbial epoxidation, and the product of this reaction, dieldrin, is both insecticidal and persistent. Some species of bacteria can apparently metabolize dieldrin to a still more toxic product, photodieldrin. Aldrin disappears slowly with time, whereas the epoxide persists for years. Numerous other chlorinated molecules are subject to microbial modification, and some of the metabolites that are generated are extremely toxic and long lasting. Herbicides and fungicides can also be biotransformed into more toxic products and products affecting nonnuisance species.

The list of halogenated pesticides that can be modified to yield environmental pollutants is large. In many cases this transformation is merely the consequence of nonspecific microbial enzyme capabilities. Microorganisms have evolved these capabilities, and the solution to this problem, if such a solution is attainable, must be sought through more rigid examination of these transforming abilities coupled with increased scrutiny of those pesticides used.

25.3.2. Toxic Mercury Products

The toxicity of mercury is unquestionable, and, in addition, microorganisms have been found that use this material to generate more toxic products than mercury itself. Micoorganisms in sediments, where mercury ions are present, can transform these to produce methylmercury ($Ch_3 Hg^+$). This can enter fish and accumulate in their tissues; consumption of such contaminated fish is ill advised. Methylmercury stands out as an environmental hazard because it is more poisonous to man and other mammals than inorganic mercury ions and is excreted slowly. Microbial metabolism of mercury is not limited to aquatic systems but also occurs widely in soils. Some bacteria can also cleave the C–Hg bond in several organomercurial compounds; for example, a *Pseudomonas* species can volatilize mercury from phenylmercuric acetate, ethylmercuric phosphate, and methylmercuric chloride, which all occur in industrial wastes.

25.3.3. Toxic Products of Arsenic Metabolism

Arsenic has a long and notorious history as a poison and is toxic to most living forms. Volatile trimethylarsine [$(CH_3)_3As$] is also a notable human toxicant. Small amounts of arsenic occur in many natural materials, with trace amounts occurring in soil and water. Before 1960, organic arsenicals were widely applied as herbicides, and lead arsenate was once used to spray fruit trees. Microbial transformations of this element first became evident when human poisonings were reported in rooms containing wallpaper colored with arsenic-containing pigments. The pigment itself was not the lethal agent, but the wallpaper served as a support for the growth of fungi that liberated the volatile poison, trimethylarsine. Arsenic-containing gases, characterized by their garlic odor, are liberated by many fungi and microorganisms growing in media containing this element. Arsenic volatilization that occurs in soil is also attributable to microbiological activities. Other microorganisms in the laboratory are able to reduce arsenate to the more toxic arsenite or to oxidize trivalent arsenic to the pentavalent arsenate.

25.3.4. Acid Mine Water

Major sources of microbiologically induced pollution are sulfide (pyrite) ores. If these ores are exposed to air they undergo a series of alterations, in which microorganisms play a crucial role, leading to serious consequences in coal mining areas such as the Appalachian mountain range and the Netherlands and other countries where soils were reclaimed from the sea for agriculture. The acid drainage from these coal mines often has a pH less than 4.0 and in addition contains large amounts of soluble sulfate and iron. In many cases the pollution, originating in the mine, extends for many miles downstream, destroying aquatic communities and the like. It is hardly surprising that highly acid waters are totally unsuitable for human and industrial use. In 1969 it was estimated that 2900 acres of reservoirs and impoundments and 4800 miles of streams in the United States were polluted by surface coal mining. Metal can be corroded and even concrete structures may be damaged. Highly acid waters have a disastrous effect on microorganisms as well as other biota. The surviving bacterial populations are typically acid tolerant, with fungi and yeasts predominating. Sulfur and iron-oxidizing autotrophs proliferate extensively, and their numbers become extraordinarily large. The sulfides in waste materials can be oxidized, with the release of sulfuric acid and soluble forms of calcium, zinc, and nickel.

The role of autotrophs in the production of acid waters from pyrite ores has aroused considerable interest and controversy. The process is thought to consist of three steps: (a) the oxidation of sulfide to sulfate; (b) the conversion of Fe^{2+} to Fe^{3+}; and (c) the precipitation of ferric hydroxide. The final products from FeS_2 and O_2 would then be $Fe(OH)_3$ and H_2SO_4. The formation of acid waters, however, is not a simple and straightforward bacterial oxidation of pyrite FeS_2, and much debate has centered around delineating the bacterial steps from the nonbacterial. Some bacteria are abundant in acid waters, and they undoubtedly proliferate at the expense of oxidizable inorganic substrates. Moreover, the inoculation of pyrite with particular bacteria enhances the rate of acid formation from the ore. On the other hand, FeS_2 is oxidized, albeit slowly, in the absence of microorganisms. It has been suggested that the rate-limiting step is pyrite oxidation. Acid formation is ferrous (Fe^{2+}) oxidation, and it is probably here that bacteria play their crucial role by accelerating a reaction that is normally slow at a pH below 4.5.

Attempts have been made to counteract acid production in coal mines. The methods used have included the stimulation of sulfate-reducing organisms in an attempt to reprecipitate sulfur as sulfide, the addition of antimicrobial agents, and the precipitation of sulfur by treating effluents with limestone to elevate the pH.

25.3.5. Other Sulfur Compounds

Microbial metal corrosion seems to follow logically from a discussion on acid mine water, and, although not thought of as pollution per se, its consequences can be harmful to other living systems. Sulfur bacteria are the culprits in the corrosion of metal, in that sulfate-oxidizing bacteria produce H_2SO_4, and sulfate-reducing bacteria evolve H_2S, both of which have a direct corrosive effect on metal surfaces. Formed in many ecosystems, H_2S has long been noted for its toxicity to humans, plants, animals, and microorganisms. The quantity of biologically evolved H_2S is much greater than that generated by industry. It is effectively formed by the reduction of sulfate by the bacteria *Desulfovibrio* and by the cleavage of sulfur-containing organic molecules. Sulfate-reducing microorganisms are ubiquitous in muds, swamps, and poorly drained soils, where they proliferate, using sulfate as their terminal electron acceptor. An array of organic compounds can be converted to H_2S by many heterotrophs in culture, and an almost equally large array of microorganisms cleave sulfur from organic molecules and release it as H_2S. The rate of H_2S evolution can be markedly increased if sulfite is present and the environment becomes anaerobic. The production of H_2S is also pronounced during the decay of algae in water, and it is a common transformation in lake and ocean bottom sediments, swamps, bogs, marshes, raw sewage, and industrial effluents, where one can hardly fail to notice its rotten egg aroma.

This rather common metabolite is an extremely effective toxicant for humans. *Desulfovibrio* can proliferate in the anaerobic environment of deep sea oil pipelines, and in the North Sea operations fatalities have occurred when divers sent down to free microbiologically fouled pipelines have been overcome by H_2S fumes. In addition, higher plants are remarkably susceptible to free H_2S, and economic losses of some magnitude have occurred after the roots of rice and fruit crops have come into contact with toxic quantities.

25.3.6. Carcinogens

25 3.6.a. Nitrosamines

Much time and research has been centered on nitrosamines since it has been found that these compounds are carcinogenic as well as teratogenic and mutagenic at very low concentrations. Secondary and tertiary amines that are potentially subject to N-nitrosation are widespread in regions inhabited by microorganisms. Such amines are found in the tissues of algae and higher plants. Manure containing diphenylamine and trimethylamine is not uncommon, and many pesticides contain amines.

Nitrosamines can be generated in the gastrointestinal tract provided that both the amine and either nitrate or nitrite is present. Evidence suggests that microorganisms are implicated in this process, although nitrosamine formation can also occur by nonbiological methods. However, several microorganisms studied in isolation have been shown to be capable of synthesizing nitrosamines, and thus their role in the production of these toxic compounds should not be underestimated.

25.3.6.b. Other Carcinogens

At first sight it might seem a little farfetched to suggest a role for microorganisms in carcinogenesis, but it has been suggested that environmental factors may be involved in the etiology of 80–90% of cancers in humans. Considering the sheer ubiquity of bacteria, fungi, and the like, and the many substances that they may excrete in nature, it is not too unrealistic to postulate that they are involved, directly or indirectly, in the induction of cancerous growths.

Diet might well be implicated in cancer (the low incidence of colon cancer in African countries where the diet is mainly vegetarian testifies to this). Gross differences in diet alter the composition of the bacterial community of the intestine. The different bacteria, which have a variety of substrates available to them as foodstuffs, pass through the alimentary tract and the colon and may then synthesize carcinogens such as the sterols deoxycholic acid, cholenic acid, and apocholic acid in situ. Experimental findings do disclose a difference between both bacteria and sterols in the intestinal contents of people residing in areas with a low incidence of cancer and those residing in areas with a high incidence.

Carcinogenic aromatic hydrocarbons have been previously mentioned and are found in many locales, sometimes in disturbingly high amounts. Their ubiquity must be due, in part, to their production by microorganisms in waters, soils, and sediments. As an example of such production, cycasin (methylazoxy-methanol-D-glucoside) is a constituent of the nut of the fern known as cycad and is itself harmless. However, when given to animals, members of the intestinal bacterial community hydrolyze the molecule to the free carcinogen, methylazoxymethanol. Similar examples can be found in the literature. A few substances produced by microorganisms in culture act as carcinogens, but it is not known if they are synthesized outside the laboratory.

It should be apparent that water, soil, and the air itself are being constantly contaminated with products derived from microbial activities in natural ecosystems. Some of these metabolites may never reach levels that threaten man, animals, crops, wildlife, etc. Others have already attained and exceeded these danger levels in particular regions, causing injury to higher organisms.

25.4. Effects of Microorganisms on Environmental Pollutants

As well as creating pollutants, microbes have the ability to detoxify many potential pollutants, preventing their accumulation. Many of the compounds mentioned in this section should by now be familiar to the reader.

25.4.1. Hydrocarbon Metabolism

It has been known for many years that microorganisms can degrade hydrocarbons. The degradative ability of microorganisms is the reason we are not all knee deep in hydrocarbons today. The first account of this phenomenon was in 1895, and since then the metabolism of hydrocarbons has been extensively studied. It has been estimated that about 20% of all microbial species examined in the laboratory have some capacity to degrade hydrocarbons, the most expert being species of *Pseudomonas, Nocardia,* and *Mycobacteria.* Microbes have been shown to metabolize all types of hydrocarbon. *n*-Alkanes are the most readily degraded, while branched-chain compounds are less easily metabolized. The number of microorganisms that degrade aromatic hydrocarbons is more limited, and organisms that degrade alicyclic hydrocarbons are the lowest in number.

The various metabolic pathways will not be discussed in any detail here; excellent discussions of these pathways are found in several reviews. However, some aspects of the reactions involved are worthy of brief mention. The initial reaction in the microbial degradation involves the incorporation of molecular oxygen into the substrate; this reaction is catalyzed by oxygenase enzymes. Although the mechanistic details of this reaction vary for the different types of hydrocarbons, the end result is the same—an oxygen-containing intermediate is formed. In the case of n-alkanes the initial product is the corresponding alcohol, which can be further degraded to yield products that can enter the central metabolic pathways. The inclusion of the double bond in n-alkenes allows other possible reactions (e.g., epoxidation), but the major pathway is thought to resemble that for n-alkanes. The initial oxidative attack on aromatic hydrocarbons has been fully elucidated only in the past decade. The main distinguishing feature between this reaction and that for alkanes is that both atoms of oxygen are incorporated into the aromatic ring, whereas only one atom of oxygen is incorporated into alkanes. Alicyclic hydrocarbons are the most resistant to microbial attack, but evidence to date suggests that the initial reaction involves the incorporation of one atom of molecular oxygen.

It has recently been suggested that major crude oil spills could be removed by the addition of various hydrocarbon-utilizing microbes. This suggestion seems, for a number of reasons, rather impractical for the dispersal of large-scale oil spills, but it may be feasible in some small-scale mopping-up operations. It is unlikely at the moment that microorganisms will be the panacea that major oil companies have been waiting for.

25.4.2. Pesticide Metabolism

It is clear that the disappearance of many organic pesticides from the soil is largely due to the activities of microorganisms. The conditions that favor bacterial growth often coincide with the most rapid rates of pesticide disappearance. Moreover, there is often a relationship between actual numbers of bacteria in the soil and the rate of disappearance of a pesticide. More direct evidence of microbial detoxification of pesticides has come from experiments in which the inhibition of microbial activity results in much reduced rates of degradation.

For a long time the final proof of the dominant role of soil microbes has been the isolation of the organism responsible and its growth in pure culture using the pesticide as its sole source of carbon or nitrogen. This is perhaps not the best approach since mixed cultures of microbes may degrade a particular compound whereas no single species is able to. In recent years it has become evident that pesticides can be substantially altered by cometabolism (see Section 25.4.3.). A number of microorganisms have been shown to grow with pesticides as the sole carbon, energy, and sometimes nitrogen source. This capacity is widespread among species of *Pseudomonas*, *Nocardia*, and *Aspergillus*. It is quite remarkable that so many microorganisms can metabolize these complex, often chlorine-containing, organic molecules since these are relatively novel substances in the evolutionary time scale and have had little contact with microbes. This faculty may have arisen in two ways: induction of enzymes that the organism already has the genetic competence to produce and mutations leading to altered control mechanisms.

Microbes catalyze a number of basic chemical alterations to pesticide molecules that can be summarized as follows:

1. *Dehalogenation:* This usually involves the removal of chlorine.
2. *Dealkylation:* This occurs to several pesticides that have alkyl groups attached to nitrogen, oxygen, or sulfur atoms; alkyl groups attached to carbon atoms are in general resistant to microbial attack.
3. *Amide and ester hydrolysis:* Many pesticides are esters of inorganic acids, such as the phosphate ester insecticides, or are amides, such as the phenylamine herbicides. Several microbes have been shown to hydrolyze the amide and ester bonds in these compounds.
4. *Ring cleavage:* Aromatic rings are degraded by many soil bacteria and fungi. Initially the rings are oxidized by oxygenases, forming catechols, which can then be cleaved further.

25.4.3. Cometabolism

Many detoxification reactions occur while the microbe is utilizing the pesticide or other recalcitrant molecule as its sole source of carbon and energy, but microbes can also bring about chemical alterations of pesticides and other organic molecules without deriving sufficient carbon or energy for growth from them. This process has been called cometabolism and is thought to reflect a lack of substrate specificity on the part of some of the microbial transport mechanisms and enzymes. Clearly, for cometabolism to occur, the microbes must obtain the bulk, or all, of their carbon and energy from other substrates.

The phenomenon of cometabolism is important in relation to environmental pollution, because it presents the possibility that a series of cometabolic reactions involving several microorganisms can lead to the total degradation of a particular organic compound, such as DDT, that has been described as recalcitrant, partly because it has not been possible to isolate any microbe capable of utilizing it as the sole carbon and energy source. There is evidence suggesting that two microorganisms can together convert DDT to *p*-chlorophenylacetic acid by cometabolism, although it is not yet known whether this occurs in the environment.

The lesson that cometabolism teaches is that it is not an essential criterion of a pesticide's biodegradability that it be capable of serving as the sole source of carbon and energy for microbial growth.

25.5. Conclusion

The statement at the beginning of this chapter that life on earth would cease without microbial activities should now seem clearly justified. Microbes can be our enemies and our friends in the context of pollution—in this case man is master of his fate to a certain extent. If he continues to use the environment as a convenient sink for noxious waste, microbes will either fail to degrade or will merely partially degrade this waste to even more noxious compounds. The balance that has to be maintained may seem rather tenuous, but it is not unattainable and can be achieved if a sufficient commitment is made by everyone.

Suggested Reading

Alexander, M. Microbial formation of environmental pollutants. Adv. Appl. Microbiol. 18, pp. 1–73, 1974.

Bollag, J. M. Microbial transformation of pesticides. Adv. Appl. Microbiol. 18, pp. 75–130, 1974.

Dagley, S. Biochemistry and pollution. In Campbell, P. N., Aldridge, W. N. (Eds). Essays in Biochemistry. London: Academic Press, 1975.

Higgins, I. J., Burns, R. G. The Chemistry and Microbiology of Pollution. London: Academic Press, 1976.

McKenna, E.J., Kallio, R.E. The biology of hydrocarbons. Annu. Rev. Microbiol. 19, pp. 183–208, 1965.

Van der Linden, A. C., Thijsse, G. J. E. The mechanisms of microbial oxidation of petroleum hydrocarbons. Adv. Enzymol. 27: 469–546, 1965.

Roger D. Wyatt

26

Mycotoxins

26.1. Introduction

Mycotoxin is a term applied to a broad class of highly toxic secondary metabolites resulting from mold growth occurring on a specific substrate. The formation of mycotoxins in grain and animal feeds represents a potential economic threat to agriculture from unacceptability of grain for animal use or decreased performance of livestock and poultry consuming such contaminated grain or feed. In addition, if this situation goes unnoticed, human health could be adversely affected by mycotoxin residues in the edible portions of animals. Furthermore, mycotoxin contamination of cereal grains and oil seeds could have a direct impact on human health since a substantial portion of our diet comes directly from cereal grains, oil seeds, or their derivatives.

26.2. History

The problems associated with mycotoxin formation in agricultural commodities came to the forefront in the early 1960s as the result of a disease outbreak in Great Britain. This disease of unknown etiology caused the death of thousands of cattle, swine, sheep, chickens, and turkeys. Turkeys were among the first animals to be noticed as having the disease, and a high percentage of the losses occurred in this species—consequently the disease syndrome was called "turkey X disease." Within a short time after the disease occurred, British scientists found that the agent responsible was associated with feed, specifically, imported groundnut meal. In addition, a chemical compound formed as a result of mold growth on the meal, when given to healthy animals, would reproduce the disease symptoms. Shortly thereafter this chemical was found to be produced by a strain of *Aspergillus flavus* and was given the trivial name aflatoxin (Figure 26.1). Within a couple of years, aflatoxin was found to be a potent carcinogen in certain species of animals and much of the scientific attention directed toward aflatoxin was centered on its carcinogenic potential.

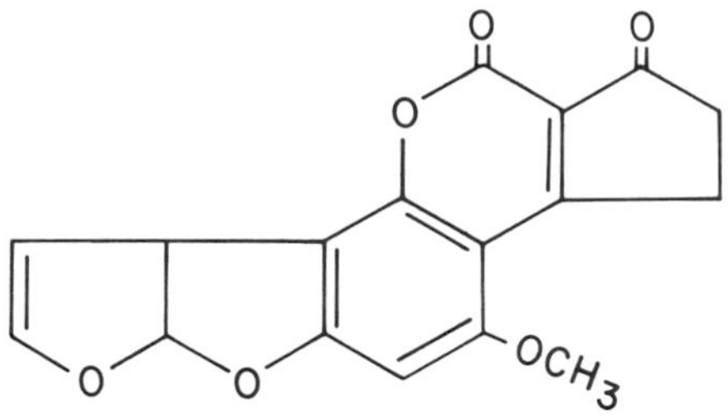

Figure 26.1   Chemical structure of aflatoxin B₁.

Simultaneously, efforts were initiated to determine the prevalence of other mycotoxins that might contaminate feed. Numerous research efforts were also initiated to determine the relationships between dietary mycotoxins and animal and human health. Currently about 200 different mycotoxins are known to be produced by numerous genera of fungi either under laboratory conditions or naturally in various agricultural commodities. Aflatoxin is generally regarded as the most toxic and most prevalent mycotoxin and is the one mycotoxin that routinely causes losses in animal production year after year. Aflatoxin is now recognized as the most potent carcinogen in rats, and epidemical data strongly suggest that aflatoxin is involved either directly or indirectly in human health problems. The molds that produce mycotoxins are ubiquitous in nature and can grow over a wide range of environmental conditions. In the words of one mycotoxin researcher, " Everything fit for consumption by man or beast has the potential to be contaminated with at least one mycotoxin at some time from production to consumption" (P.B. Hamilton, personal communication).

26.3. Mycotoxin Formation

Whether or not a mycotoxin is formed and the amount formed in a substrate are dependent upon several factors. One factor is the genetic capacity of the fungus to code for the necessary enzymes, metabolic pathways, and cellular processes required for formation of the mycotoxin. Without this inherent ability for mycotoxin formation, regardless of the status of all other factors, no mycotoxin will be formed.

It is also essential that conditions for fungal growth be met before mycotoxin formation can take place. Fungi are strict aerobes; consequently, a supply of free oxygen is necessary for growth and subsequent mycotoxin formation. Fungi must be able to derive a source of carbon, energy, and necessary nutrients from their substrate to support their growth. Additionally, certain nutrients are specifically required for mycotoxin formation, independent of growth. Therefore, it is possible in certain instances to affect mycotoxin formation by manipulation of essential nutrients without affecting the growth pattern of the organism. For example, *A. flavus*, the primary fungal producer of aflatoxin, has a rather stringent requirement for zinc. Without adequate availability of zinc, abundant mold growth will occur; however, significant amounts of aflatoxin will not be formed. In raw soybeans the zinc appears to be in bound form and unavailable for mold utilization. Consequently, aflatoxin formation in raw soybeans is usually not considered a severe problem even though this substrate can become obviously moldy with *A. flavus*.

As with most microorganisms, each mold species has an optimum growth temperature. Usually this temperature will coincide with the temperature at which maximum levels of its respective mycotoxin(s) will be formed; however, a few exceptions do exist. One such exception is that of *Fusarium tricinctum* and its most widely studied mycotoxin, called T-2 toxin. The optimum temperature for growth of this mold is about 20°C; however, at this temperature little if any T-2 toxin is formed. At a temperature of about 5–10°C the mold grows very slowly, but maximal formation of T-2 toxin results. Hence, temperature has a direct impact on both mold growth and mycotoxin formation; however, the relationships among temperature, mold growth, and mycotoxin formation are complex and not yet fully understood.

These findings indicate that mycotoxin production in a given commodity can vary with differences in environmental conditions such as seasonal variation of temperatures and humidity and the subtle differences encountered from one year to the next. In a similar fashion, the formation of a given mycotoxin in various substrates may be altered due to differences in nutrient composition or availability.

Perhaps the single most limiting factor for growth of mycotoxin is moisture. A rather high water activity is required before mold growth will occur. As with temperature, a specific mold has an optimum water activity for growth. This requirement varies between genera and species. Consequently, if a given substrate is contaminated with a variety of toxigenic molds, which one will grow and produce a mycotoxin is primarily dependent upon the water activity in the substrate.

Table 26.1 lists the major mold organisms and their respective mycotoxins generally considered to pose a threat to animal production and human health. It is apparent that a wide assortment of molds possess the capability to produce mycotoxins. Since each mold has its own unique requirements for moisture, temperature, and substrate, it is logical to assume that in almost any environment the probability of at least one toxigenic mold growing and producing a mycotoxin is rather substantial.

26.4. Types of Mycotoxins and Relationship to Human Disease

Although mycotoxins are often referred to collectively as a single group of compounds, the biological activities of the individual mycotoxins are extremely diverse. For example, aflatoxin is a highly stable mycotoxin that is currently recognized as the most potent carcinogen in rats. Other mycotoxins, such as ochratoxin, are unstable and may not be carcinogenic.

One unique class of mycotoxins is the trichothecenes (Table 26.2). Most trichothecenes possess a potent inflammatory and tissue-irritating activity. These mycotoxins, if ingested by livestock or poultry, will cause an oral inflammation and necrotic lesions about the mouth parts. The trichothecenes have also been implicated as the cause of a disease in humans known as alimentary toxic aleukia (ATA). ATA was widespread in the USSR during World War II and lasted until the late 1940s. The disease was characterized by leukopenia, hemorrhages, degenerated bone marrow, alimentary tract disturbances, and often death. The etiological agents associated with this disease were toxigenic fungi found in various grains. The grains that were consumed by individuals affected with these fungi were allowed to remain in the field long

Table 26.1 Major Mycotoxigenic Fungi and Their Principal Mycotoxins

Genus	Species	Major mycotoxins produced
Aspergillus	flavus, parasiticus	Aflatoxin
	ochraceus, sulphurus, melleus, sclerotiorum, alliacius, ostianus	Ochratoxin, penicillic acid
	clavatus	Patulin
	niveus	Citrinin
	virdi-nutans	Viriditoxin
	chevalieri	Gliotoxin
	versicolor and nidulans	Sterigmatocystin
	terrus	Patulin and citrinin
Penicillium	rubrum	Rubratoxin
	viridicatum	Ochratoxin, penicillic acid
	citrinum	Citrinin
	purpurogenum	Rubratoxin
	oxalicum	Oxalic acid
	expansum	Patulin
	martensii	Penicillic acid
	cyclopium	Ochratoxin
	puberulum	Aflatoxin, tremorgens
	urticae	Patulin
	palitans	Ochratoxin, tremorgens
	commune	Ochratoxin
	variabile	Ochratoxin
Fusarium	poae, sporotrichoides tricinctum, solani, nivale	Trichothecenes[a]
	moniliforme, equiseti	Moniliformin
	avenaceum, roseum	Zearalenone (F-2 toxin)
Claviceps	purpurea, paspali, fusiformis, gigantea	Ergot alkaloids
Stachybatrys	alternans	Unknown
Pithomyces	chartarum	Sporodesmin
Phoma	herbarum var. medicaginis	Brefeldin A and cytochalasin B
Myrothecium	roridum, leucotrichum, verrucaria	Verrucarin A[a], roridin A[a]
Rhizoctonia	leguminicola	Slaframine

[a]See Table 26.2.

after the normal harvest time. As a result of this late harvest, the grain was subjected to a variety of temperatures, rain, snow, etc. The fungi present had an opportunity to grow and produce mycotoxins. The population of this area was "forced" to consume this grain since conditions during and after the war were not conducive to farming, and food was in short supply.

Aflatoxin has also been suggested as a cause of disease in humans; however, conclusive data are lacking. Several disease conditions have been linked to aflatoxin, including primary liver cancer, Indian childhood cirrhosis, and Reye-

Table 26.2   Naturally Occurring Trichothecenes

Scirpene	Calonectrin	Triacetoxyscirpendiol
Trichodermol (roridin C)	Acetoxyscirpendiol	Verrucarin A
Trichodermin	Diacetoxyscirpenol	Dehydroverrucarin A
Scirpen-4,8-diol	Neosolaniol	Verrucarin B
Trichothecolone	HT-2 toxin	Verrucarin J
Trichothecin	T-2 toxin	Roridin A
Crotocin	Nivalenol	Roridin D
Diacetylverrucarol	Fusarenone X	Roridin E
Diacetylcalonectrin	Diacetylnivalenol	Roridin H

Source: Smalley, E. B., Strong, F. M. In Purchase, I.F.H. (Ed.). Mycotoxins. Amsterdam: Elsevier, 1975.

Johnson syndrome. The evidence for the possible involvement of aflatoxin in these diseases is circumstantial, and no definitive basis for a cause and effect relationship has been established.

In theory, mycotoxicoses should pose more of a problem in the underdeveloped countries of the world, where storage conditions of food for both animal and human consumption are more lax than in countries where a high level of technology prevails. Numerous in-depth scientific investigations have failed to confirm this theory; however, certain countries with a low level of agricultural technology do appear to have a high incidence of aflatoxin-related disease in farm animals and humans alike. For example, correlations between hepatocellular carcinoma and the incidence of aflatoxin in human foods reveal a possible link between the two. Such correlations have been made in Uganda, Swaziland, Thailand, Kenya, and India. Results from studies of this type are often difficult to interpret due to possible errors in sampling, mycotoxin analyses, diagnosis of liver carcinoma, and medical records; however, the current consensus is that a reasonably strong correlation exists between average dietary aflatoxin intake and the incidence of liver cancer in humans. It is of interest to note that attempts to find such a correlation in humans from various regions of the United States have been unsuccessful.

Perhaps the best known human disease caused by ingestion of a mycotoxin is ergotism. This disease, affecting humans and farm animals, results from ingestion of grains, such as rye and wheat, and certain grasses overgrown with *Claviceps purpurea* and *C. paspali*. The toxic principles associated with ergotism are often referred to as the ergot alkaloids. These alkaloids possess a biological activity that affects the nervous system and results in vasoconstriction. The vasoconstriction, if not corrected, can result in necrosis of tissue and ultimately gangrene.

26.5. Government Regulations

Of all the mycotoxins known to be produced, only aflatoxin is regulated by the FDA. The maximum allowable level of aflatoxin that can be present in any commodity entering channels of interstate commerce is 20 ppb. This regulation applies to any commodity, whether intended for consumption by humans or animals. Milk is also regulated by the FDA in regard to aflatoxin contamination. After a lactating dairy cow consumes aflatoxin, the aflatoxin is metabolized to yield several by-products. One such metabolic by-product is called aflatoxin M_1 and is excreted via the milk. The maximum allowable level for aflatoxin M_1 in raw or processed milk is 0.5 ppb.

26.6. Prevention and Control of Mycotoxin Formation

The need to control mold growth and mycotoxin formation in our environment is obvious. Mycotoxins can adversely influence animal health, leading to poor performance and production. Mycotoxins of all types can pose a threat to human health as well.

In order to maintain maximal grain quality, whether the grain is destined for animal or human consumption, certain practices must be initiated during grain production to ensure freedom from mycotoxin contamination. Genetic hybrids of grain with high vigor, an ability to tolerate environmental stresses, and inherent insect resistance should be those chosen. Early planting of these varieties with the appropriate plant density, irrigation, insecticide application, and fertilization rates have been demonstrated to reduce the probability of preharvest mycotoxin problems while increasing yields and overall acceptability of grain.

Harvesting of the grain at the appropriate time is the next critical consideration. The grain should be harvested as soon as possible and dried immediately. Provided the mold is present, storage of undried corn for as little as 8 hr can result in detectable grain deterioration, and mycotoxin formation can result in 48 hr. Recent studies have revealed that undried corn, when stored in a hopper wagon overnight, can become contaminated with aflatoxin in concentrations such that consumption by livestock would result in heavy losses. As mentioned previously, moisture is generally the single limiting factor for mold growth; consequently, grain should be dried to a moisture content as low as practical. Corn dried to a moisture content of 13–17% will not mold rapidly, although mold growth will occur at a relatively slow rate. A moisture content of 13% is generally considered to be safe. Rapid drying is advantageous, as the faster the grain can be dried, the less the microbial growth and the greater the nutrient value of the grain.

Grain and feed should be stored in clean and structurally sound containers. Caked, moldy, or wet material should be removed from storage containers prior to placing grain or feed in such containers. Moldy or moist material can serve as a reservoir for bacteria, yeasts, molds, and insects. These organisms can contaminate grain or feed placed into the bin. If feed or grain suspected of containing a mycotoxin has been previously stored in the bin, the bin should be disinfected with a commercial disinfectant prepared according to the manufacturer's recommendations. After disinfection, sufficient time should be allowed for drying of the bin before grain or feed is introduced. Once a food product or feed is manufactured, every effort should be made to minimize the time from manufacture to consumption. As mentioned previously, microbial deterioration of feed can occur in a matter of hours.

The microbes responsible for grain, feed, and food deterioration are ubiquitous in nature. *A. flavus* can infect corn prior to harvest, and aflatoxin can be formed in the field, during storage, and/or after feed manufacture. Proper drying and storage will greatly reduce the likelihood of deterioration. The use of chemical preservatives can also help ensure food or feed quality.

Various chemical additives are routinely added to foods, animal feed, and grain to prevent microbial deterioration. These compounds can retard or prevent mycotoxin formation as well. Calcium propionate, sorbic acid, and benzoic acid are examples of additives used in various human foods to retard spoilage. Propionic acid, acetic acid, and calcium propionate are common additives used in grain and animal feed. In general, rigid quality control practices to avoid the introduction of mycotoxins into human or animal foods will minimize the chances of mycotoxins contaminating our food chain. These practices include chemical analyses to detect the presence of these compounds, appropriate management practices to minimize mold growth and subsequent mycotoxin formation during food or feed manufacture, and continual monitoring for mycotoxin production during the shipment or storage of such products.

Suggested Reading

Rodricks, J. V., Hesseltine, C. W., Mehlman, M. A. (Eds.). Mycotoxins in Human and Animal Health. Park Forest South, Ill. Pathotox, 1977.

Wyllie, T., Moorehouse, L. G. (Eds.). Mycotoxin Fungi, Mycotoxins, Mycotoxicoses: An Encylclopedic Handbook, Vols. 1–3. New York: Dekker, 1978.

W. T. Blevins

27

Geosmins and Other Odorous Metabolites of Microbial Origin

27.1. Occurrence of Odorous Metabolites

27.1.1. Environmental Significance

The quality of the environment in which we live is often judged by the olfactory system; the sense of smell may further serve as an early warning mechanism that potentially toxic materials may be present in harmful concentrations. The occurrence of undesirable tastes and odors in the environment, especially in water supplies, is an old problem and is of concern to biologists, water treatment plant operators, and the general public. Taste and odor are frequently used synonymously, but most so-called tastes are actually odors.

Odors in surface waters may be due to industrial and municipal sewage effluents, but many odors are of biological origin and may be attributed to the decomposition of organisms or to microbial metabolites. Cities and towns throughout the world that obtain their water from streams, rivers, natural lakes, overflow reservoirs, canals, or impoundments are periodically plagued with objectionable odors in their drinking water. This problem has been experienced in the United States, Egypt, Russia, Israel, England, Japan, the Netherlands, and other countries. These odors not only reduce the quality of recreational and drinking water, but may also be absorbed and concentrated in tissues of aquatic animals. Odors in the flesh of fresh-water fish may persist even after cooking and thus impart an undesirable and unpalatable taste to the product. The accumulation of odorous compounds in the flesh of salmon, carp, and catfish has been reported world wide. An earthy flavor (odor) frequently found in intensively cultured catfish in the southeastern United States at times renders the fish unmarketable; thus the problem can become an economically important one.

Various methods used in efforts to remove odorous compounds from water supplies have met with limited success. Ozone, bromine, chlorine, and potassium permanganate have had little effect, and chlorination reportedly intensifies some odors. Chlorine dioxide has been relatively effective in eliminating odors from untreated water, but water containing chlorinated derivatives of these metabolites may require five times as much chlorine dioxide for oxidation as the nonchlorinated compounds, and some chlorinated substances are potential health hazards. Odors in water have also been diminished by γ-irradiation. Adsorption of odorous metabolites from water onto activated carbon is presently the most successful method for elimination of odors, although on a large scale there is no universally acceptable method. This adsorption process can be prohibitively expensive. Therefore, for economic reasons, it may have to be limited to those periods when odor episodes occur.

27.1.2. Prevalent Odors and Microorganisms Responsible

Odors in water supplies have been described as earthy, musty, woody, potato bin, leathery, fishy, camphoric, peachy, tennis shoe, etc. Since the first reports in the 1890s, numerous articles have been published on the earthy or musty odors in soils, vegetables, fruits, and water supplies.

Odors of biological origin may be produced by various bacteria, fungi, and algae. Aquatic actinomycetes (filamentous bacteria) of the genera *Micromonospora*, *Nocardia*, and especially *Streptomyces* are known to produce a variety of volatile metabolites, several of which are odorous. These heterotrophic bacteria are abundant in shallow bottom muds of lakes and streams and are ubiquitous in soil. The earthy odors of garden soil and certain vegetables such as beets have been attributed to odorous metabolites produced by actinomycetes. Certain blue-green algae (or cyanobacteria), including *Anabaena circinalis*, *Oscillatoria tenuis* and other *Oscillatoria* species, *Symploca muscorum*, *Lyngbia* species, *Microcystis* species, and *Aphanizomenon* species reportedly produce earthy odors. The alga *Synura petersenii* produces fishy and cucumberlike odors, and the fungus *Trichoderma viride* produces a coconutlike odor.

27.2. Chemical Nature of Odorous Metabolites

Biologically and industrially produced compounds can play an important role in taste and odor problems in the environment. The composition of odorant mixtures, especially in water supplies, may vary considerably and is usually very complex. Phenol and its chlorinated products constitute the best known examples of taste and odor compounds of industrial origin. Among other important industrially derived odorous compounds are formaldehyde, methylamine, dichloroisopropyl ether, ethylbenzene, 2-methyl-5-ethylpyridine, naphthalene, phenylmethylcarbinol, 1,2,3,4-tetrahydronaphthalene, various chlorinated and nonchlorinated terpenes and sesquiterpenes, alkyl-substituted benzenes, and bicyclic aromatics.

Considerable progress in the chemical characterization of odorous metabolites of biological origin has been made in the past decade. As stated previously, the earthy smelling compound which is the major odorous substance produced by numerous actinomycetes has been isolated and identified as geosmin (*trans*-1,10-dimethyl-*trans*-9-decalol) (Figure 27.1). The name is derived from the Greek *ge*, meaning "earth", and *osme*, meaning "odor." This volatile terpenoid is also produced by a few species of autotrophic blue-green algae. Geosmin is a clear

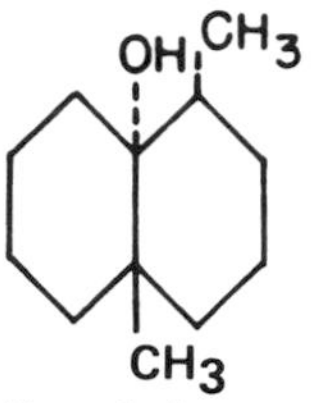

Trans–1, 10–dimethyl–trans–9–decalol
(GEOSMIN)

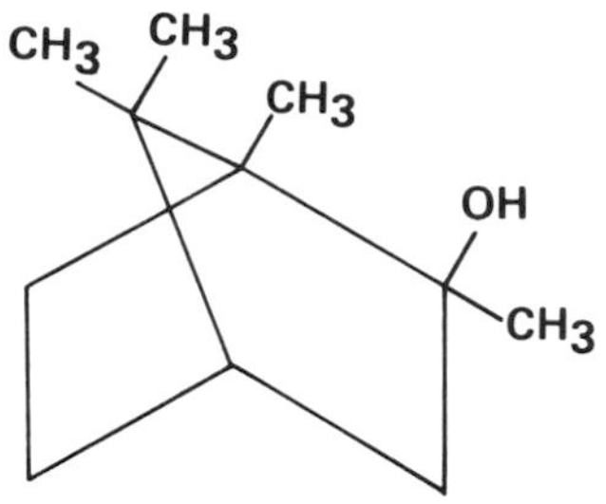

2–Methylisoborneol

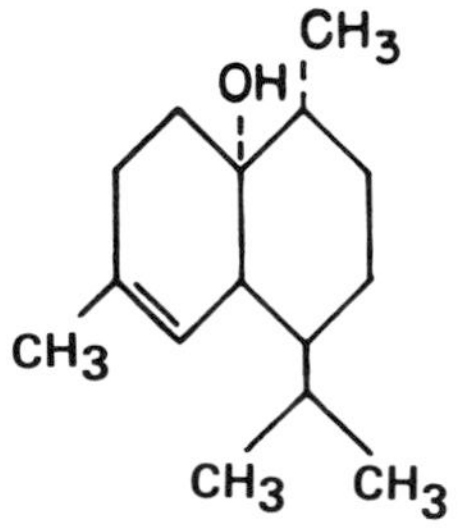

Cadin-4-ene-1-ol

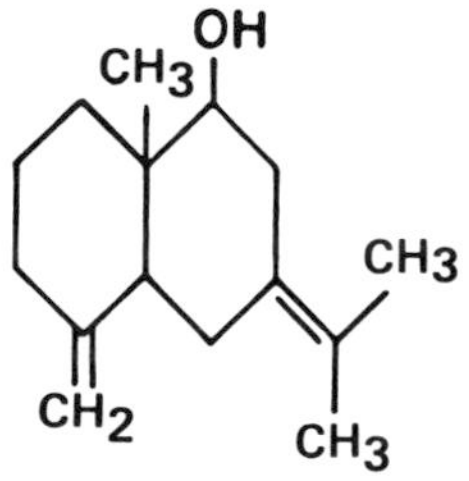

Selina-4(14),7(11)-diene-9-ol

Figure 27.1 Chemical structures of important odorous metabolites of microorganisms.

neutral oil that has an extremely low odor threshold concentration of 0.2 ppm or less. The compound has a molecular weight of 182 and the empirical formula $C_{12}H_{22}O$. The widespread occurrence of odor problems caused by geosmin is well documented. Geosmin can be extracted from the spent growth media of several *Streptomyces* species and blue-green algae, and in most instances has been the major chemical adsorbed onto activated carbon from water having the typical earthy odor. In addition, the compound has been extracted from the flesh of fish having a muddy or earthy taint, where the threshold taste level was established at 0.6 μg geosmin/100 g flesh.

In addition to geosmin, a volatile camphor/menthol smelling compound, identified as 2-methylisoborneol (1,2,7,7-tetramethyl-2-norbornanol) (Figure 27.1), is produced by a few *Streptomyces* species, a species of *Actinomadura*, and two species of the blue-green alga *Lyngbia*. Extracts of earthy smelling soil and of raw water have been reported to contain 2-methylisoborneol in addition to geosmin. This compound has a molecular weight of 168 and the empirical formula $C_{11}H_{20}O$ and is a white crystalline solid with a threshold odor concentration of 0.1 ppm. The occurrence of 2-methylisoborneol in nature is rare, although borneol has been isolated from fermentations to which α-pinene or camphene has been added, and a very small amount of isoborneol can be formed by the reduction of D-camphor in rabbit liver cytosol.

The involvement of 2-methylisoborneol in an odor problem in natural water systems was reported in 1970 in Grand Lake, Ohio, where the compound was found to be responsible for 68% of the odor in the water, while in Indian Lake,

Ohio, it contributed 75% of the odor. This compound has since been isolated from waters in Europe and Japan.

Several other odorous compounds have been isolated and identified. Two odorous sesquiterpene monoalcohols from *Streptomyces* species have been identified as cadin-4-ene-1-ol, which has an earthy or woody odor, and selina-4(14), 7(11)-diene-9-ol, which is a faintly odorous compound reportedly very similar to the compound that gives hops their characteristic odor (Figure 27.1). The coconutlike smelling compound 6-pentyl-α-pyrone was identified as a major metabolite of *Trichoderma viride* and has also been isolated from peaches. The cucumberlike, watermelonlike odorous compound produced by *Synura petersenii* has been tentatively identified as *n*-heptanal. A chemical agent, originally called mucidone, which caused a severe musty odor in the Cedar River near Cedar Rapids, Iowa, was identified as 6-ethyl-3-isobutyl-2-pyrone, and a potatolike odor from a geosmin-producing *Streptomyces* is caused by 2-isopropyl-3-methoxypyrazine. Two odorous compounds, 1-phenyl-2-propanone and 2-phenylethanol, have been identified from *S. platensis*. A *S. cinnamoneus*-like strain of *Streptomyces* produces 5-methyl-3-heptanone as a major odorous metabolite. Other less complex microbially produced compounds that may contribute to odors in the environment are butyric acid and other fatty acids, aldehydes, alcohols, esters, amines, hydrogen sulfide, isopropyl mercaptan, and other sulfur-containing compounds. The major odorous compounds and responsible organisms are listed in Table 27.1.

Table 27.1 Major Types of Odorous Compounds and the Microorganisms That Produce Them

Chemical compound	Odor	Organism
Trans-1,10-dimethyl-*trans*-9-decalol (geosmin)	Earthy	*Streptomyces* spp. *Micromonospora* spp. *Anabaena circinalis* *Oscillatoria* spp. *Symploca muscorum* *Microcystis* spp. *Aphanizomenon* spp.
1,2,7,7-tetramethyl-2-norbornanol (2-methylisoborneol)	Camphor/menthol (musty)	*Streptomyces* spp. *Actinomadura* spp. *Lyngbia* spp.
Cadin-4-ene-1-ol	Earthy or woody	*Streptomyces* spp.
Selina-4(14),7(11)-diene-9-ol	Hopslike	*Streptomyces* spp.
6-Pentyl-α-pyrone	Coconutlike	*Trichoderma viride*
2-Isopropyl-3-methoxypyrazine	Potatolike	*Streptomyces* spp.
n-Heptanal	Cucumber- or watermelon like	*Synura petersenii*
6-Ethyl-3-isobutyl-2-pyrone (mucidone)	Musty	*Streptomyces* spp.
1-Phenyl-2-propanone	—	*Streptomyces platensis*
2-Phenylethanol	—	*Streptomyces platensis*
5-Methyl-3-heptanone	—	*Streptomyces cinnamoneus*

27.3. Environmental Factors Promoting Microbial Production of Odorous Metabolites

In most untreated water, the microbial population is heterogeneous and well balanced. However, the influx of extraneous nutrients from fertilizers, agricultural runoff, and domestic and human wastes can result in increased availability of organic compounds, phosphorus, nitrogen, and other minerals in the water. These chemical factors can stimulate microbial growth and may cause an increase in the production of odorous metabolites by these organisms. In addition, such factors as pH, temperature, and dissolved oxygen may be critical for optimal growth of microorganisms and production of odorous compounds.

Studies on geosmin production by a *Streptomyces* species have shown that environmental conditions affect the growth of these organisms and odor production. Actinomycete populations and geosmin production increase in streams and lakes following excessive rainfall, which causes increased agricultural runoff and an influx of domestic wastes from the watershed area. *Streptomyces* populations are usually much higher in muds or soils containing high organic content, and the amount of nitrate, ammonia, and organic nitrogen also directly affects the growth of these organisms and subsequent geosmin production. *Streptomyces* species are aerobic organisms; therefore, adequate dissolved oxygen is required for growth and/or odor production to be significant. It has been reported that the metabolic activities of actinomycetes are greatly enhanced by the oxygen production that occurs during algal blooms, so that odor production might erroneously be attributed to the metabolic activities of the algae. In addition, senescing algae following a significant bloom may serve as nutritional substrates for actinomycetes. Other decomposing plant materials may also serve as nutrients for actinomycetes, and thus these microorganisms often flourish during the warm season in reservoirs having large areas of shallow water with prolific vegetation.

Growth and geosmin production by *Streptomyces* species increase directly with increasing alkalinity of the water; poor growth and low odor production are usually reported for impoundments on acid soils. Water temperatures ranging from a minimum of 15°C to a maximum near 38°C are necessary for geosmin synthesis, with optimal geosmin production occurring near 30°C. Thus in the United States geosmin production in water is usually a problem in spring to early summer and in the fall, when the water temperature is favorable. If extensive rainfall precedes a period of favorable temperature, intense odors may follow. Control of domestic and industrial waste effluents and agricultural runoff into streams may prevent or limit odor pollution of recreational and drinking water supplies; furthermore, control of water depths to limit the amount of shallow water in impoundments and subsequent growth of vegetation could be important in reducing the intensity of odor episodes.

27.4. Biological Studies

27.4.1. Toxicity

No thorough studies have been done on the toxicological aspects of odorous compounds. Geosmin reportedly inhibits early stages of heterocyst formation in the blue-green alga *Anabaena circinalis* but stimulates heterocyst maturation later in the life cycle. In one study, 5 mM 2-methylisoborneol in nutrient broth had no effect on the growth of various species of bacteria associated with soil, water, and humans. Mice force fed low concentrations of 2-methylisoborneol suffered no ill effects. An LD_{50} of 1310 mg/kg has been reported for camphor administered to mice, and an LD_{50} of 1059 mg/kg for borneol; these levels indicate that both compounds are relatively nontoxic. Both of these compounds are structurally very similar to 2-methylisoborneol. Camphor is readily absorbed at the site of contact in humans, and large doses can induce nausea and vomiting. Camphor can act as a central nervous system stimulant and can cause mild and transient hepatic derangements. Decahydronaphthalene (decalin), which is the bicyclic structure of the geosmin molecule, is normally considered to be nontoxic. However, it can cause mucous membrane and skin irritation, and vapor exposures can cause cataracts and kidney lesions in guinea pigs. Inhalation of 1.8 mg decahydronaphthalene/liter air for 8–23 days has caused deaths in rabbits, with liver and kidney damage evident. In rats, orally administered decahydronaphthalene had an LD_{50} of 4710 mg/kg and a low lethal concentration of 500 ppm for 2 hr. Decahydronaphthalene has an aquatic toxicity rating of 100–1000 ppm. These values indicate that decahydronaphthalene is not a potent toxic substance.

Various toxicological effects of other terpenoid compounds and derivatives have been observed. Some terpenoids inhibit the development of field and storage fungi on wheat seed without affecting seed germination. Heptanal, which is an odorous metabolite produced by *Synura petersenii*, has been investigated as a possible seed treatment because of its antifungal properties. In mice, orally administered heptanal had an LD_{50} of 500 mg/kg. Pentacyclic triterpenes have been shown to be cytotoxic to sea urchin embryos, and foam from lagoons of pulp effluents contains diterpenes that are toxic to juvenile sockeye salmon. Terpenoids and phenols that accumulate in plant tissue have toxic effects on microorganisms and may play a role in phytoimmunity. Some sesquiterpene lactones have been reported to be antitumorigenic; effects such as inhibition of DNA polymerase, protein synthesis, energy metabolism, and cholesterol synthesis have been observed in Ehrlich ascites tumor cells in mice. Microorganisms degrade camphor, producing various sesquiterpene lactones as intermediates. 2-Methylisoborneol may be metabolized in a similar fashion; however, the intermediates in 2-methylisoborneol degradation have not been identified.

The results of the study conducted by the EPA on New Orleans, Louisiana, drinking water in 1974 prompted a National Organics Reconnaissance Survey after President Ford signed the Safe Drinking Water Act in December 1974. Subsequent analyses of the water supplies of several major cities revealed that a large percentage of the pollutants were halogenated organic (aliphatic and aromatic) compounds. Experimental data indicate that chlorination of water containing various nonchlorinated compounds will result in a mixture of halogenated organic compounds. In one study, chlorination resulted in increased production of chloroform, dichloronitromethane, nitrotrichloromethane, chloroxylene, and chlorotoluene. Halogenation may affect the toxic, carcinogenic, or odorous properties of various organic compounds. Halogenation increases the bacteriostatic or verminoxious activity of some terpenes and, as mentioned previously, may alter or enhance water odor. The specific compounds that may be formed by chlorination of odorous metabolites have not been determined and any toxicological effects are therefore unknown. Photolysis, ozonation, and γ-irradiation reportedly degrade or alter various organic compounds, but specific effects on odorous metabolites have not been reported.

27.4.2. Metabolism

Very little is known about the metabolism of biologically produced odorous compounds. In one study a strain of *Bacillus cereus* at a concentration of 10^5–10^6 cells/ml reportedly altered or destroyed 86% of the geosmin present in the medium. No information on degradative intermediates or products was given. It is not known whether geosmin that accumulates in the tissues of fish is metabolized, but a 10–14-day period in odor-free water reduces the concentration below the threshold taste level.

The metabolism of decahydronaphthalene, structurally very similar to geosmin, has been studied in mammalian systems. The urine of dogs fed decahydronaphthalene contained an unidentified decahydronaphthol representing 37.7% of the decahydronaphthalene administered. Approximately 60% of the decahydronaphthalene administered orally to rabbits was excreted in the urine as ether-linked glucuronides, with a mixture of two racemic 2-decalols. *Trans*-decahydronaphthalene was mostly metabolized to ($\pm$)-*trans-cis*-decalol, and *cis*-decahydronaphthalene was hydroxylated to ($\pm$)-*cis-cis*-2-decalol. Hydroxylation was postulated to occur through the activity of a mixed-function oxidase.

A *Pseudomonas* species degrades camphene via the intermediate isoborneol and camphor, and camphene-grown cells rapidly oxidize isoborneol. Since 2-methylisoborneol is structurally similar to camphor, degradative pathways may be similar, although no specific studies with 2-methylisoborneol have been reported. Microbial degradation of camphor proceeds via various terpenoid lactones, the chemistry of which varies with different microorganisms.

In one study, a strain of *Pseudomonas putida* oxidized 2-methylisoborneol at very low rates, but breakdown products were not identified. In mice force fed ^{14}C-labeled 2-methylisoborneol, most of the compound was metabolized, as evidenced by the relatively high levels of radioactivity found in the feces and urine. Aqueous extracts of feces and urine contained an unidentified compound more polar than 2-methylisoborneol. The very small amount of total radioactivity found in tissues was greatest in the lungs, with aqueous extracts of liver containing the highest activity of the aqueous fractions. Hydroxylation of other terpenoids by rabbit liver has been reported, and isoborneol can be formed by reduction and hydroxylation of camphor by rabbit liver cytosol.

The widespread occurrence of geosmin, 2-methylisoborneol, and other odorous metabolites in soils, water, and foods should warrant more thorough studies on the toxicity and metabolism of odorous compounds and their derivatives.

Suggested Reading

Buttery, R.G., Garnibaldi, J.A. Geosmin and methylisoborneol in garden soil. J. Agric. Food Chem. 24:1246–1247, 1976.

Dougherty, J.D., Morris, R.L. Studies on the removal of actinomycete musty tastes and odors in water supplies. J. Am. Water Works Assoc. 59:1320–1326, 1967.

Gerber, N.N. Geosmin, from microorganisms, is *trans*-1,10-dimethyl-*trans*-9-decalol. Tetrahedron Lett. 25:2971–2974, 1968.

Gerber, N.N. Three highly odorous metabolites from an actinomycete: 2-isopropyl-3-methoxy-pyrazine, 2-methylisoborneol and geosmin. J. Chem. Ecol. 3:475–482, 1977.

Lovell, R.T., Sackey, L.A. Absorption by channel catfish of earthy–musty flavor compounds synthesized by cultures of blue-green algae. Trans. Am. Fisheries Soc. 102:774–777, 1973.

Medsker, L.L., Jenkins, D., Thomas, J.F. Odorous compounds in natural waters: An earthy-smelling compound associated with blue-green algae and actinomycetes. Environ. Sci. Technol. 6:461–464, 1968.

Piet, G.J., Zoetman, B.C.J., Draaywveld, A.J.A. Earthy-smelling substances in surface waters of the Netherlands. Water Treat. Exam. 21:281–286, 1972.

Rudd, R.L. Environmental Toxicology. Detroit: Gale Research Co., 1977.

Silvey, J.K.G., Henley, D.E., Wyatt, J.R. Planktonic blue-green algae: Growth and odor production studies. J. Am. Water Works Assoc. 64:35–39, 1972.

Weete, J.D., Blevins, W.T., Wilt, G.R., et al. Chemical, biological, and environmental factors responsible for the earthy odor in the Auburn city water supply. Auburn Univ. Agric. Exp. Station Bull. 490:1–46, 1977.

W.C.Dauterman
E. Hodgson

28

Chemical Transformations and Interactions

28.1. Introduction

Most chemicals released into the environment do not remain in a static situation. Just as animal wastes are converted to breakdown products by a variety of reactions, so are most chemicals and pollutants altered. Heavy metals are not degraded but are interconverted between available and nonavailable forms. Other organic compounds, such as some PCBs, are degraded extremely slowly over a period of many years to less harmful compounds, while compounds such as the organophosphate insecticides may break down in only a few hours.

Chemical transformations may increase or decrease the toxicity of the parent compound. Elemental mercury is methylated to form methylmercury; the parent compound, which has low toxicity, is thus converted to a very hazardous toxicant. Parathion is a fairly nontoxic insecticide until either a living system or photooxidation oxidizes the parent compound to paraoxon, one of the more toxic materials in use today. These reactions are called intoxication reactions, as opposed to detoxication reactions, in which compounds are degraded to less toxic substances (e.g., hydrolysis of parathion).

When a lipophilic (fat-soluble) compound enters a living animal, the xenobiotic-metabolizing enzymes alter the toxicant to polar metabolites that can be excreted rapidly from the body. However, very lipophilic compounds may be deposited in the fatty constituents of tissues and organs and partitioned away from metabolic activity. Thus sequestered, they resist breakdown and tend to remain stored in the fat of animals for a long period of time. High fat solubility and chemical stability are properties that are associated with compounds that easily enter food chains and subsequently pass throughout the environment, as in the case of many chlorinated hydrocarbons.

If a chemical is toxic enough to kill an animal the toxicant becomes a part of the biomass that is decomposed after the death of the animal. Thus, all chemicals are circulated throughout the environment in one form or another. The products are acted upon (slowly or rapidly) and converted progressively to smaller molecules and eventually utilized in various cycles (e.g., the carbon cycle). Nonbiological reactions, such as those mediated by light, pH changes, hydrolysis, etc., are also a part of this type of transformation. However, in the final analysis, the action of microorganisms is probably the ultimate cause of biochemical transformation to small molecules that are utilized in the various cycles. Many microorganisms use pollutants as a source of food and energy.

Certain chemicals are localized in situations in which little transformation occurs. Elements such as mercury, lead, copper, arsenic, etc. are deposited as minerals deep within the earth's crust in forms that are basically nontoxic. Only after mining and smelting and subsequent manufacture are these compounds exposed to the environment and possible incorporation into biological systems. There is some possibility that we have created a problem that will not be reversible for many thousands of years unless such elements find safe storage via chelation or other processes that bind them to nonusable substrates.

Chemical transformations may be catalyzed by enzymes in organisms or may occur wherever appropriate physicochemical conditions are present in the environment. The reactions that degrade a toxicant or pollutant usually involve a number of different chemical reactions, proceeding simultaneously, which involve the parent compound as well as the metabolites formed. The various metabolites formed may alter the transformation of other metabolites by inhibition, induction, etc. (see Section 28.3).

28.2. Major Chemical Reactions

The major types of reactions involve oxidation, hydrolysis, reduction, conjugation, dehydrohalogenation, ring scission, hydration, chelation, or combustion. Of these reactions, conjugation is the only one mediated strictly by enzymes, whereas chelation is strictly nonenzymatic. The remaining reactions are all known to occur both enzymatically and nonenzymatically.

28.2.1. Oxidation

Oxidation reactions utilize energy in the incorporation of molecular oxygen in the molecule. In most mammalian systems a monoxygenase (mixed-function oxidation) system utilizing molecular oxygen, NADPH, and cytochrome P-450 is involved in these reactions.

28.2.1.a. Monoxygenase System

Hydroxylation. Hydroxylation by microsomes, NADPH, and one atom of molecular oxygen results in the addition of a hydroxyl group to the substrate, which usually decreases toxicity, increases water solubility, and provides a reaction group for further transformations such as conjugation. Both aromatic hydroxylations (Reaction 28.1) and aliphatic hydroxylations (Reaction 28.2) occur:

$$\xrightarrow[\text{NADPH}]{\overset{\text{microsomes}}{\underset{}{O_2}}}$$

(28.1)

(28.2)

Desulfuration. Replacement of sulfur with oxygen is a very important reaction for thiophosphate insecticides. Many of these insecticides, such as parathion, contain P = S groups and are rather nontoxic until the P = S is oxidized to the P = O, paraoxon; the toxicity is increased many thousandfold over the parent compound:

(28.3)

Nitrogen and oxygen dealkylation. When short-chain alkyl groups are attached to nitrogen or oxygen, the alkyl groups can be easily hydroxylated with a subsequent removal of the alkyl group:

$$RNHCH_3 \xrightarrow[\text{NADPH}]{\substack{\text{microsomes} \\ O_2}} [RNHCH_2OH] \longrightarrow RNH_2 + H_2CO.$$

(28.4)

A similar reaction occurs for O-dealkylation.

Epoxidation. Addition of an oxygen atom to an olefinic bond results in epoxide formation. Some carcinogens are formed by epoxidation (e.g., benzo[a]pyrene). In general, the arene oxides formed are quite reactive, but a few, such as dieldrin, are rather stable. One important example of an epoxidation reaction is the initial activation of benzo[a]pyrene (also see Reaction 28.20):

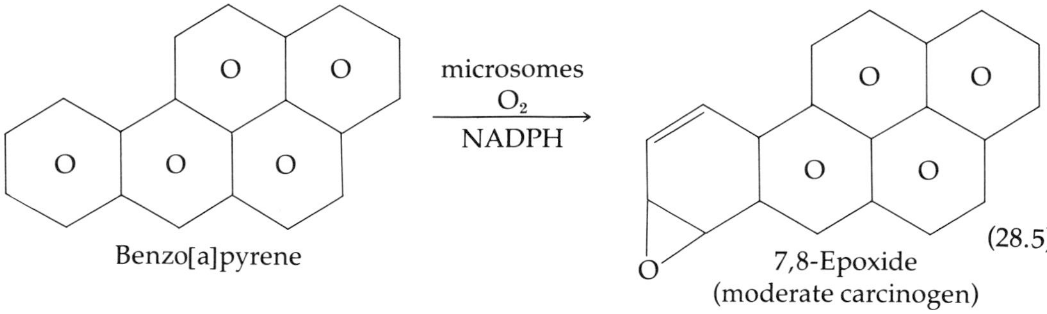

Benzo[a]pyrene

microsomes
O_2
NADPH

7,8-Epoxide
(moderate carcinogen)

(28.5)

Epoxides are further degraded by epoxide hydrase and by conjugation with glutathione.

28.2.1.b. Dioxygenase System

Microorganisms appear to lack a functional monoxygenase system. In order to oxidize various aromatic hydrocarbons, both atoms of molecular oxygen are added to the double bond:

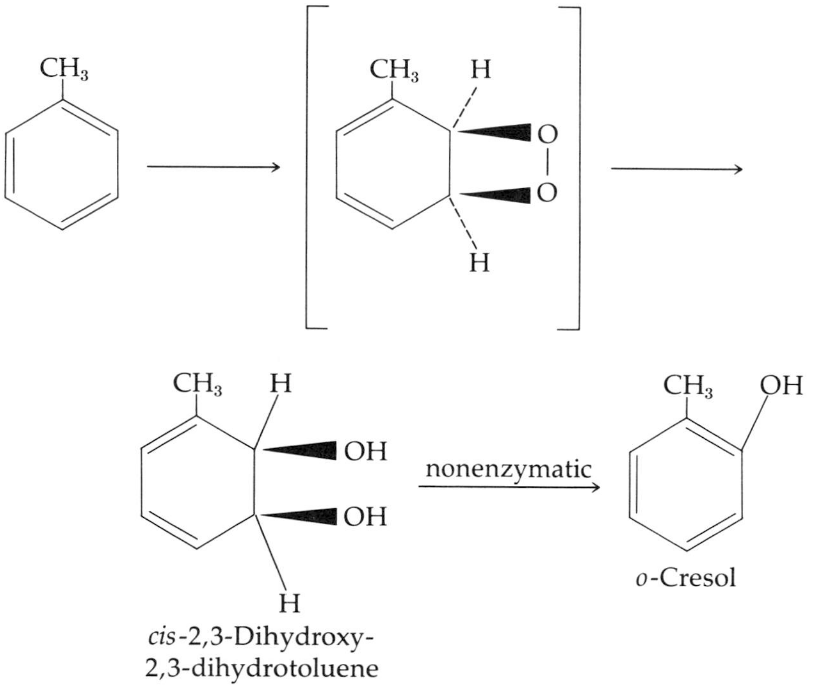

(28.6)

cis-2,3-Dihydroxy-
2,3-dihydrotoluene

nonenzymatic

o-Cresol

28.2.1.c. Mitochondrial System

β-Oxidation. As the result of β-oxidation (fatty acid oxidations), long-chain, unbranched alkyl groups (such as many detergents) are oxidized to 2-carbon units by most biological organisms:

$$RCH_2CH_2CH_2COOH \longrightarrow RCH_2COOH + CH_3COOH \qquad (28.7)$$

Oxidative deamination. Aliphatic amines and aryl-substituted aliphatic amines are metabolized by amine oxidases forming the corresponding aldehyde and ammonia. Two types of amine oxidases are found in mammalian tissue, i.e., monoamine oxidases and diamine oxidases:

$$RCH_2NH_2 \xrightarrow{\text{monoamine oxidase}} RCHO + NH_3 \tag{28.8}$$

$$H_2N(CH_2)_nNH_2 \xrightarrow{\text{diamine oxidase}} H_2N(CH_2)_{n-1}CHO + NH_3. \tag{28.9}$$

28.2.1.d Photooxidation

In addition to the various biologically mediated oxidations within organisms, oxidation also occurs in the atmosphere and on the surface of plant material, soil particles, etc. These transformations are mechanistically complex and fairly slow. Both intoxication and detoxication may occur. Photons of light ($h\nu$) provide the necessary energy to mediate the reactions with oxygen. The high-energy intermediate from fluorocarbons (aerosols) that ultimately results in destruction of the ozone layer is postulated as follows:

$$CCl_2F_2 \xrightarrow{h\nu} CClF_2 + Cl$$
$$Cl + O_3 \longrightarrow ClO + O_2 \tag{28.10}$$
$$ClO + O \longrightarrow Cl + O_2.$$

An interesting photooxidation of parathion occurs on plant surfaces. This is an important hazard to farm workers in certain regions of the country and not in others. In most regions of the United States, parathion is rapidly degraded on plant surfaces due to moist conditions (see Section 28.2.2). However, in California conditions are extremely dry in the citrus growing areas and parathion is photooxidatively converted to paraoxon (Reaction 28.3). The treated foliage can be quite toxic. Thus, during the past 20 years more than 500 accidental poisonings seem to have occurred in California due to this type of mechanism, while none has been reported in the eastern United States.

28.2.2. Hydrolysis

This is an important detoxication mechanism in which water is added to an ester bond. This reaction can occur either enzymatically, or nonenzymatically under acid or alkaline conditions. Compounds that undergo hydrolysis include esters, carbamates, and substituted phosphates:

$$RCOR + H_2O \longrightarrow RCOH + HOR$$

(where the carbonyl groups are as shown, $RC(=O)OR$ and $RC(=O)OH$)

$$R-OCNH_2 + H_2O \longrightarrow ROH + CO_2 + NH_3 \tag{28.11}$$

$$(RO)_2POR' + H_2O \longrightarrow (RO)_2POH + R'OH.$$

Phosphate insecticides are degraded rather easily by hydrolysis. This is the reason phosphate triesters do not survive in the environment longer than a few weeks. Rates of hydrolysis are drastically affected by pH. Diazinon has a half-life of 4435 hr at pH 7 but only 750 hr at pH 5 and 150 hr at pH 10.

28.2.3. Reduction

A variety of xenobiotics and pollutants are reduced enzymatically by certain mammals as well as by microorganisms. The following are some examples:

$$RNO_2 \longrightarrow RNH_2$$

$$RCCl_3 \longrightarrow RCHCl_2$$

$$R-S-S-R \longrightarrow 2RSH \tag{28.12}$$

$$R_2SO \longrightarrow R_2S.$$

Reduction reactions usually proceed under anaerobic conditions; one well-known example is the production of H_2S by microorganisms.

28.2.4. Conjugation

Conjugation reactions involve the combination of foreign compounds with endogenous compounds to form conjugates that are water soluble and can be easily eliminated from the organism. The endogenous compounds utilized in the biosynthesis are sugars, amino acid residues, phosphates, sulfur compounds, etc. Compounds that have hydroxyl, amino, and mercapto groups are the common aglycones.

28.2.4.a. Glycosides

Glucuronides are formed in animals, whereas glucosides are produced in plants and animals:

$$\text{Glucuronic acid} + \text{C}_6\text{H}_5\text{OH} \longrightarrow \text{Phenyl glucuronide} \tag{28.13}$$

$$\text{Glucose} + \underset{\text{OH}}{\bigcirc} \longrightarrow \text{Phenyl glucoside.} \qquad (28.14)$$

28.2.4.b. Peptide Conjugates

Glycine is probably the most common amino acid utilized in peptide conjugation. Aromatic acids are especially reactive:

$$\underset{\text{COOH}}{\bigcirc} + NH_2CH_2COOH \longrightarrow \underset{\text{CONHCH}_2COOH}{\bigcirc} \qquad (28.15)$$

28.2.4.c. Sulfate Conjugates

Sulfate residues from other biochemical reactions are utilized in conjugation of certain phenolic-type toxicants:

$$\bigcirc\!\!-OH + SO_4^{2-} \longrightarrow \bigcirc\!\!-OSO_3^- \qquad (28.16)$$

28.2.4.d. Glutathione Conjugates

Glutathione, a natural constituent of biological tissues, will conjugate with compounds containing halogens, epoxides, cyano groups, olefinic bonds, etc.:

$$\bigcirc\!\!-Br + \begin{array}{c}\text{reduced}\\\text{glutathione}\end{array} \longrightarrow$$

$$(28.17)$$

$$\bigcirc\!\!-\text{glutathione} + HBr$$

28.2.5. Dehydrohalogenation

DDT is dehydrochlorinated to DDE by a glutathione-dependent enzyme that removes HCl. Although the enzyme-mediated reaction requires glutathione, it is not a conjugation reaction:

(28.18)

28.2.6. Ring Scission

Aromatic ring compounds are fairly stable in the environment. However, certain microorganisms are able to open aromatic rings by oxidation:

(28.19)

After opening of the aromatic rings, the compounds may be further metabolized. The number, type, and position of substituents on the ring may appreciably retard scission as these substituents may protect the ring from enzymatic attack.

28.2.7. Hydration

Epoxide rings of certain arene and alkene compounds are hydrated enzymatically with the addition of water to form the corresponding *trans*-dihydrodiols. Hydration of the initial epoxidation of benzo[a]pyrene (Reaction 28.5) illustrates formation of a dihydrodiol, which is further epoxidized to the ultimate carcinogen:

7,8-Epoxide

$$\xrightarrow{\hspace{2cm}}$$

7,8-Dihydrodiol

$$\xrightarrow[\text{NADPH}]{\substack{\text{microsomes} \\ O_2}}$$

(28.20)

7,8-Diol-9,10-epoxide
(potent carcinogen)

28.2.8. Chelation

Many metals (copper, zinc, manganese, and so on) form complexes with organic compounds by sharing electrons:

(28.21)

This usually serves to solubilize the metal involved; however, these complexes may be insoluble or nonavailable, particularly in the environment, thus preventing a potential toxicant from reaching the site of action. Amino acid residues have the appropriate ligands for this action.

Metal chelation may also take place in vivo; e.g., penicillamine (β,β-dimethylcysteine) is used to remove copper from body tissue and EDTA is used in lead poisoning.

28.2.9. Combustion

Combustion of chemicals involves the oxidation of compounds with the accompanied release of energy. Under normal environmental conditions, combustion is not usually complete, resulting in the formation of pyrolysis products. Combustion products are released via emissions from power plant stacks, home fireplaces, automobile exhausts, etc. Thus, sulfur compounds are released by combustion of coal, nitrogen oxides by automobile engines, and trace amounts of dioxins in flue gases from municipal incinerators—all environmental pollutants. An example of very toxic combustion products released into the environment as a result of a relatively minor change in temperature occurred in Senesco, Italy, in July 1976. The desirable temperature for manufacture of hexachlorophene from trichlorophenols ($\cong 150°C$) was mistakenly raised to approximately 200°C, and a very toxic compound, TCDD, was released into the environment as a result of a plant explosion.

28.3. Interactions

28.3.1. Metabolic Interactions

Man and other living organisms are exposed to many xenobiotics simultaneously, involving different portals of entry, modes of action, and metabolic pathways. The effect of chemicals on the metabolism of other exogenous compounds is becoming one of the most important areas of toxicology, since it concerns toxicity-related interactions between different xenobiotics.

Only a very small number of toxicants have been studied extensively in several organisms, have had all of their principle metabolic intermediates and end products characterized, or have had the enzymes involved identified, purified, and characterized. It is not surprising that our knowledge of the mechanisms of chemical interactions is even more rudimentary. The magnitude of the problem can be appreciated by considering the following estimates of the number of chemical additives in use today (the source of the estimates is given in parentheses):

1500	Active ingredients of pesticides (EPA)
4000	Active ingredients of drugs (FDA)
2000	Drug additives to improve stability, inhibit bacterial growth, etc. (FDA)
2500	Food additives with nutritional value (FDA)
3000	Food additives to promote product life (FDA)
50,000	Additional chemicals in common use (EPA).

Xenobiotics, in addition to serving as substrates for a number of enzymes, may also serve as inhibitors or inducers of these or other enzymes. In fact, many examples are known of compounds that first inhibit, and subsequently induce, enzymes such as the microsomal mixed-function oxidases. The situation is further complicated by the fact that whereas some substances have an inherent toxicity and are detoxified in the body, others, without inherent toxicity, can be metabolically activated to potent toxicants. The following examples are illustrative of situations that might occur involving two compounds:

1. Compound A, without inherent toxicity, is metabolized to a potent toxicant. (a) In the presence of an inhibitor of its metabolism there would be a reduction in toxic effect. (b) In the presence of an inducer of the activating enzymes, there would be an increase in toxic effect.
2. Compound B, a toxicant, is metabolically detoxified. (a) In the presence of an inhibitor of the detoxifying enzymes there would be an increase in the toxic effect. (b) In the presence of an inducer of the detoxifying enzymes there would be a reduction in toxic effect.

In addition, the toxicity of the inhibitor or inducer as well as the time dependence of the effect must also be considered, since many xenobiotics that are initially enzyme inhibitors become inducers.

28.3.1.a. Inhibition

As indicated above, inhibition of xenobiotic-metabolizing enzymes can cause either an increase or a decrease in toxicity. Inhibitory effects can be demonstrated in a number of ways at different organizational levels.

In vivo symptoms. The measurement of the effect of an inhibitor on the duration of action of a drug is the commonest of these methods, and the most frequently used involve the measurement of effects on the hexobarbital sleeping time and the zoxazolamine paralysis time. Both of these drugs are fairly rapidly deactivated by the hepatic microsomal mixed-function oxidase system, and thus inhibitors of this system prolong their action.

The well-known inhibitor of drug metabolism, SKF-525A, causes an increase in both hexobarbital sleeping time and zoxazolamine paralysis time in rats and mice, as do the insecticide synergists piperonyl butoxide and tropital, the optimum pretreatment time being about 0.5 hr before the narcotic.

In the case of activation reactions, such as the activation of the insecticide azinphosmethyl to its potent anticholinesterase oxon derivative, a decrease in toxicity is apparent when rats are pretreated with SKF-525A.

Cocarcinogenicity may also be an expression of inhibition of a detoxication reaction, as in the case of the cocarcinogenicity of piperonyl butoxide and Freons 112 and 113.

Distribution and blood levels. Treatment of an animal with an inhibitor of foreign compound metabolism may cause changes in the blood levels of an unmetabolized toxicant and/or the levels of its metabolites. This procedure, carried out on the intact animal, has an advantage over in vitro methods in that it yields results of direct physiological or toxicological interest. The time sequence of the effects can also be followed in individual animals, which is a factor of importance when inhibition is followed by induction—a common event.

Effects on metabolism in vivo. A further refinement of the previous technique is the determination of the effect of inhibition on the overall metabolism of a xenobiotic in vivo, usually by following the appearance of metabolites in the urine and/or feces, or in some cases in the blood or tissues. The use of the intact animal has practical advantages over in vitro methods although it tells little of the mechanisms involved.

Effects on in vitro metabolism. Since the preparation of enzymes usually involves dilution with the preparative medium during homogenization, centrifugation, and resuspension, in vitro measurements following in vivo treatment may not be reliable, as inhibitors that are not tightly bound to the enzyme are lost. Thus negative results can have little utility, although positive results do provide an indication of excellent binding to the enzyme.

Microsomal mixed-function oxidase inhibitors that form stable inhibitory complexes with cytochrome P-450, such as SKF-525A, piperonyl butoxide, and other methylenedioxyphenyl compounds, and amphetamine and its derivatives can be readily investigated in this way since the microsomes isolated from pretreated animals have a reduced capacity to oxidize many xenobiotics.

In vitro measurement of the effect of one xenobiotic on the metabolism of another is the most useful method for the study of inhibitory mechanisms, particularly when purified enzymes are used. This method is of more limited utility in assessing the toxicological implications for the intact animal since it does not assess the effects of factors that affect absorption, distribution, and prior metabolism.

Although the kinetics of inhibition of xenobiotic-metabolizing enzymes can be investigated in the same ways as any other enzyme mechanism, there are a number of problems that may lessen the value of this type of investigation. They arise from the fact that many of the enzymes involved are particulate and part of multienzyme systems, and both substrate and inhibitor are lipophilic.

Various types of reversible inhibition are known but, because the inhibitors can be displaced by the substrate, are of less importance.

Irreversible inhibition is frequently much more important toxicologically. In the majority of cases either covalent binding or disruption of the enzyme structure is involved. In neither case can the effect be reversed in vitro by dialysis or by dilution.

Covalent binding may involve the prior formation of a metabolic intermediate that then interacts with the enzyme. An excellent example of this type of inhibition is the effect of piperonyl butoxide on hepatic microsomal mixed-function oxidase activity. This compound forms a stable inhibitory complex that blocks carbon monoxide binding to cytochrome P-450 and also prevents substrate oxidation.

The terms synergism and potentiation have been variously defined and used but, in any case, involve a toxicity that is greater when two compounds are given simultaneously or sequentially than that which would be expected from a consideration of the toxicities of the compounds when given alone. Some toxicologists have used the term synergism for cases that fit the above definition, but only when one compound is toxic alone while the other has little or no intrinsic toxicity. This is the case with the toxicity of insecticides to insects and mammals and the effects of methylenedioxyphenyl compounds such as piperonyl butoxide and sesamex. The term potentiation is then reserved for those cases in which both compounds have appreciable intrinsic toxicity, such as in the case of malathion and EPN. Unfortunately, other toxicologists have used the terms in precisely the opposite manner, while even more use the terms interchangeably, without definition, leading to such statements as "potentiation of the toxicity of X by the synergist Y."

Antagonism may be defined as that interaction in which the toxicity of two or more compounds administered either together or sequentially is less than that which might be expected from a consideration of their toxicities when administered individually.

Antagonism not involving induction (Section 28.3.1.b) is a phenomenon often seen at a marginal level of detection and is, consequently, both difficult to explain and of marginal significance. Several different types of antagonism of importance to toxicology but not involving xenobiotic metabolism are also known. These include competition for receptor sites, such as the competition between carbon monoxide and oxygen in carbon monoxide poisoning, or situations in which one toxicant combines nonenzymatically with another to reduce its toxic effects, such as in the chelation of metal ions. Physiological antagonism, in which two agonists act on the same physiological system but produce opposite effects, is also of importance.

28.3.1.b. Induction

Some 25 years ago, during the course of studies on the N-demethylation of aminoazo dyes, it was observed that the pretreatment of mammals with the substrate or, more remarkably, with other xenobiotics, caused an increase in the ability of the animal to metabolize these dyes. It was subsequently shown that this is due to an increase in the microsomal enzymes involved. Since that time it has become clear that this phenomenon is widespread and quite nonspecific. Several hundred compounds of diverse chemical structure have been shown to induce mixed-function oxidase and other enzymes. These compounds include drugs, insecticides, polycyclic hydrocarbons, and many others; their only obvious common denominators are that they are organic and lipophilic.

The many inducers of mixed-function oxidase activity fall into two principle classes: one, exemplified by phenobarbital, contains many drugs, insecticides, etc., of diverse chemical classes; and the other, exemplified by 3-methylcholanthrene and benzo[a]pyrene, contains primarily polycyclic hydrocarbons. Some overlap between classes does appear to occur, however. Many inducers require either fairly high doses, frequently greater than 10 mg/kg and some as high as 100–200 mg/kg, or repeated dosing to be effective. However, some insecticides, such as Mirex, can induce at dose levels as low as 1 mg/kg, while the most potent inducer known, TCDD, is effective at $1\mu g/kg$ in some species.

In the liver, phenobarbital-type inducers cause a marked proliferation of the smooth endoplasmic reticulum and induction of cytochrome P-450 with approximately the same spectral characteristics as that of the liver of uninduced mammals. A wide range of oxidative activities is induced, including

O-demethylation of p-nitroanisole, N-demethylation of benzphetamine, pentobarbital hydroxylation, aldrin epoxidation, and many others, but increases in aryl hydrocarbon hydroxylase activity are minimal.

Induction by polycyclic hydrocarbons, on the other hand, causes no increase in smooth endoplasmic reticulum and results in the appearance of cytochrome P-448, characterized by a shift in the λ_{max} of the reduced cytochrome–CO complex to 448 nm. This cytochrome also shows a shift in the pH equilibrium point of the reduced cytochrome–ethyl isocyanide complex. Unlike phenobarbital-type induction, there is no increase in the type I binding of hexobarbital concomitant with the increase in cytochrome level. The appearance of a type I optical difference spectrum with benzo[a]pyrene or 3-methyl-cholanthrene and a marked drop in the K_m values for aryl hydrocarbon hydroxylase substrates is further evidence for the formation of a cytochrome P-450 (P-448 or P_1-450) of different physical and substrate-binding characteristics. A relatively narrow range of oxidative activities, primarily aryl hydrocarbon hydroxylase, is induced by polycyclic hydrocarbons. The extremely potent inducer TCDD appears to fall in this class.

Although the majority of published investigations on induction of mixed-function oxidase enzymes deal with mammalian liver, it should be pointed out that induction has been observed in other mammalian tissues and in nonmammalian species, both vertebrate and invertebrate.

Although stress can affect the level of mammalian mixed-function oxidase activity, the effect is secondary, since induction has been demonstrated in isolated perfused liver and also in isolated hepatocytes. Induction of mixed-function oxidase activity is a true induction, involving synthesis of new enzyme, and not the activation of enzyme already synthesized, since it is prevented by inhibitors of protein synthesis. For example, aryl hydrocarbon hydroxylase induction is inhibited by puromycin, ethionine, and cycloheximide.

The use of inhibitors of RNA and DNA metabolism has shown that the inductive effect is at the level of transcription and that DNA synthesis is not required.

The effects of inducers are usually the opposite of those of inhibitors, and thus their effects can be demonstrated by much the same methods, that is to say, by their effects on pharmacological or toxicological properties in vivo or by the effects on enzymes in vitro following prior treatment of the animal with the inducer. In vivo effects are frequently reported, the most common being the reduction of the hexobarbital sleeping time or zoxazolamine paralysis time. For example, in the rat the paralysis time resulting from a high dose of zoxazolamine can be reduced from 11 hr to 17 min by pretreatment of the animal with benzo[a]pyrene 24 hr before the administration of zoxazolamine.

Induction of mixed-function oxidase activity may also protect from the effect of carcinogens by increasing their rate of detoxication. This has been demonstrated in the rat with a number of carcinogens, including benzo[a]pyrene, N-2-fluorenylacetamide, and aflatoxin. Effects on carcinogenesis may be expected to be complex since some carcinogens are both activated and detoxified by mixed-function oxidase enzymes, while epoxide hydrase, which can also be involved in both activation and detoxication, may also be induced. For example, the toxicities of the carcinogen 2-naphthylamine, the hepatotoxic alkaloid monocrotaline, and the cytotoxic cyclophosphamide are all increased by phenobarbital induction, an effect mediated via the increased production of active intermediates.

The effects of inducers on the metabolic activity of hepatic microsomes subsequently isolated from treated animals have been reported many times. The polycyclic hydrocarbons primarily induce aryl hydrocarbon hydroxylase activity and a few related activities, which are probably all catalyzed by cytochrome P-448. The more general inducers, however, such as phenobarbital, DDT, etc., have been shown to induce many oxidative reactions, including benzphetamine N-demethylation, p-nitroanisole O-demethylation, N-demethylation of ethylmorphine, aldrin epoxidation, and many others. Some enzyme activities are induced by both types of inducers, such as zoxazolamine hydroxylase, chlorpromazine N-demethylation, and aniline hydroxylation.

Although less well studied, xenobiotic-metabolizing enzymes other than the microsomal mixed-function oxidases are also known to be induced, frequently by the same inducers. These include glutathione S-transferases, epoxide hydrase, and UDP glucuronyltransferase.

Many inhibitors of mammalian mixed-function oxidase activity can also act as inducers. Inhibition of microsomal mixed-function oxidase activity is fairly rapid and involves a direct interaction with the cytochrome, while induction is a slower process. Therefore, following a single injection of a suitable compound, an initial decrease due to inhibition would be followed by an inductive phase. As the compound and its metabolites are eliminated, the levels would be expected to return to control values. Some of the best examples of this type of compound are the methylenedioxyphenyl synergists.

28.3.2. Chemical Interactions

Nonenzymatic interaction of foreign compounds may take place either inside the body or outside, in the environment. In either case an increase or a decrease in toxicity may ensue. For example, nitrosamines, a class of compounds that includes several potent carcinogens, can be formed by the interaction of nitrites with primary or secondary amines. Since nitrites are used as food additives, the formation of nitrosamines, particularly in foods such as smoked fish and meats, is of particular concern.

An example of a nonenzymatic interaction that may take place either in vivo or in the environment is metal chelation (Section 28.2.8).

28.3.3. Physiological Interactions

28.3.3.a. Modes of Toxic Action

Interaction of toxicants with physiological or biochemical systems in the body includes all of the modes of toxic action. This area is one of great importance in toxicology and has been the subject of innumerable reports. Present space limitations permit only a brief summary.

Acute toxicity is usually exerted through the nerve synapse or the neuromuscular junction, or through inhibition of oxidative phosphorylation in the mitochondria. The best known example of a toxic effect at the synapse is that of the inhibition of cholinesterase by organophosphate and carbamate insecticides, while other insecticides, such as rotenone and 2,4-dinitrophenol, either inhibit mitochondrial electron transport or uncouple oxidative phosphorylation.

Chronic toxicity is commonly expressed following the interaction of toxicants or their reactive metabolites with DNA, as in the case of carcinogenesis, mutagenesis, and teratogenesis. A well-known example of carcinogenesis caused by a reactive metabolite is that caused by the dihydrodiol epoxide of benzo[a]pyrene, formed by the action of the cytochrome P-448–dependent mixed-function oxidase system. This metabolic sequence is probably typical of the formation of proximate carcinogens from polycyclic hydrocarbons.

Hepatotoxicity can be either acute or toxic, depending upon the toxic agent and the dose involved; in either case, it involves either fatty infiltration or necrosis of the liver cells. Hepatotoxicity also involves the formation of reactive intermediates and their interaction with cellular macromolecules, in this case cellular proteins. Although carbon tetrachloride is the best studied hepatotoxicant, the problem is now recognized as being both widespread and of considerable human health importance.

The endocrine system is also a target for toxic effects. An example of environmental interest is that of the decrease in egg shell thickness in certain raptorial bird species as a result of the accumulation of DDT and its metabolite DDE in the tissues. Although the precise mechanism is not known, it is believed to be an effect on the metabolism of steroids resulting from the ability of DDT and DDE to induce the enzymes of the microsomal mixed-function oxidase system.

28.3.3.b. Displacement

Foreign compounds primarily exist in the body bound to macromolecules. These may be the lipoproteins of the body fluids involved in their distribution, lipoprotein membranes, or receptor sites. In theory, any compound not covalently bound could be displaced by another compound that binds more strongly to the same binding site. There are several examples of this action in drug therapy, but its importance in environmental toxicology is yet to be determined. It has been suggested that dieldrin will displace DDT from blood proteins and will also reduce the body burden of DDT and DDE.

28.3.3.c. Penetration

Penetration through the skin is frequently facilitated by other compounds, particularly organic solvents, and thus the solvent in which a toxicant is dissolved, even though it may have little toxicity alone, can play an important role in the expression of a toxic effect. For this reason, the toxic hazard to humans of a pesticide formulated in an oil is much greater than that of the same compound in a dry formulation or as an aqueous suspension.

28.3.3.d. Nutrition

The expression of toxicity can be greatly affected by the diet and nutritional state of the organism. Some of these effects are nonspecific, such as the increased incidence of cancer of the large intestine in populations who have a diet high in meat; while others appear more specific, such as the decrease in breast cancer in women on a high-selenium diet.

28.3.4. Physical Interactions

The effect of physical factors on enzymatic reactions in vitro will not be considered since it has little direct relationship to environmental toxicology. Temperature changes, ionizing radiation, light, moisture, altitude, and noise have all been shown to affect, in vivo, the systems that metabolize foreign compounds.

Changes in temperature, which frequently affect toxicity, even in homeothermic animals, appear to do so via a stress mechanism, and an intact pituitary–adrenal axis is necessary. Other environmental effects, such as noise, which has been shown to cause a slight increase in the rate of metabolism of 2-naphthylamine, are probably also mediated through a stress mechanism.

The effect of light is essentially one of photoperiod rather than light intensity. Many enzymes, including those involved in xenobiotic metabolism, show a diurnal cycle of activity, and as a result the toxicity of a particular toxicant varies with the time of day.

Altitude can cause either an increase or a decrease in toxicity. For example, an altitude of 5000 ft or more causes a decrease in the toxicity of digitalis or strychnine to mice, while it causes an increase in the toxicity of d-amphetamine. Depending upon the experimental design, stress, as well as oxygen deficit, can play a role in altitude effects on toxicity.

28.4. Conclusions

The metabolism of toxicants is complex, involving both single enzymes and multienzyme systems, as well as many cell types, tissues, and organs. Since the enzymes in question are induceable as well as nonspecific, many interactions among xenobiotics are possible, in addition to the interactions between xenobiotics and physiological systems. Although in the laboratory many of these interacting compounds and systems can be separated and their effects determined separately, this cannot be done easily at the level of environmental toxicology, the level at which the interactions are most important. One of the keys to future progress in environmental toxicology is an increase in our ability to understand the complex interactions touched upon in this chapter.

Suggested Reading

Cicerone, R. J., Stolarski, R. S., Walters, S. Science 185:1165, 1974.

Conney, A. H. Pharmacological implications of microsomal enzyme induction. Pharmacol. Rev. 19:317, 1967.

Hodgson, E., Guthrie, F. E. (Ed.). Introduction to Biochemical Toxicology. New York: Elsevier North Holland, 1980.

Hodgson, E., Philpot, R. M. Interaction of methylenedioxyphenyl (1,3-benzodioxole) compounds with enzymes and their effects on mammals. Drug Metabol. Rev. 3:231, 1974.

National Academy of Sciences. Degradation of Synthetic Organic Molecules in the Biosphere. Proceedings of a Conference, San Francisco, Calif., June 12–13, 1971. Washington, D.C., 1972.

Wilkinson, C. F. Insecticide interactions. In: Wilkinson, C. F., (Ed.). Insecticide Biochemistry and Physiology. New York: Plenum Press, 1976, Chapter 15.

R. B. Leidy

29

Detection: Analytical

29.1. Introduction

Rarely can one read a newspaper or listen to the news without some mention being made of the discovery of some form of environmental pollution that might affect the quality of life in a particular region of the world. These news features generally list the extent of the pollution, the amounts found, and the length of time that the region will be contaminated. In most cases these values are accurate to levels that were unattainable 20 years ago, and the primary reason for this improvement is the increased sensitivity of modern analytical instruments. However, instrumentation is but one part of the analytical process, which consists of a series of six operations culminating in the determination of the extent and quantity of the pollutant present.

The first step of the analytical process is a definition of the goal. If there is reason to suspect that a pollutant has been released into the environment, one must consider, based on the nature of the pollutant, what should be determined and how should it be done. Sampling is the second and most important step, because if one cannot obtain either representative samples or one containing the pollutant, the resulting data will not present accurate information as to concentration and extent of contamination. Isolation of the pollutant, the third step, involves extraction of the compound from the sample. Generally, other interfering materials are released during this step and must be separated (the fourth step) from the pollutant. The separation step precedes the actual identification of the pollutant, which is done by an analytical instrument, and its quantitation. The last step is an evaluation of the data to determine if additional samples are required, if other types of materials should be sampled, and if additional areas should be sampled.

This chapter is concerned with the sampling, isolation, separation, and measurement of a pollutant. Each of these will be subdivided into more detailed sections so that a general knowledge can be obtained as to the complexity of the analytical processes.

29.2. Sampling

One can have the most sophisticated analytical equipment in the world, but the resulting data are only as representative as the samples from which the results are derived. Care must be taken to assure that the sample is representative of the object of study. Often, special attention to sampling procedures is necessary. Sampling accomplishes a number of objectives, depending on the type of area being studied. In environmental areas (e.g., wilderness regions, lakes, or rivers) it can provide data on not only the concentration of pollutants but also the extent of contamination. In urban areas sampling can provide information on the types of pollutants one is exposed to, either by inhalation or perhaps by ingestion over a given period.

In industrial areas, unsafe conditions can be detected and sources of pollution identified. Sampling is used in the process of designing pollution controls and can provide a chronicle of changes in operational conditions as these controls are implemented. Another important application of sampling in industrial areas is the documentation of compliance with existing OSHA and EPA regulations. The many methods available for sampling the environment can be divided into air, soil, tissue, and water sampling.

29.2.1. Air Samples

Most pollutants entering the atmosphere come from fuel combustion, industrial processes, and solid waste disposal. Additional miscellaneous sources, such as atomic explosions, forest fires, soil dusts, volcanoes, natural gaseous emissions, and agricultural burning, contribute to the level of atmospheric pollution. In order for pollutants to affect terrestrial animals and plants, the pollutant must be in a size range that allows it to get into a body and remain there. In other words, the pollutant must be in an aerosol, which can be defined as an air-borne suspension of liquid droplets or solid particles small enough to possess a low settling velocity. Suspensions can be classified as liquids—including fogs (small particles) and mists (large particles) produced from atomization, condensation, or entrainment of liquids by gases—and solids—including dusts, fumes, and smokes produced by crushing, metal vaporization, and combustion of organic materials, respectively.

At rest an adult human inhales 6–8 liters air/min (1 liter = 0.001 m³) and during an 8-hr work day, one can inhale anywhere from 5 to 20 m³ depending on the level of physical activity. The optium size range for aerosol particles to get into the lungs and remain there is 0.5–5 μm. Thus air samplers have been designed to collect the particular matter in the size range most detrimental to humans.

An air sampler generally consists of an inlet to direct air into a collector, a filter to screen out larger particles that might interfere with an analysis, the collector where the sample is deposited, a flowmeter and valve to calibrate airflow, and a pump to pull air through the system (Figure 29.1). In recent years samplers have been miniaturized so that they can be connected to individuals while they are working, walking, or riding in a given area, thus allowing an estimation of exposure of the individual.

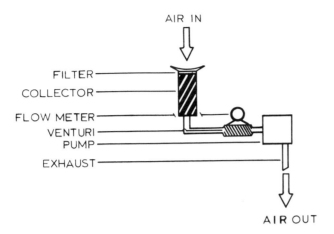

Figure 29.1 Typical air sampler.

Many air samplers use various types of filters to collect solid particulate matter, such as asbestos, which is collected on glass fiber filters with pores 20 μm in diameter or less. Membrane filters with pores 0.01–10 μm in diameter are used to collect dusts and silica. Liquid-containing collectors called impingers are used to trap mineral dusts and pesticides. Mineral dusts are collected in large impingers that have flow rates of 10–50 liters air/min passing through them, and insecticides can be collected in smaller "midget" impingers that handle flows of 2–4.5 liters air/min. Depending upon the pollutant being sought, the entrapping liquid might be distilled water, alcohol, ethylene glycol, hexylene glycol, or some other solvent. Small glass tubes approximately 7 cm × 0.5 cm in diameter containing activated charcoal are used to entrap organic vapors in air. A large-volume air sampler has been developed recently by the EPA for detection of chlorinated hydrocarbon insecticides and PCBs: air flows through a polyurethane foam pad at a rate of 225.0 liters/min and the insecticides and PCBs are trapped in the foam. Direct reading instruments are being developed rapidly, and mention will be made of their principles of operation in Section 29.5.3.e. These direct reading instruments take the place of the collector in the sampling system.

29.2.2. Soil Samples

When environmental pollutants become deposited on land areas, their behavior is complicated by a series of simultaneous interactions with organic and inorganic components, the existing liquid–gas phases, and the living and nonliving components of the soil. Depending upon its chemical and physical structure, the pollutant might remain in one location for long or short periods, might be absorbed into plant tissue, or might move into the soil by diffusion resulting from random molecular motion. Movement is also affected by mass flow as a result of external forces, such as the pollutant being dissolved or suspended in water or adsorbed onto inorganic and organic soil components. Thus, sampling for pollutants in soils can be simple or quite difficult.

In order to obtain representative samples, one must take into consideration the chemical and physical characteristics of the sampling site(s), possible reactions of the pollutant with the soil components, and the degree of variability in the sampling area. With these types of data, the site(s) can be divided into homogeneous areas and the required number of samples can be collected. The number of samples would depend upon the functions of variance and the degree of accuracy required. Once the correct procedure has been determined, sampling can proceed by random or systematic means.

Many types of soil samplers are available, but the various coring devices are preferred because this method of collection allows vertical determination of a pollutant's distribution. These devices can be either steel tubes, which vary from 2.5 to 7.6 cm in diameter and 60–100 cm in length (for hand use), or large boring tubes that are 10×200 cm (operated mechanically). It is possible to sample to uniform depths with devices such as these. Another type of coring equipment is a wheel to which small tubes are attached so that large numbers of small subsamples can be taken, thus allowing more uniform sampling over a given site. Specialty samplers with large diameters (about 25 cm) incorporate a blade to slice a core of soil after reaching the desired depth.

29.2.3. Tissue Samples

When environmental areas are suspected of being contaminated, surveys of plants and animals are conducted. Many of the surveys, conducted during hunting and fishing seasons, determine the number of animals killed, and organs and other tissues are removed for analysis for suspected contaminants by federal and state laboratories. Sampling is conducted randomly throughout an area; the analysis can help determine the concentration, extent of contamination within a given species, and areas of contamination.

29.2.3.a. Plant Tissue

When plant material is gathered for analysis, it might be divided into roots, stems, leaves, and flowers and/or fruit, or the whole plant could be analyzed as a single entity. Pooling of samples from a site could also provide a single sample for analysis. This choice would depend upon the characteristics of the suspected contaminant.

29.2.3.b. Animal Tissue

Many environmental pollutants are known to concentrate in bone, certain organs, or specific tissue (e.g., adipose). These organs are removed from recently killed animals for analysis. In many instances the organ system would not be pooled with others from the same species but would be subsampled and analyzed as a single sample.

There are many methods of subdividing both plant and animal tissue to obtain representative fractions. The reader is directed to the Suggested Reading section at the end of the chapter.

29.2.4. Water Samples

In order to obtain representative samples of water, many factors must be considered; the most important are the nature of the pollutant and where it entered the aquatic environment. Pollutants may be contributed by agricultural, industrial, municipal, or other sources, such as spills from wrecks or train derailments. The prevailing wind direction and speed, the velocity of stream or river flow, temperature, thermal and salinity stratification, and sediment content are other important factors.

Two important questions are where to monitor or sample and what type of device to use. The answers would depend upon the type of data required and the best way to obtain a representative sample.

The simplest method of collecting water is the "grab" technique, whereby a container is lowered into the water, rinsed, filled, and capped. A Van Dorn type sampler is frequently used to obtain water at greater depths.

With the implementation of the EPA Clean Water Act of 1977, continuous monitoring is required to obtain data for management decisions. There are a number of continuous monitoring devices in operation. These consist of a pump (floating, peristaltic, submersible, or tank mounted) to draw water into collecting devices (generally glass or plastic bottles), metering devices to determine flow rates, and timers to implement periodic sampling. Because large numbers of samples can be generated by such devices, collectors containing membranes with small pores (about 0.45 μm) to entrap metal-containing pollutants, or ion-exchange resins or resin-loaded filter paper to bind organic pollutants, are used to diminish the number and bulk of the samples by allowing water to pass through and leave only the pollutants entrapped in a small cylinder or container.

Once samples have been collected, they should be frozen immediately and returned to the laboratory. If they are not analyzed at that time, they should be stored in a freezer.

29.3. Isolation

In most cases the analysis of a pollutant depends upon its physical removal from the sample medium. This process is called extraction and involves bringing a suitable solvent into intimate content with the sample, generally in a ratio of 5–25 volumes of solvent to 1 volume of sample. One or more of four different procedures can be used, depending upon the chemical and physical characteristics of the pollutant and the sample matrix.

29.3.1. Blending

The use of an electric or air-driven blender is currently the most common method of extraction of biological materials. The weighed sample is placed in a container and solvent is added, and the tissue is homogenized by motor-driven blades. Blending for 5–15 min and then a repeat blending will remove most environmental pollutants. The homogenate can be filtered through anhydrous sodium sulfate to remove water which might cause problems later.

29.3.2. Exhaustive Extraction

This procedure is performed on solid samples (e.g., soil) and involves the use of an organic solvent or combination of solvents. The sample is weighed into a cup called a thimble, which is made of specialized porous materials (e.g., cellulose or fiberglass). A specialized apparatus called a Soxhlet extractor is used to remove the pollutant from the sample matrix. The apparatus consists of a boiling flask in which the solvent is placed, an extractor, which holds the thimble, and a water-jacketed condensor. When heated to boiling, the solvent vaporizes, is condensed, and fills the extractor, thus bathing the sample and removing the pollutant. A siphoning action drains the solvent back into the flask and the cycle begins again. Depending upon the nature of the pollutant and sample matrix, the extraction can be completed in as little as 2 hr but might take 3–4 days.

29.3.3. Shaking

Pollutants are generally extracted from water samples, and in some cases soils, by shaking with an appropriate solvent or solvent combination. Mechanical shakers have been developed to handle several water or soil samples at one time, although the separatory funnel is used widely. Two or more shakings normally are required to remove the pollutant.

29.3.4. Washing

With some environmental samples such as plants or fruits, a simple surface washing with water and a detergent or with solvent is sufficient to determine surface contamination.

29.3.5. Other Methods

Other extraction methods are boiling, grinding, or distilling the sample with appropriate solvents, but these are not used to the same extent as the above-mentioned methods.

29.4. Separation

During the extraction process many undesirable components are released from the sample matrix, and these must be removed in order to obtain quantitative results from certain instruments. These components include plant and animal pigments, lipids, organic material from soil and water, and inorganic compounds. If not removed, the impurities decrease the sensitivity of the detectors and columns in the analytical instrument, mask peaks, or produce extraneous peaks on chromatograms. Instruments have been developed in recent years that automatically remove these substances and concentrate the pollutants to small volumes for quantitative analysis. However, many laboratories cannot afford these devices and rely on more classical, yet relatively inexpensive, methods. These methods include adsorption chromatography, thin-layer chromatography (TLC), and solvent partitioning. Before the separation step is conducted, the solvent containing the extracted pollutant must be concentrated to a small volume (approximately 5–10 ml). This is accomplished by removal of the solvent by distillation, evaporation under a stream of air or inert gas such as nitrogen, or evaporation under vacuum. Once the working volume is reached, extracts can be cleaned up by one or more procedures.

29.4.1. Adsorption Chromatography

This procedure involves column chromatography using a glass column and Teflon stopcock to control flow rate. The adsorbent might be activated charcoal, aluminum oxide, Florisil, silica, silicic acid, or mixed adsorbents. Of course, the adsorbent would depend upon the characteristics of the pollutant. Once the concentrated extract is placed on the column, the pollutant can be removed selectively by passing one or more solvents through the column while the coextracted materials remain. In some instances, selected solvents are used to remove interferences first; then the pollutant is eluted by another solvent system. Once removed, the eluate containing the pollutant is reduced to a small volume for quantitation.

29.4.2. Thin-Layer Chromatography

Many pollutants can be separated from interfering substances with TLC. This is a form of chromatography in which the adsorbent is spread as a thin layer (250–2000 μm) on a glass plate, resistant plastic, or fiberglass backings. When the extract is placed near the bottom of the plate, and the plate is placed in a tank containing a solvent system, the solvent migrates up the plate and the pollutant or interferences move with the solvent; differential rates of movement result in separation. The pollutant can be scraped from the plate and eluted from the adsorbent with a suitable solvent. It should be mentioned that recent developments in TLC adsorbents allow pollutants and other materials to be quantitated at the nanogram (10^{-9} g) and picogram (10^{-12} g) levels.

29.4.3. Solvent Partitioning

Many organic pollutants will distribute between two immiscible solvents (e.g., hexane and acetonitrile). When shaken in a separatory funnel and then allowed to equilibrate into the two original solvent layers, some of the pollutant will have transferred from the extracting solvent into the other layer. With repeated additions (e.g., 4–5 volumes), mixing, and removal, most or all of the pollutant will have been transferred, leaving interferences in the original extracting solvent.

Regardless of the separation method or combination of methods used, the pollutant will be in a large volume of solvent in relation to its amount; the volume of solvent can be reduced by an evaporation step. The final volume should be such that dilutions can be made readily, if required. For example, 1 ml can be removed from a 10-ml total volume and placed in another tube to which 9 ml solvent is added. The resulting volume, 10 ml, would be equivalent to 100 ml. Of course, this will depend upon the concentration of the material, type of instrument used, and method of data calculation.

29.5. Identification

Once the pollutant has been extracted and separated from extraneous materials, the actual identification procedure can begin. Recent advances in circuit miniaturization and column technology, the development of microprocessors, and new concepts in instrument design have allowed sensitive measurement at the parts per billion and parts per trillion levels for many pollutants. This increased sensitivity has focused public attention upon the extent of environmental pollution, because many toxic materials present in minute quantities could not be detected until technological advances reached the present state of the art. At present most environmental pollutants are identified and quantified by chromatography, spectroscopy, and bioassays (discussed in Chapter 30).

29.5.1. Chromatography

All chromatographic processes (e.g., TLC or gas–liquid) utilize an immobile and a mobile phase to effect a separation of components. In TLC, the immobile phase is a thin layer of adsorbent placed on glass, resistant plastic, or fiberglass and the mobile phase is the solvent. The mobile phase can be a liquid or gas, whereas the immobile phase can be a liquid or solid. Chromatographic separations are based upon the interactions of these phases on surfaces. All chromatographic procedures use the differential distribution or partitioning of one or more components between the phases, based on the absorption, adsorption, ion-exchange, or size exclusion properties of one of the phases.

29.5.1.a. Gas–Liquid Chromatography (GLC)

GLC has become the most common instrument used for the analysis of organic pollutants. It consists of an injector port, oven, detector, amplifier (electrometer), and supporting electronics (Figure 29.2). Contained within the oven is a column of glass, nickel, stainless steel, or perhaps a polymer, filled or coated with the immobile phase. The immobile or stationary phase is a liquid coated on an inert support material. The mobile phase is an inert gas (called a carrier gas), such as helium or nitrogen, which passes through the column.

When a sample is injected into or onto the column, the injector port is at a temperature sufficient to vaporize the sample components. Based on the solubility and volatility of these components with respect to the stationary phase, the components separate and are swept through the column by the carrier gas to a detector, which responds to the concentration of each component. It should be mentioned that the detector might not respond to all components. The electric signal produced as the component passes through the detector is amplified by the electrometer and the resulting signal is sent to a recorder, computer, or electronic data-collecting device for quantitation.

29.5.1.b. Column Technology

Increased sensitivity has resulted from new advances in solid-state electronics, column, and detector technology. In the field of column technology, the capillary column has revolutionized pollutant detection in complex samples.

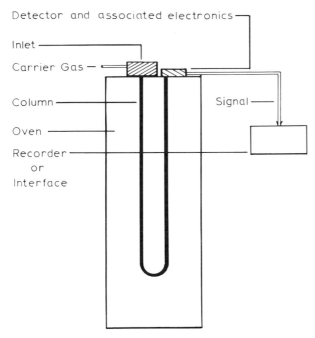

Figure 29.2   Gas chromatograph.

Capillary columns differ from conventionally packed ones in three ways: (a) there is an open, unrestricted path through the column rather than the obstructed path in conventional columns that are filled with material; (b) the diameter of tubing varies from 0.2 to 0.5 mm inner diameter compared to 2–6.3 mm in conventional columns; and (c) the length varies from 15 to 100 m as opposed to 0.6–6.7 m in packed columns.

Two types of capillary columns are receiving widespread use: the support-coated, open tubular (SCOT) and the wall-coated, open tubular (WCOT) columns. The SCOT column has a very fine layer of diatomaceous earth coated with liquid phase which is deposited on the inside wall. The WCOT column is pretreated and then coated with a thin film of liquid phase. Of the two columns, the SCOT is claimed to be more universally applicable because of large sample capacity, simplicity in connecting it into the chromatograph, and lower cost. For difficult separations or highly complex mixtures, the WCOT is the more efficient type. Water samples chromatographed on capillary columns routinely separate 400–500 compounds, compared to 90–120 resolved compounds from conventional columns.

29.5.1.c. Detector Technology

The other advance in GLC has been detector technology. Five detectors are used widely in pollutant detection: the flame ionization (FID), flame photometric (FPD), electron capture (ECD), alkali flame, and conductivity detectors (Figure 29.3). However, new detectors are being introduced that could have an impact on pollution analysis, including the Hall conductivity detector, the nitrogen–phosphorous detector, and the photoionization detector.

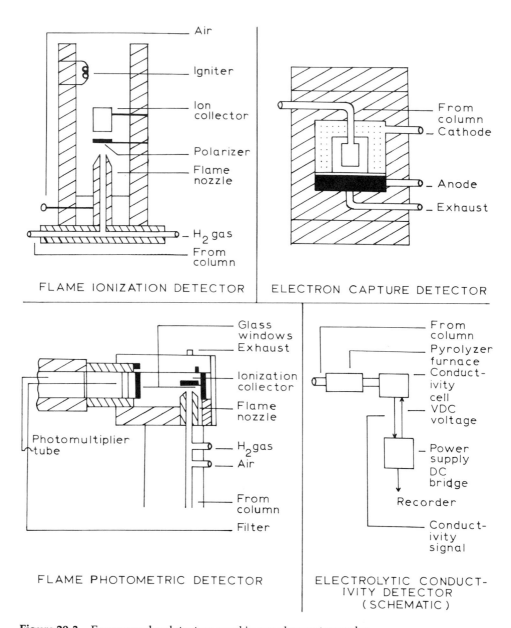

Figure 29.3   Four popular detectors used in gas chromatography.

The FID operates on the principle of ion formation from compounds being burned in a hydrogen flame as they elute from a column. The concentrations of ions formed are several orders of magnitude greater than those formed in the uncontaminated flame. The ions cause a current to flow between two electrodes held at a constant potential, thus sending a signal to the electrometer.

The FPD is a specific detector in that it detects either phosphorous or sulfur-containing compounds. When atoms of a given element are burned in a hydrogen-rich flame, the excitation energy supplied to these atoms produces a unique emission spectrum. The intensity of the wavelengths of light emitted by these atoms is directly proportional to the number of atoms excited. Larger concentrations cause a greater number of atoms to reach the excitation energy level, thus increasing the intensity of the emission spectrum. The change in intensity is detected by a photomultiplier, amplified by the electrometer, and recorded. Filters that allow only the emission wavelength of phosphorous (526 nm) or sulfur (394 nm) are inserted between the flame and the photomultiplier to give this detector its specificity.

The ECD is used to detect halogen-containing compounds, although it will produce a response to any electronegative compound. When a negative DC voltage is applied to a radioactive source (e.g., ^{63}Ni or ^{3}H), low-energy beta particles are emitted which produce secondary electrons by ionizing the carrier gas as it passes through the detector. The secondary electron stream flows from the source (cathode) to a collector (anode), where the amount of current generated (called a standing current) is amplified and recorded. As electronegative compounds pass from the column into the detector, electrons are removed or "captured" and the standing current is reduced. The reduction is related to both the concentration and electronegativity of the compound passing through, and this produces a response that is recorded. The sensitivity of the ECD is greater than that of any of the other detectors currently available.

Early electrolytic conductivity detectors operated on the principle of component combustion, which produced simple molecular species that readily ionized, thus altering the conductivity of deionized water. The changes were monitored by a DC bridge circuit and recorded. By varying conditions the detector could be made selective for different types of compounds (e.g., chlorine- or nitrogen-containing).

The alkali flame detector can also be made selective. Enhanced response to compounds containing arsenic, boron, halogen, nitrogen, and phosphorous results when the collector (cathode) of an FID is coated with different alkali metal salts such as KBr, KCl, Na_2SO_4, and Rb_2SO_4. As with conductivity detectors, by varying gas flow rates, type of salt, and electrode configuration, enhanced responses are obtained.

New detectors are also being utilized in the field of pollutant analysis. The Hall electrolytic conductivity detector uses advanced designs in the conductivity cell, furnace, and an AC conductivity bridge to detect chlorine, nitrogen, and sulfur-containing compounds at sensitivities of 0.01 ng. It operates on the conductivity principle described previously. A nitrogen–phosphorous alkali detector was introduced recently. In this detector the alkali salts are embedded in a Silica Gel matrix and are heated electrically. The detector allows routine use of chlorinated solvents and derivatizing reagents to prevent contamination of the salts. It will also reduce a response to phosphorous by 30% while maintaining the normal response to nitrogen for confirmation purposes. Another new detector, the photoionization detector, uses a UV light source to ionize molecules by absorption of a photon of UV light. The ion formed has an energy greater than the ionization potential of the parent compound, and the formed ions are collected by an electrode. The current, which is proportional to concentration, is amplified and recorded. The detector can measure a number of organic and inorganic compounds in air, biological fluids, and water.

29.5.2. High-Performance Liquid Chromatography (HPLC)

Although it is a relatively new instrument in the field of analytical chemistry, HPLC has become very popular for the following reasons: it can be run at ambient temperatures; it is nondestructive to the compound, which can be collected intact; in many instances derivatization is not necessary for response; and columns can be loaded with large quantities of the material for detection of low levels.

The instrument consists of a solvent reservoir, gradient-forming device, high-pressure pumping device, injector column, and detector. The principle of operation is very similar to GLC except that the mobile phase is a liquid instead of a gas. It is the composition of the mobile phase and its flow rate that effect separations. The columns being developed for HPLC are too numerous to discuss in detail. Most use finely divided packing (5–10 μm in diameter), some have bonded phases, and others are alumina or silica. The columns normally are 25–50 cm in length with small diameters (approximately 4.6 mm inner diameter). A high-pressure pump is required to force the solvent through this type of column. The major detectors presently used for HPLC are UV fluorescent spectrophotometers or differential refractometers, although others are being developed.

29.5.3. Spectroscopy

In order to discuss spectroscopy a short review of radiation is necessary. In certain experiments involving radiation, observed results cannot be explained on the basis of the wave theory of radiation. One has to assume that radiation comes in discrete units, called quanta. Each quantum of energy has a definite frequency v, and the quantum energy can be calculated by the equation $E = hv$, where h is Planck's constant (6.6×10^{-27} erg-sec). Matter absorbs radiation one quantum at a time, and the energy of radiation absorbed becomes greater as either the frequency of radiation increases or the wavelength decreases. Therefore, radiation of shorter wavelength brings about more drastic changes in a molecule than that of longer wavelength.

Spectroscopy is concerned with the changes in atoms and molecules when electromagnetic radiation is absorbed or emitted. Instruments have been designed to detect these changes, and these instruments are important to the field of pollution analysis. Atomic absorption (AA) spectroscopy, mass spectroscopy (MS), and infrared (IR) and ultraviolet (UV) spectrophotometry are discussed below.

29.5.3.a. Atomic Absorption Spectroscopy

One of the more sensitive instruments utilized to detect metal-containing pollutants is the AA spectrophotometer. Samples are vaporized either by aspiration into an acetylene flame or by carbon rod atomization in a graphite cup or tube (flameless AA). The atomic vapor formed contains free atoms of an element in their ground state, and when illuminated by a light source that radiates light of a frequency characteristic of that element, the atom absorbs a photon of wavelength corresponding to its atomic absorption spectrum, thus exciting it. The amount of absorption is a function of concentration. The flameless instruments are much more sensitive than conventional flame AA. For example, arsenic can be detected at levels of 0.1 ng/ml and selenium at 0.2 ng/ml, which represent three orders of magnitude greater sensitivity than conventional flame AA.

29.5.3.b. Mass Spectroscopy

The MS is an outstanding instrument used for the identification of compounds. In pollution analysis the MS is used widely as a highly sensitive detector for GLC and is increasingly used with HPLC since these instruments can be interfaced to the MS. The GLC or HPLC is used to separate individual components as previously described. A portion of the column effluent passes into the MS, where it is bombarded by an electron beam. Electrons or negative groups are removed by this process, and the ions produced are accelerated. After acceleration, they pass through a magnetic field, where the ion species are separated by the different curvatures of their paths under gravity. Normally, only single positive ions are detected. The resulting pattern is characteristic of the molecule under study. By interfacing the detector with a computer system, data reduction, analysis, and quantitation are performed automatically. Large libraries of mass spectra have been developed for computing systems, and with technological advances substances in femtogram (10^{-15} g) quantities are detected and quantitated.

29.5.3.c. Infrared Spectrophotometry

Within molecules, atoms are in constant motion, and associated with these motions are molecular energy levels that correspond to the energies of quanta of IR radiation. These motions can be resolved into rotation of the whole molecule in space and into motions corresponding to the vibration of atoms with respect to one another by bending or stretching of covalent bonds. These vibrational motions are very useful in identifying complex molecules, because functional groups (e.g., OH, C = O, and S–H) within the molecule have characteristic absorption bands. The principle functional groups can be determined and used to identify compounds where chemical evidence permits relatively few possible structures. Standard IR spectrophotometers cover the spectral range from 2.5 to 15.4 μm (wave number equivalent to 4000–650 cm^{-1}) and utilize a source of radiation that passes through the sample and reference cells into a monochromator (a device used to isolate spectral regions). The radiation is then collected, amplified, and recorded. Current instruments utilize microprocessors, allowing a number of refinements that have increased the versatility of IR instruments so that more precise qualitative and quantitative data can be obtained.

29.5.3.d. Ultraviolet/Visible Spectrophotometry

Transitions occurring between electronic levels of molecules produce absorptions and emissions in the visible (VIS) and UV portions of the electromagnetic spectrum. Many inorganic and organic molecules show maximum absorption at specific wavelengths in the UV/VIS range, and these can be used to identify and quantitate compounds. Instruments designed to measure absorbance in the UV/VIS portions of the spectrum (200–800 nm) have been used in many disciplines for years. Today's instruments are being designed to be used for specific purposes, such as detectors used in HPLC. Basic spectrophotometers have the same components as the IR instruments described previously, including a source (usually a tungsten lamp for VIS measurements or a hydrogen discharge lamp for UV), sample chamber, monochromator, and detector.

29.5.3.e. Other Analytical Methods

As mentioned previously, the above instruments are the primary ones employed in pollution analysis, but an enormous number of analytical techniques are employed in the field. Many of the instruments are expensive (e.g., Raman spectrometer and X-ray emission spectrometer), and few laboratories possess them. However, many other instruments are available, such as the specific ion electrode, which is both sensitive and portable. Specific ion electrodes have many other advantages in that sample color, suspended matter, turbidity, and viscosity do not interefere with analysis; therefore, many of the sample preparation steps are not required. Some of the species that can be detected at ppb levels are ammonia, carbon dioxide, chloride, cyanide, fluoride, lead, potassium, sulfide, and urea. Analytical pH meters or meters designed specifically for this application are used to calculate concentrations.

Finally, an increasing number of portable, direct reading instruments are now available to detect and quantitate environmental pollutants. Most of these measure air-borne particulates and dissolved molecules and operate on such diverse principles as aerosol photometry, chemiluminescence, combustion, and polarography. Striking advances are being made in this area, and these instruments can be interfaced to remote samplers and automatic data collection systems.

29.6. Data Collection

Automatic data handling systems are used widely with current instruments. Many of the more sophisticated systems such as GC/MS are connected directly to computers to facilitate rapid identification and quantitation. Integrating calculators are used to handle data from GLCs, and, as mentioned previously, microprocessor-equipped IR and UV spectrophotometers ease data manipulation.

Many data are calculated by hand, by measuring either peak heights or areas; by comparing these to known standards, one can quantitate amounts. Although many data are based on either external or internal standards, the calculated values are only as good as the efficiency of the analytical method. In other words, does the method employed in extracting and analyzing give a true concentration? This can be determined to a great extent by adding known amounts of the material being analyzed to a sample matrix known to be free of the pollutant. Analyzing these "recovery" or "spiked" samples with the unknown will allow the analyst to determine the efficiency of the analytical method. Adding the same amount of material to solvent and analyzing it without performing the extraction and cleanup allows a further check on efficiency. Generally, at least 80% recovery is considered necessary for an analytical method to be adequate, although some analytical methods effect only 50–60% recovery. Recovery samples, in addition to indicating efficiency, can tell an analyst how well the instruments are functioning. Thus one can correct data from a particular set of samples to reflect daily variation.

29.7. Confirmation

Scientists involved with chromatographic analyses of biological and environmental samples have had problems in the past with "artifact" peaks whose retention times corresponded to certain chlorinated hydrocarbons (e.g., aldrin, DDT, and dieldrin). From initial work done in Sweden, it became apparent that the artifact peaks were really PCBs. Although PCBs have been used for 45 years, it was not until 1966 that these compounds were detected in our environment. In addition to PCBs, decomposition products or metabolites might interfere with an analysis and make data interpretation impossible. Thus, it is important to confirm that the peaks seen on a recording chart indeed represent the suspected pollutant.

Confirmation can be done in a number of ways. One can use another chromatographic column whose characteristics differ from the first, thus causing the material to elute at a different retention time. When rechromatographed, the artifact normally would elute at a time different from the reference standard. Changing flow rates and temperatures could produce the same results. Thin layer chromatography might be used to confirm by developing the material along with the reference standard. The mass spectrometer can confirm the identity of the material as can the infrared spectrophotometer. The infrared spectrophotometer requires a relatively pure material in μg quantities. Derivatization is another popular technique to confirm a material. Many derivatizing materials are on the market and many of the procedures require only a few minutes of preparation.

Suggested Reading

Frei, R. W., Hutzinger, O. (Eds.). Analytical Aspects of Mercury and Other Heavy Metals in the Environment. New York: Gordon and Breach, 1975.

Keith, L. H. Identification and Analysis of Organic Pollutants in Water. Ann Arbor, Mich.: Ann Arbor Science, 1976.

Pickering, W. F. Pollution Evaluation: The Quantitative Aspects. New York: Dekker, 1977.

Zweig, G. (Ed.). Analytical Methods for Pesticides and Plant Growth Regulators. New York: Academic Press. (This is a multivolume series that contains analytical methods for the analysis of food and food additives, fungicides, herbicides, nematocides, pheromones, rodenticides, and soil fumigants.)

Gary M. Rand

30

Detection: Bioassay

30.1. Introduction

The problem of toxic substance control is important and of immediate concern to everyone. In the past few years we have witnessed a number of major catastrophes resulting from the misuse of such toxic substances as asbestos, chlordecone (Kepone), polyvinyl chloride, mercury, etc. These substances have produced deleterious effects not only on humans but also on many other nontarget organisms. In an attempt to cope with the toxic substance crisis the federal government, since 1970, has put into law several acts to regulate and control potentially toxic substances. The primary objective is essentially to eliminate any further environmental damage by preventing chemicals from entering the environment that pose an unreasonable hazard or imminent risk. This means that for each compound manufactured, a series of rigid and extensive tests will be performed prior to use of the compound.

There has been a proliferation of approaches to evaluating the toxicity of compounds, but the most extensively used is the bioassay. Bioassay is the "determination of the relative strength of a substance by comparing its effect on a test organism with that of a standard preparation." The scale or degree of response may be the rate of growth or decrease of a population, colony, or individual; a behavioral, physiological, or reproductive response; or simply an alive or dead response. The bioassay, therefore, allows us to determine safe levels for compounds in the environment, that is, concentrations that do not produce adverse effects on organisms.

This chapter is concerned with some of the general bioassay techniques that have been used to detect and evaluate the nature of chemically induced changes in organisms. The discussion will include different types of acute and chronic laboratory-controlled bioassay procedures and special bioassay techniques of ecosystem response to chemicals. Because many of the major bioassays used in environmental toxicology involve aquatic organisms, much of the methodology section will pertain to these organisms.

30.2. Terminology

One of the current problems in environmental toxicology is the overwhelming variety of terms used to describe a particular response or toxicological effect. Consequently, some of the standard and widely used terminology of bioassay/ toxicity testing is presented in this section.

The following terms may be used to describe the harmful effect of an agent or the type of bioassay test being conducted:

Acute: A severe and rapid response to a stimulus, usually within 4 days for fish and other aquatic organisms. Acute responses in mammalian species may occur within 24 hr to 2 weeks. Acute bioassays are usually mortality tests to determine the lethality of a potentially toxic agent.

Subacute: A response to a stimulus that is less severe than an acute response, is produced after a longer time, and may become chronic.

Chronic: A response to a stimulus that continues for a long time, often periods of about one-tenth or more of the total life span. In a chronic bioassay with aquatic organisms, the test species is usually exposed for its entire life cycle to determine the effects on growth, reproduction, and development. In a chronic bioassay with mammals, exposure is for 1 year or more to determine the carcinogenic potential of a compound in addition to its effects on growth, reproduction, and development. Chronic toxicity may be lethal or sublethal.

Lethal: A stimulus in a concentration that causes death by direct action.

Sublethal: A stimulus in a concentration that is below the level that directly causes death.

Aquatic bioassay: A toxicity test that uses aquatic organisms to evaluate the effects of a toxic agent and/or environmental factor (pH, dissolved oxygen, temperature, etc.).

An aquatic bioassay may be conducted to determine (a) whether environmental conditions are suitable for aquatic life, (b) concentrations or levels of environmental factors favorable and unfavorable for aquatic life, (c) the effects of these environmental factors on the toxicity of compounds, (d) the relative toxicity of different compounds to a selected species or a number of species, (e) the relative sensitivity of aquatic organisms to a toxicant, (f) the amount of waste treatment needed to meet water pollution control requirements if the toxic agent is an effluent, (g) water quality requirements for aquatic life, (h) safe concentrations for all toxic agents, and (i) compliance with water quality standards.

Some of the following terms are employed in acute bioassay tests in which mortality is being measured:

LD_{50}: The median lethal dose of a compound that will kill 50% of the test organisms. Although appropriate when rats, mice, or dogs are the test species, it is not appropriate for aquatic organisms since it indicates the amount of drug or toxicant administered into the body via injection or ingestion rather than concentrations in the surrounding water.

LC_{50}: The median lethal concentration or the quantity of toxic substance in the surrounding water that produces 50% mortality when fish or other aquatic organisms are used as test species.

Both LC_{50} and LD_{50} express the lethal toxicity of a given compound to the average or typical group of organisms. When effects other than death are measured, the expressions effective concentration (EC) and effective dose (ED) are used:

EC_{50}: The effective concentration of a toxic substance that produces a change in a sublethal behavioral or physiological response in 50% of the test organisms. For example, the EC_{50} is used with the invertebrate species *Daphnia magna* when immobility is evaluated.

ED_{50}: The effective dose of a drug or toxic substance that produces a change in a behavioral or physiological response in 50% of the test organisms.

Acute bioassay results with aquatic organisms may also be expressed in terms of tolerance limits. Tolerance bioassays are measured in terms of survival rate:

TL_{50}: The median tolerance limit or the concentration at which 50% of the test organisms survive.
Most acute bioassays with aquatic organisms, however, use LC_{50} instead of TL_{50}.

Another important value that may be determined in an acute bioassay with aquatic organisms is the concentration at which acute toxicity ceases or the concentration at which 50% of the population can live for an indefinite period of time. Incipient LC_{50} is the term generally accepted to describe this:

Incipient LC_{50}: The lethal concentration for 50% of the test organisms on long-term exposure or the concentration at which 50% of the population can live indefinitely.

The effects of toxic substances in the environment depend upon both the concentration of toxic substance and the length of exposure. Therefore, in an acute bioassay an indication of exposure time should be designated with each test and included in the results. For example, the results of an acute bioassay may be expressed as the 96-hr LC_{50}, 24-hr LD_{50}, or 96-hr TL_{50}, thereby indicating the period of exposure. The results of acute bioassays may also involve other percentages, such as 20% or 80%, i.e., 96-hr LC_{20} or 24-hr LD_{80}, respectively.

There are also a number of terms associated with the results obtained from chronic aquatic toxicity tests:

Safe concentration (SC): The maximum concentration of a potential toxicant that is harmless to organisms after long-term exposure for at least one generation. The SC for substances are used in establishing water quality criteria when widely distributed, sensitive species are used in the toxicity bioassays.

Maximum allowable toxicant concentration (MATC): The concentration of a toxic substance that may be present in a receiving water without producing significant harm to the aquatic organisms.

The MATC may be determined from a partial life cycle bioassay of the organism using the sensitive life stages (e.g., egg, fry, etc.), or a complete life cycle study. However, the partial life cycle studies have been used more often to determine the MATC for toxicants as they require a few months, and a complete life cycle study may take several years depending on the species.

In general, a few studies have evaluated the MATC values for fish and other aquatic organisms. There are, however, indirect methods to estimate the MATC for toxicants. For each toxicant there is a numerical value for the ratio of the MATC to the 96-hr LC_{50}. These values are called application factors (AF = MATC/96-hr LC_{50}). In order to indirectly estimate the MATC, the assumption has been made that the application factor is constant for related groups of chemicals. Therefore, the MATC can be estimated from the ratio by conducting an acute bioassay for the toxicant to determine the (96-hr LC_{50},) and this value may then be multiplied by the application factor for that group of toxicants (MATC = 96-hr $LC_{50} \times$ AF).

In reality, an application factor should be determined for each potentially toxic compound by direct methods. This would first necessitate conducting an acute 96-hr LC_{50} test and then a thorough study on the physiological, biochemical, and behavioral effects of the compound to determine the MATC.

30.3. Principles of Bioassay/Toxicity Tests

Most of the test methods developed in environmental toxicology are a result of the need to obtain as much information as possible about the toxic effects of environmental agents on a variety of organisms in order to assess environmental hazard. Bioassay test procedures may be based upon all or some of the following principles:

1. In order for any environmental agent to elicit a toxicological effect it must come into contact and interact with some part of the living biological system under consideration. This reaction may eventually effect the structure or function of the system.
2. For each environmental agent there is some concentration that will produce no known effect on the biological system, and there is also some greater concentration of this agent at which a significant effect will be elicited on all biological systems. Between these concentrations is a range of concentrations that will produce a significant effect on some of the biological systems.
3. In general, cells and tissues that have similar functions in different species will be affected similarly by the same environmental agent.
4. Changes in the structure of an environmental agent as a result of metabolic or environmental transformation will influence the activity and action of that agent.

The general bioassay test procedures described in this section may be applied in investigations of the effects of environmental agents on nonmammalian organisms (fish, invertebrates, etc.). These species lend themselves to accurate and simple laboratory procedures in which the environmental variables may be well controlled.

In general, laboratory toxicity studies may follow a sequence similar to that presented in Figure 30.1. Testing is conducted in five stages, each of which are discussed below.

30.3.1. Characterization of the Environmental Agent

The characterization of the agent should include an evaluation of all available data on its biological, chemical, and physical properties, including toxicological effects. Knowledge of the chemical and physical properties of the agent is useful

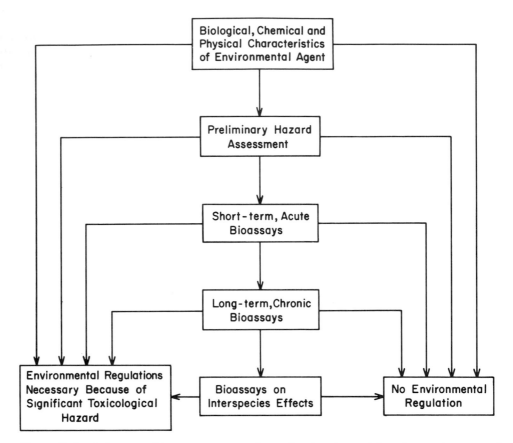

Figure 30.1 Laboratory bioassay sequence for evaluating the toxicity of an environmental agent.

in determining its distribution, transport, and concentration in the atmosphere, soil, and water after it is released. This information helps one determine which organisms (soil, water, etc.) would be most affected by the agent and which should be employed in toxicity tests. Any environmental factors that would alter the availability of the compound should be considered, as many agents are affected by changes in pH, salinity, temperature, and other parameters.

Similarities in the chemical and physical properties of the agent to known environmental toxicants may be an indication of its potential toxicity. This may also lead to an understanding of the environmental factors that should be considered when conducting the toxicity tests.

30.3.2. Preliminary Assessment

A preliminary assessment of the agent's hazard and toxicity can be estimated after the available data are evaluated with respect to environmental concentrations, chemical and physical properties, and toxicological effects. It is possible that present regulatory controls are sufficient to maintain the integrity of the environment with respect to this agent. However, if there are no adequate controls for the agent, further toxicity testing should be pursued.

A decision should be made regarding the degree of testing to be undertaken for determination of the effects on the biota. This decision is related to the biological impact and dispersal of the agent in the environment. The factors that contribute to the biological impact of the agent are its availability, biomagnification, stability, dispersal, persistence, and all aspects of toxicity.

An agent with a high biological impact (available, persistent, and stable, with ecosystem effects) that is proposed for widespread dispersal in relatively significant quantities requires extensive testing. Agents that produce insignificant or no acute effects and whose dispersal is localized with low release are usually not tested extensively.

30.3.3. Short-Term (Acute) Tests

Short-term or acute toxicity tests are the first bioassays performed. These bioassays may be categorized as range finding, exploratory, or short-term definitive tests. The exploratory tests are used to determine the approximate range of concentrations of the toxicant or waste to be employed in the full-scale definitive tests. The short-term definitive tests will determine the LC_{50}, EC_{50}, etc. The results of the definitive tests may also indicate the concentrations that should be tested in the partial life cycle or complete life cycle studies.

The range-finding tests are 24-hr bioassays. The test organisms are usually exposed to a range of concentrations based on a logarithmic scale. In order to determine the concentration required in the definitive acute tests, the highest concentration that has killed none or only a few of the test organisms and the lowest concentration that has killed most or all of the test organisms are selected from the range-finding tests. A series of concentrations is then determined based on the progressive bisection of intervals on a logarithmic scale (Table 30.1).

In the short-term definitive toxicity test the organisms are exposed to at least four different concentrations of the toxicant with one control and the tests are

Table 30.1 Concentrations to be Used Based on the Progressive Bisection of Intervals on a Logarithmic Scale

Col. 1	Col. 2	Col. 3	Col. 4	Col. 5
10.0				
				8.7
			7.5	
				6.5
		5.6		
			4.2	
				3.7
	3.2			
				2.8
			2.4	
				2.1
		1.8		
				1.55
			1.35	
				1.15
1.0				

run in duplicate. The duration is determined by the toxicant under consideration, but most acute bioassays are limited to 96 hr. Tests may be conducted for longer periods of time, however, as acute toxicity may not always occur within the 96-hr period.

Acute toxicity tests with aquatic organisms can be conducted in a static or flow-through system. In a static system the test organisms and test solution are placed in test chambers for the duration of the experiment. Although this procedure is uncomplicated and inexpensive, there are disadvantages:

1. The toxicant may be degradable and volatile.
2. The toxicant may be masked by high BOD.
3. The toxicant may be progressively adsorbed on the chambers or fish slime, metabolized, or otherwise changed so that actual concentrations in the chambers change with time.
4. The excretory products of the test organisms may react with the toxicant being tested, producing a greater or smaller toxic response.

If any of these conditions exists the results of the static bioassay may indicate a condition that does not actually exist. Therefore, the alternative continuous flow-through procedure should be used, in which test solutions flow into and out of the test chamber on a "once through" basis for the duration of the test. This results in stable test conditions in which the toxicant concentration, dissolved oxygen content, and other water quality characteristics remain constant.

Short-term bioassays may also provide useful information on the rate of degradation of an agent. For example, a decrease in the observed toxicity of a test solution to fish over the time of the acute test would indicate removal of the toxicant by degradation or some other means. Similarly, an increase in toxicity may indicate the formation of a more toxic agent as part of the degradation process. However, only long-term bioassays can give reliable information on the rates of degradation and transformation.

Analysis of the concentration of the agent in different parts of the organisms before and after acute exposure may reveal the tendency toward bioaccumulation, even at concentrations that do not produce adverse effects.

If the agent and its degradation products are of low acute toxicity, and the bioconcentration potential is minimal, additional testing may not be necessary. This decision may be supported if the estimated environmental concentrations do not exceed the acute toxicity concentrations. However, agents that are persistent, accumulate within an organism, and disperse in large quantities should be tested further.

30.3.4. Long-Term (Chronic) Tests

Although acute bioassays are useful as initial bioassay techniques, they have some serious limitations. One major limitation is that values obtained from these tests do not indicate concentrations that are safe after long-term sublethal exposure. In most instances organisms are not confronted with acute (lethal) concentrations unless they are at the actual impact site of the toxicant. Due to dilution factors (air, water, etc.), organisms are generally confronted with sublethal levels. These levels may not directly lead to death but nonetheless may cause behavioral and/or physiological disturbances of major biological significance. Effects on these parameters go unnoticed in acute tests. Therefore, substantial testing on chronic exposure to low levels is important. This type of testing leads to a better understanding of safe limits that permit normal life processes to continue with little or no adverse effects.

Partial or complete life cycle bioassays with aquatic organisms are performed with a flow-through system. In those instances in which the life cycle can be carried out readily, the tests are continued from egg to egg or beyond, or for several life cycles in smaller organisms.

The toxicological effects that can be measured with long-term studies are innumerable, but measurements of growth, reproduction, maturation, spawning, hatching, survival, behavior, and bioaccumulation are of primary importance regarding the confidence that can be placed on their interpretation.

Four or more concentrations are used, based upon the results of the short-term tests. Exposure chambers, spawning chambers, hatching containers, growth chambers, and other equipment are varied to meet the needs of the different organisms.

From the chronic tests a safe level may be determined for the environmental agent under investigation so that an application factor can be calculated.

30.3.5. Interspecies Effects

Those agents that reach the environment should be subjected to toxicity tests that involve different organisms. This is especially important in cases in which persistent agents or stable metabolites accumulate and magnify in the food chain. Bioassays with environmental agents should include studies on diverse aquatic species, plant–plant interactions, wildfowl, transport through the food chains, and alteration of the toxicant as a result of chemical, photochemical, or microbial activity. The most sensitive and vulnerable nontarget species must be determined in order that future recommendations for environmental concentrations may protect these organisms from any adverse effects.

30.4. Statistical Procedures

A concept to be considered in measuring toxicity is that no environmental agent is completely safe, and no environmental agent is completely harmful. This is based on the assumption that an agent may come into contact with a biological membrane without producing an affect on the membrane (structure or function) if the concentration of that agent is below some effective level. One can also assume that any agent can produce a deleterious effect if a great enough concentration of the agent comes into contact with the biological membrane. Therefore, the most important factor in toxic action, which determines whether the agent is potentially harmful or safe, is the relationship between the concentration (or dose) of the agent and the effect produced in the biological system.

The extreme effects of any agent on an individual animal (cell or tissue) may be manifested as an all-or-none response (or quantal response), such as alive or dead. However, the effects may vary within a group of animals (cell or tissues) from very intense (death) to minimal (no effect) on exposure to equivalent concentrations of the agent. These effects are therefore graded with respect to the entire group of animals. The differences in response to an equivalent concentration of an agent are attributed to biological variation. This variation is normally small within members of the same species but generally greater between species.

30.4.1. Dose–Response Curve

The object in measuring toxicity is a determination of the concentration at which the agent produces some harmful response on a population of test organisms under controlled conditions of exposure. The results are plotted in terms that relate the concentration of the agent to the percentage of test organisms exhibiting the defined response.

   The data can be represented in a graph that relates the concentration and the number of test subjects in the group exhibiting a quantitatively identical effect (Figure 30.2). The results indicate that at the mean concentration (X) a large percentage of the subjects respond similarly, while the deviations in either direction indicate that some show an equivalent response to a lower concentration, and others require a higher dose.

   Toxicological data are generally plotted in the form of a curve relating the concentration to the cumulative percentage of animals exhibiting the response (Figure 30.3, linear scale); these curves are called dose–response curves. In such a curve, the concentration (or dose) at which 50% of the individuals react (the median) is used as a measure of the activity or toxicity (LC_{50}) of the agent.

30.4.2. Calculating the LC_{50}

When the dose–response relationship is expressed on a logarithmic scale of the concentration, an estimation of the LC_{50} may be interpolated (Figure 30.4). This involves plotting the data on semilogarithmic coordinate paper with the concentrations on the logarithmic scale and the percent, mortality on the arithmetic scale. A straight line is usually drawn between the points representing the percentage dead at two successive concentrations that were lethal to more than

Figure 30.2   Dose–frequency plot following exposure of a group of test organisms to an agent.

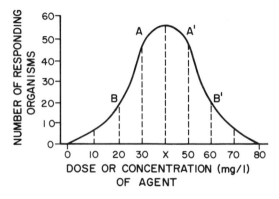

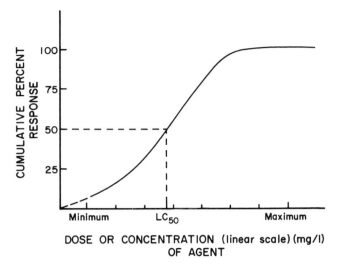

Figure 30.3 Dose–response curve for an agent administered to a group of test organisms.

Figure 30.4 Estimation of LC$_{50}$ for an agent by straight line interpolation.

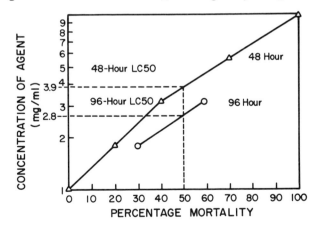

Experimental Data (Hypothetical) Plotted Above

No. of Test Animals	Concentration of Agent	48 hr No.	48 hr %	96hr No.	96hr %
10	1.0	0	0	1	10
10	1.8	2	20	3	30
10	3.2	4	40	6	60
10	5.6	7	70	9	90
10	10.0	10	100	10	100

50% and to less than 50% of the test organisms. The LC$_{50}$ may be estimated by drawing a line from the 50% mortality point to where it intersects the curve. It is evident from the curves that the LC$_{50}$ values for 48- and 96-hr exposures are 3.9 and 2.8 mg/ml, respectively.

The LC$_{50}$ may also be estimated by probit analysis (Figure 30.5). This involves plotting the data on logarithmic probability paper. To construct the graph, the concentrations are plotted on the horizontal-logarithmic scale and the percent mortality is plotted on the vertical-probability or "probit scale." The probit scale never reaches 0 or 100% mortality, so any points must be plotted with an arrow indicating their true position. A line is then fitted to the points by eye. Emphasis should be given to points between 16 and 84% mortality, and an effort should be made to minimize the total vertical deviations of the line from the points. If there is a doubt about the placement of the line, it should be rotated to a flatter slope (made more horizontal), since this acknowledges more variability in the data.

The LC$_{50}$ concentration causing 50% mortality for a specified exposure time is read from the fitted line. This is reported as the result of the acute bioassay. In our example, the estimated 96-hr LC$_{50}$ is 8.0 mg/ml. This signifies the estimated concentration that would kill the "average" or typical organism in 96 hr.

The estimated LC$_{50}$ value interpolated by graphic procedures is accurate and similar to that obtained by probit analysis.

In order to estimate the LC$_{50}$ with reasonable accuracy, each concentration of toxic substance should be at least 50% of the next highest one. It is also important to have several partial mortalities at different concentrations. In research, at least one of the responses should be in the range of 16–84% mortality because these represent ± 1.0 probit about the median response. The LC$_{84}$ represents +1 standard deviation (S.D.) from the LC$_{50}$, and the LC$_{16}$ represents −1 SD from the LC$_{50}$. The percent mortality can be converted to probits, which are simply values assigned to percentages, so for the 50% mortality response the probit value 5 has been used.

Figure 30.5 Estimation of LC$_{50}$ by probit analysis for a given exposure time. The line is drawn by eye to fit the results plotted on logarithmic probability paper.

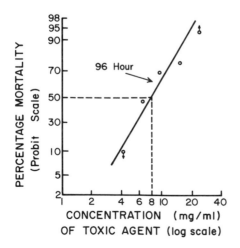

30.4.3. Plotting Toxicity Curves

If a 96-hr LC_{50} test is conducted, it is of interest to estimate the LC_{50} for the various time periods before 96 hr (e.g., 24, 48, and 72 hr). The series of LC_{50}'s can then be used to construct a toxicity curve (Figure 30.6) to give the experimenter an overall idea of the progress of the test. It may also indicate when acute lethality has ceased. This would be indicated where the curve became asymptotic to the time axis. For example, for *a* in Figure 30.6, the vertical asymptote after about 300 min indicates that acute mortality was all over, and the experiment may have ended earlier. However, for *b* in Figure 30.6, the lack of an asymptote at 48 hr indicates that acute mortality was continuing, and one would probably wish to continue the bioassay to 96 hr. The LC_{50} for a specific exposure time that is in the asymptotic part of the curve is called the threshold or incipient LC_{50}. Sometimes straight line relationships have been found with no evidence of a lethal threshold even at low concentrations of prolonged exposure.

The toxicity curves may assume a variety of shapes and provide information about the mode of action of an agent or indicate the presence of more than one toxic agent.

30.4.4. Final Estimate of the LC_{50} and Confidence Limits

When the bioassay has been completed, an estimate of the LC_{50} should be determined for each exposure period, including the longest time period of the toxicity test. The confidence limits for each LC_{50} should also be calculated. The confidence limits indicate the accuracy of the estimate that would be expected from replicate bioassays carried out at the same time with exactly the same conditions. Accuracy within 10% is usually attainable. If the asymptote has been reached in the toxicity curve (where acute lethality has ceased), the incipient LC_{50} or threshold lethal concentration should also be expressed. This threshold value of acute lethality has more theoretical significance than an LC_{50} for some arbitrary time period.

Figure 30.6 Toxicity curve for two agents (a,b) using a series of LC_{50}s that were estimated as the experiment progressed for 48 hr.

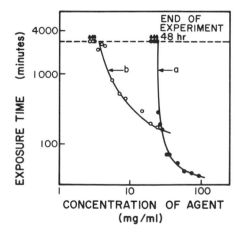

30.4.5. Alternative Methods for Calculating the LC_{50}

Alternative methods for calculating the LC_{50} include the nomographic methods of Litchfield-Wilcoxon and the computer methods based on Finney's method for probit analysis.

30.5. Reporting Results

The LC_{50}, the exposure time, the confidence limits, and the slope of the probit line (or slope function of Litchfield-Wilcoxon) should be reported. From this, future investigators can reproduce the probit line. In addition, a figure of the toxicity curve should be presented. The mortality at each concentration at the end of each time period is also important, including mortality in the control group.

Descriptions should also be presented of the following (a) the species (source, weight, number used, etc.); (b) the toxic agent (its source, physical and chemical properties, etc.); (c) the concentrations used; (d) the test conditions (temperatures, dissolved oxygen concentration and pH if aquatic bioassays are performed, etc.); and (e) the behavior of animals during the test.

30.5.1. Results of Quantitative Bioassays

Quantitative or graded bioassays are tests in which each organism elicits a response that is variable in degree, such as change in growth, body weight, behavior, or reproductive success. These responses are measured on a graded scale for each test concentration using standard techniques. The final result that is obtained in these tests is the concentration that would cause a significant change in response in the typical or average animal.

30.5.2. Limitations of the Bioassay

The accuracy and precision of the bioassay is limited by many factors, but many of these can be controlled in the laboratory. However, normal biological variation within and between species cannot be controlled. Therefore, toxicity studies with one selected species do not necessarily yield accurate information on the toxicity of that agent to other species and life stages. A bioassay with one species gives an estimate of the toxicity only to others of that species of similar size, age, and physiological condition.

One of the major drawbacks is the lack of bioassays for combined effects of two or more toxicants on organisms. In addition, the effects of various modifying factors and fluctuating concentrations on toxicity require further investigation.

30.6. Special Bioassays Used to Evaluate Environmental Agents

One technique that has been used more recently is the simulated microecosystem approach. This, and similar systems, are designed to model the processes involved in a terrestrial–aquatic ecosystem. A typical model may include soil organisms, benthic fauna, a plant, an insect, a snail, an alga, a crustacean, and a fish species maintained under controlled exposure conditions for 1 month or more. The model ecosystem may be as diversified as the natural environment under investigation and may range from observations in small flasks or tanks to more complex systems contained in large environmental chambers. These systems are designed to study the fate, transport, metabolism, and accumulation of persistent compounds as well as biochemical and physiological effects of toxic agents on organisms.

The model ecosystem thus acts as an early warning system to screen potentially toxic substances. Effects on individual organisms and food webs may be studied for quantitative as well as qualitative assessments of environmental agents.

Suggested Reading

Adriens, E. J., Simonis, A. M., Offermeier, J. Introduction to General Toxicology. New York: Academic Press, 1976.

American Public Health Association, American Water Works Association, and Water Pollution Control Federation. Standard Methods for the Examination of Water and Wastewater, 14th edition. New York: American Public Health Association, 1976.

Cairns, J., Dickson, K. L. Biological Methods for the Assessment of Water Quality. ASTM Special Technical Publication 528. Philadelphia: American Society for Testing and Materials, 1973.

Glass, G. E. Bioassay Techniques and Environmental Chemistry. Ann Arbor, Mich.: Ann Arbor Science, 1973.

Loomis, T. A. Essentials of Toxicology. Philadelphia: Lea & Febiger, 1974.

Metcalf, R. L., Sangha, G. K., Kapoor, I. P. Model ecosystem for the evaluation of pesticide biodegradability and ecological magnification. Environ. Sci. Technol. 5:709, 1971.

National Academy of Sciences. Principles for Evaluating Chemicals in the Environment. Washington, D. C., 1975.

Michael J. Matteson

31

Control of Industrial Air Pollution

31.1. Introduction

Air pollution is an environmental problem that dates back to the discovery of fire. Today we recognize it as the introduction into the atmosphere of material, both gaseous and particulate, in such quantities as to cause ill effects on man's health and on nature in general. These effects can involve the impairment of breathing, a reduction in visibility, and a deterioration of structures. Other ill effects include eye irritation, breakdown of synthetic materials, and destruction of crops. Air pollution, seen over most of our major cities in the past 2 decades, shields some of the sun's radiation, changing heat absorption patterns on the earth's surface, and modifies rainfall over large metropolitan areas and downwind from these cities.

31.1.1. Classification of Pollutants

Pollutants that exist in the atmosphere may be gaseous, liquid, or solid and may be converted from one state to another by chemical or physical interaction. The primary pollutants (emitted directly to the atmosphere) regulated by the Clean Air Amendments of 1970 are particulate matter (PM), SO_2, CO, NO_x, and hydrocarbons (HC). Certain oxidants are classified as secondary pollutants because they are formed in the environment by interaction among primary pollutants and atmospheric consituents. Some particulates are also formed in the atmosphere, and these also would be classified as secondary pollutants.

31.1.2. Major Sources of Pollutants

The major sources of pollution from stationary operations can be divided into fuel combustion and industrial processing (Table 31.1). Most of the SO_2 and NO_x are generated by fuel combustion, and industrial processes are responsible for the majority of the CO. Combustion and industrial process sources account for

Table 31.1   Stationary Sources of Air Pollutants (10^6 tons/year), United States, 1970

Source	CO	SO_2	NO_x	HC	PM	Total
Fuel combustion	1.9	22.0	7.5	0.7	6.0	38.1
Industrial processing	7.8	7.2	0.2	3.5	5.9	24.6

about an equal amount of PM. The estimates of pollutants from all sources for 1985 (in millions tons per year) are PM 11.3, SO_2 30.9, NO_x 23.2, HC 21.2, and CO 42.1.

31.2. Control of Particulate Pollutants

Particles discharged into the atmosphere may be in the form of fly ash, soot, dust, fog, or fume, and the time they remain suspended depends on their size and density. Particles are normally classified according to equivalent spherical diameter in micrometers. A dust is a cloud of solid particles generated by grinding or some form of mechanical disintegration. A fume consists of particles formed by condensation or chemical reaction that are generally smaller than 1 μm. Smoke is usually taken to mean a cloud of particles in very high concentration consisting of condensed vapor from a combustion process.

Those particles that have a tendency to remain suspended longest in urban air are also the most hazardous in terms of depth of penetration into the lung. These are referred to as submicron (diameter less than 1 μm) particles and are weakly influenced by gravitational forces. Clean air may contain 10–20 μg/m³ PM, while 70–700 μg/m³ may be suspended in polluted air. Much of the toxic nature of PM is associated with gases adsorbed on the surface or absorbed within the particle.

31.2.1. Physical Characteristics of Particulate Matter

If a particle is large enough and possesses enough inertia, then it has the tendency to leave the streamlines of carrier gas flowing around an immersed body and to impact on the surface of the body. On the other hand, if the particles are very small, they tend to be swept along with the streamlines of gas. When the particles approach molecular dimensions they begin to behave like large gas molecules, and their motion is more erratic because of molecular collisions. At this level the likelihood of capture begins to increase due to diffusional effects. Thus there is actually a minimum observed when measuring collection efficiency versus particle size, and this usually occurs at diameters of 0.3–0.5 μm for particles of unit density. The dominant collection mechanism for particles smaller than 0.1 μm is diffusion.

One criterion used to estimate the ability of a given collector to capture a particle by inertial impaction is the Stokes number (Stk):

$$\text{Stk} = \frac{V_p d_p^2 \rho_p C_s}{18 \mu_g d_c}, \qquad \text{dimensionless} \qquad (31.1)$$

where V_p is the velocity of the particle of diameter d_p and density ρ_p, relative to the collecting body of diameter d_c, in a carrier gas of viscosity μ_g. The slip correction factor, C_s, accounts for surface–gas discontinuities when particle size approaches the mean free path, λ, of the gas molecules:

$$C_s = 1 + \frac{\lambda}{r_p}\left[1.246 + 0.420 \exp\left(-\frac{0.87\, r_p}{\lambda}\right)\right], \quad \text{dimensionless} \tag{31.2}$$

where r_p is particle radius. The Stokes number is really the ratio of the distance a particle will travel on its own inertia, in the absence of other forces, to a dimension characteristic of the collecting body (e.g., the diameter). If this number is about equal to or greater than one, the particle stands a good chance of capture due to inertial impaction (Figure 31.1).

Particles may be so large that they respond best to settling as a means of separation. Suppose a particle is settling in a gravitational field. It will accelerate vertically downward according to

$$m_p\frac{dV_p}{dt} = m_p g - \tfrac{1}{2}\rho_g A_p V_p{}^2 C_D/C_s \tag{31.3}$$

where m_p is the particle mass, g is the gravitational acceleration, A_p is the projected area of the particle ($A_p = \pi d_p{}^2/4$, for sphere of equivalent diameter), and C_D is the coefficient of drag. As the particle approaches terminal velocity, $dV_p/dt \to 0$, and hence its terminal velocity is

$$V_{pt} = \left(\frac{8r\,\rho_p g C_s}{3\rho_g C_D}\right)^{1/2} \tag{31.4}$$

Figure 31.1 Target efficiencies for spheres and cylinders, for conditions where Stokes' law applies. Target efficiency is defined as the ratio of the radius or half-thickness of that incident stream, completely swept free of particles, to the radius of the collecting sphere or cylinder.

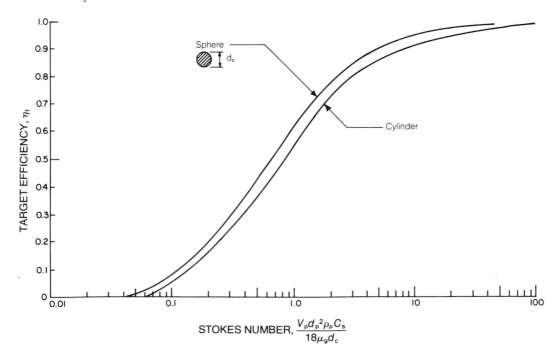

STOKES NUMBER, $\dfrac{V_p d_p{}^2 \rho_p C_s}{18\mu_g d_c}$

If the particles are susceptible to collecting an electrostatic charge, q_p, they will respond to an electrostatic field, E, and one may replace the gravitational force $m_p g$ with the electrostatic force Eq_p in Equation (31.3).

31.2.2. Filtration

The basic advantage to filtration as a means of gas–particle separation is that one may obtain almost any kind of filter for handling any type of particle with a wide range of efficiencies. There is a relatively low energy demand in filter operation when it is first installed; however, as the cake builds on the filter, the pressure drop increases, and the power consumption in the blower or compressor can become significant. Many filter media must be used at relatively low temperatures and on relatively dry gases in order to avoid early deterioration, and most filters have limited resistance to corrosion. A low mechanical strength limits the amount of handling since a single puncture can destroy the effectiveness of many square meters of filter surface. The three basic types of industrial gas filters are fabric filters (usually in the form of a bag or sleeve), panel filters (which are packed fibrous mats), and packed columns.

31.2.2.a. Filtration Theory

The main particle separation mechanisms at work in filters are inertial impaction, direct interception, and diffusion. Fabric filters have efficiencies of 99% and higher when collecting 0.5-μm particles and are able to remove a significant number of 0.01-μm particles.

The efficiency of a fibrous filter is a function of the radius of the individual fibers, treated as cylinders, the Stokes numbers of the particles, and the Reynolds number of the incident gas. Single fiber efficiencies, η_f, have been developed from the theory (Figure 31.1), and these results extended to a layer of fibers of packing density α:

$$\alpha = \frac{\text{Fiber volume}}{\text{Total volume}} = \frac{(\pi \, d_f^2/4) \, L}{A dz} = 1 - \epsilon \tag{31.5}$$

where dz is an elemental thickness of filter and d_f is an individual fiber diameter. The total fiber length within volume element $A dz$ is L, and the porosity is ϵ. The number of particles penetrating the filter is

$$N = N_0 \exp\left(-\frac{4\alpha\eta_f \Delta z}{\pi d_f (1 - \alpha)}\right) \tag{31.6}$$

where N_0 is the number entering and the overall efficiency is

$$\eta_0 = 1 - \frac{N}{N_0}. \tag{31.7}$$

Therefore, in order to define a filter efficiency it is necessary to know porosity or packing density, filter thickness, single fiber diameter, and efficiency. Equation

(31.7) describes the efficiency of a single filter. If there are n filters in series, each of equal efficiency, then the overall efficiency is

$$\eta_0 = 1 - \left(\frac{N}{N_0}\right)^n. \tag{31.8}$$

The next most important operating parameter in filtration is pressure drop. This is a combination of the pressure loss through the clean filter and the filter cake:

$$\Delta P_0 = \Delta P_f + \Delta P_c \tag{31.9}$$

where

$$\Delta P_f = \frac{2\rho_g V_\infty^2 \Delta z_f C_D \alpha}{\pi d_f (1 - \alpha)^2} \tag{31.10}$$

$$\Delta P_c = \frac{36 K_1 \mu V_\infty^2 C (1 - \epsilon) t}{\rho_p d_p^2 \epsilon^3} \tag{31.11}$$

where V_∞ is the face velocity, t is the exposure time, C is the concentration of dust, and K_1 is the filter constant.

31.2.2.b. Filter Types

Bag filters are suspended in a baghouse in long, vertical, cylindrical units. The dusty air flows through the inside open end at the bottom, upward, and out through the pores in the bags. Almost all commercial bag filter cloths remove as much as 99% of the particles from gas streams. The variety in design is found in the bag cleaning apparatus, which may be by mechanical shaking and reverse jets or sonic vibrators. The basic parameter of the baghouse is the air-to-cloth ratio or total flow rate in cubic meters per minute divided by total surface of cloth in square meters.

Fibrous mat filters may be rectangular or be produced as continuous reel-to-reel type rolls. Mat filters are replaced once the layer of dust builds up, although some can be washed with water and reused.

Mist eliminators are intended for those processes, such as sulfuric acid manufacture, in which a fine suspension of corrosive droplets escapes in the flue gas stream. A packed wire-mesh mat filter is used for fine mists, and a louver for particles larger than about 10 μm. Fluidized beds are also employed for large particle removal.

31.2.3. Centrifugal or Cyclone Separators

Centrifugal separators are able to remove particles from gases by spinning the dust-laden streams at a velocity sufficient to cause the suspended particles to diverge from the streamlines of the carrier gas and impact on the enclosing walls. The gas may be injected tangentially at the top of a cylindrical vessel and rotate downward through a conical section, executing several turns before being forced up through the core of the vortex (Figure 31.2). A second type of cyclone

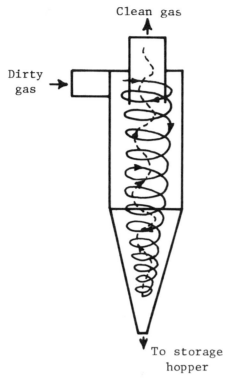

Clean gas

Dirty
gas

To storage
hopper

Figure 31.2 Cyclone separator. The particle-laden gas is injected tangentially at the top of the cylindrical vessel; the particles collect on the sides and slide down to the storage hopper. Clean air is forced up through the vortex.

allows the gas to enter vanes arranged around the periphery of the upper cylinder. The collected particles slide down the walls and enter a storage hopper. Cyclones offer the advantages of low operating and investment expenses, and have been operated at temperatures as high as 1000°C and pressures up to 500 atm.

It is possible to estimate the collection efficiency of a cyclone, assuming the gas moves in a spiral with a velocity equal to the average inlet velocity V_∞. The particle size for which the capture efficiency is 50% in a cyclone of radius R_c is

$$d_{p_{50\%}} = \left(\frac{9 \mu_g R_c}{2 \rho_p V_\infty \pi N_t} \right)^{1/2} \tag{31.12}$$

where N_t is the number of spiral turns.

From the above relation it is apparent that collection efficiency, in terms of capturing smaller particles, can be improved by increasing the inlet velocity or number of turns, or by reducing the radius of the cyclone. However, one must make a compromise between collection efficiency and pressure loss since

$$\Delta P = \frac{K Q^2 P \rho_g}{T} \tag{31.13}$$

where Q is the volumetric rate of flow of gas through the cyclone and is directly proportional to V_∞. The constant K is a design parameter based on cyclone radius.

Because the cyclone has no moving parts it is simple and highly reliable, making it the least expensive of all high-efficiency particle collectors.

31.2.4. Wet Collectors

There are a variety of designs of wet collectors; the common feature is that dust particles are impacted by water or liquid droplets. The contact may be by a vertical downward spray encountering a rising gas (spray chamber scrubber), a horizontal, radially outward spray from a vertical spindle directed at a spiraling gas (wet cyclone), or a cocurrent spray created by impact of the dirty gas on a curtain of scrubbing liquid (Venturi scrubber). Wet scrubbers are best suited for collection in the 0.1–10.0 μm particle size range when a moderately high collection efficiency is required. They have the added advantage of removing gaseous contaminants along with the particulate matter. Problems include recovery of the dissolved contaminants, disposal of sludge, and a lowering of the temperature of the exhaust gas stream.

Spray towers have been constructed to operate with countercurrent and with cross flow. Since inertial impaction is the primary mechanism of collection, efficiency improves with dust particle size and falls off rapidly for particles smaller than 2 μm; however, there is an optimum droplet size around 750 μm. Above this size, the mechanism of inertial impaction begins to lose its effectiveness.

To estimate the efficiency of a spray tower one must first calculate a Stokes number, as in Equation (31.1), based on a certain droplet and particle diameter, d_{d_i} and d_{p_j}. Then from Figure 31.1 one obtains a target efficiency $\eta_{T_{ij}}$ for individual spheres. The tower efficiency for the collection of the d_{p_j} fraction of particles by the d_{d_i} fraction of droplets is

$$E_{T_{ij}} = 1 - (1 - \eta_{T_{ij}})^{n_{ij}} \tag{31.14}$$

where n_{ij} is the number of times a particle of size d_{p_j} encounters a collecting droplet of size d_{d_i}.

The efficiency of the tower can be calculated based on the fraction of tower cross section occupied by droplets. Let w be the water injection rate (in cm³/sec), α_i the fraction of droplets with diameter d_{d_i}, A_T the tower cross section, and N_i the number of droplets per cm³ with diameter d_{d_i}

$$n_i = \frac{3}{2} \frac{w\alpha_i}{A_T d_{d_i}} \left(\frac{H_T}{v_g} + \frac{H_T}{v_1} \right) \tag{31.15}$$

where H_T is the column height and v_g and v_1 are linear velocities of gas and liquid, respectively.

This calculation must be repeated for each α_i fraction of droplets to arrive at a total efficiency for a particular particle size d_{p_j}:

$$E_{T_j} = \sum_i E_{T_{ij}}. \tag{31.16}$$

Cyclonic wet scrubbers combine a centrifugal motion of the dust stream with the inertial impaction mechanism of the injected water droplets. The centrifugal motion, aided by initial wetting, removes the larger particles. For a cyclonic wet scrubber with radial water injection the efficiency takes the form of Equation (31.14), where

$$n = \frac{3}{2} \frac{\alpha_i R w}{d_{d_i} A_T V_G} \tag{31.17}$$

R is the radius of the collector, and V_G is the velocity at the inlet.

As with the spray chamber, efficiencies of cyclonic wet scrubbers are best for particles in the greater than 2-μm diameter range.

One type of wet scrubber that can perform well in the submicron particle size range is the Venturi (Figure 31.3). This scrubber consists of a convergent section, a throat, and a divergent section. The scrubbing liquid is introduced radially at the throat and is dispersed by the high-velocity, dust-laden gas, producing a spray of droplets upon which the dust particles are impacted. The diameter of the resulting droplets has a volume–surface mean of

$$d_d = \frac{4900}{V_\infty} + 28.7 L^{1.5}, \, (\mu m) \tag{31.18}$$

where L is the number of liters scrubbing liquor per cubic meter of gas, and V_∞ is the throat velocity in meters per second.

Figure 31.3 Venturi-type gas scrubber. A scrubbing liquid is introduced at the narrow aperture of the instrument and is dispersed by the high-velocity, dust-laden gas, yielding droplets on which the dust particles impact.

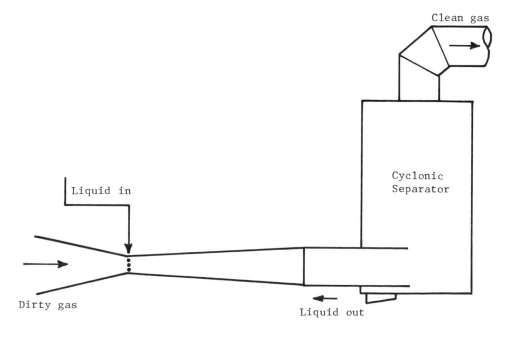

Clean gas

Cyclonic
Separator

Liquid in

Dirty gas

Liquid out

The main disadvantage of the Venturi is the high pressure loss associated with impacting and accelerating the liquid from zero velocity to that of the gas stream:

$$\Delta P = 1.03 \times 10^{-6} V_\infty^2 L, \text{ (cm H}_2\text{O).}$$ (31.19)

However, efficiencies have been measured at 100% for particles 5 μm and larger, and as high as 99% for submicron particles. The collection efficiency for a given particle size has been related to the pressure drop:

$$E_{T_i} = 1 - \exp\left(-\frac{6.1 \times 10^{-9} \rho_L \rho_p C_D d_{p_i}^2 f^2 \Delta P}{\mu_g^2}\right)$$ (31.20)

where ρ_d and ρ_p are the droplet and particle specific gravities, respectively, and f is a constant between 0.1 and 0.4.

31.2.5. Gravity Separators

Gravity settling chambers are applicable for collection of dust when particles are larger than 50 μm and of unit density. A general rule is that the settling or terminal velocity should be greater than 10 cm/sec. The dusty gas is fed horizontally over a series of hoppers that collect the falling particles.

Since volume is usually a limitation, one can estimate the required length of the chamber if something is known about the flow pattern of the gas. If the gas is moving through a wide rectangular duct of height 2B at low velocities, the minimum length required to capture a particle of diameter d_{p_i} with 100% efficiency is

$$L = \left(\frac{6\Delta P B^3}{d_{p_i}^2 \rho_p C_s g}\right)^{1/2}.$$ (31.21)

31.2.6. Electrostatic Precipitators (ESP)

Particles in the submicron size range are best collected by electrostatic techniques, provided they are capable of holding a charge. In modern ESPs the dust is exposed to a corona discharge and collects negatively charged gas ions. The dust particles then migrate to a collector electrode in the presence of the electrostatic field, E_c, between the wire where the corona is produced and the collector plates. One of the expressions frequently used to measure ESP efficiency is the Deutsch equation:

$$E_T = 1 - \exp\left(-\frac{A V_p}{G}\right)$$ (31.22)

where A is the area of the collector electrodes and G is the gas throughput. The drift velocity, V_p, is determined from a balance of the electrical force on the particle and the drag force $F_e = q_p E_c = F_d$:

$$V_p = \frac{q_p E_c}{3\pi\mu_g d_p V_p} \qquad (31.23)$$

and the particle charge is estimated from

$$q_p = \frac{3\epsilon_p}{\epsilon_p + 2} \cdot \frac{E_c d_p^{\,2}}{4}. \qquad (31.24)$$

ESPs are costly to install but have relatively low operating costs. They have the advantage of almost zero pressure loss and have been operated at temperatures as high as 650°C and pressures up to 150 psi (10 bars). Gas volume flow rates can range from 100 to 4×10^6 ft³/min and particles varying in size from 0.05 to 200 μm are removed with efficiencies close to 100%. Another advantage to the ESP is that the gas stream remains physically and chemically unchanged, since the separation mechanism is acting only on the particles.

Problems may arise with some dusts because of their high electrical resistance, that is, inability to accept charge. ESPs are most effective on dusts with resistance in the 10^4–10^{10} ohm-cm range. When this is not the case, the dust may be conditioned by adding moisture or hygroscopic gases that adsorb on the dust surface.

31.2.7. Summary

In summary, the choice of particle collection device depends upon

1. Dust loading and size of particles to be removed and with what efficiency.
2. Volume of gas to be cleaned and its temperature, pressure, and dew point.

Settling chambers will handle high volumes of gas with high dust loads and very little pressure drop, but operate best with large ($> 50 \mu$m) particles. Fabric filters can remove all ranges of particle size but are limited to low temperature, low humidity, and low dust-loading and volumetric flow rates. Wet scrubbers can operate with high flow rates but are limited to particles above 2 μm. The exception here is the Venturi scrubber, which can remove particles below 1 μm, but at reduced efficiencies. Wet scrubbers will alter the temperature and humidity of the gas, and corrosion problems and pressure drop are drawbacks. ESPs can scrub with large flow rates and remove submicron particles with high efficiencies, but the dust must be able to accept a charge and may require pretreatment.

31.3. Control of Gaseous Pollutants

Problems associated with the control of gaseous pollutants are somewhat more complex than those associated with particulate removal in that one is relying on both chemical and physical mechanisms for separation. In terms of mass, the gaseous pollutants comprise the major portion of the air contaminants. However, the technology for dealing with gases has lagged behind particulate removal systems, and only relatively recently has equipment been made available for large-scale gas scrubbing. Because it has been shown to have toxic effects, SO_2 has received much attention in the literature; new information and techniques for control are constantly being reported. Therefore, this discussion will include both proven and emerging scrubbing systems that appear to offer dependable control for some time to come. On the other hand, CO, NO_x, and HC control is still mainly limited to combustion modification techniques, but some attempts are being made at stack gas separation.

31.3.1. Sulfur Dioxide

The concentration of SO_2 in polluted air is in the range of 0.02–2 ppm. The primary man-made source of SO_2 in the atmosphere is the combustion of fossil fuels for power. Sulfur is present in coal and oil in amounts ranging from less than 1% up to 5% by weight. While desulfurization of fuel oil is relatively economical, removal of sulfur from coal prior to combustion has been difficult. When the coal is burned, sulfur is oxidized to SO_2 and leaves as a gaseous component of the combustion products. A modern 1000-MW power plant consumes 8500 tons coal/day and emits 600 tons SO_2/day. Removal of the SO_2 from the stack gases is difficult since it is usually present in concentrations of 500–2000 ppm, and the gas flow rates are on the order of 3×10^6 ft³/min at 150°C. The presence of noncombustible fly ash at 1000 tons/day further complicates the picture. Other sources of SO_2 include smelting of ores and petroleum refining.

The major efforts in desulfurization are in the following areas: (a) coal gasification, to remove sulfur prior to combustion; (b) fluidized bed combustion, to remove sulfur during combustion; and (c) flue gas desulfurization, to remove sulfur after combustion. Relative costs for representative processes are shown in Table 31.2. Flue gas desulfurization, in conjunction with conventional coal cleaning, is now commercially available; coal gasification and fluidized bed combustion should be available by 1985.

31.3.1.a. Coal Gasification

Gasification is attractive because it both removes the sulfur and provides a high heating value ($3.36–3.73 \times 10^7$ J/m³) pipeline quality fuel. Lower heating value pipeline gases ($0.56–1.87 \times 10^7$ J/m³) are also obtainable for use in utility boilers.

Table 31.2 Cost Comparison of Major SO_2 Control Technologies

Process	Capital cost[a] ($/kW$_e$)	Total annual cost[b] (mills/kW$_e$)
Gasification (open cycle)	395–555	19–23.5
Fluidized bed (atmospheric)	389–409	18.5–21.5
Flue gas desulfurization (lime/limestone)	366–476	21–24

[a]Complete installation.
[b]Includes cost of coal and SO_2 control.

Coal consists mainly of carbon (75%), and the hydrogen content is only about 5%. The object of gasification is to produce as pure a stream of methane as possible (75% carbon and 25% hydrogen by weight). Therefore, the coal must be reacted with hydrogen to form methane while rejecting the other reaction products.

Coal is heated to 500–800°C via partial combustion to produce some methane directly plus carbon as char. This char is then treated with steam at high ($> 900°C$) temperatures:

$$C + H_2O \rightleftharpoons CO + H_2 \tag{31.25}$$

$$C + 2H_2 \rightleftharpoons CH_4 \tag{31.26}$$

$$CO + H_2O \rightleftharpoons H_2 + CO_2. \tag{31.27}$$

The last reaction is frequently used downstream at temperatures of 400–600°C to produce more hydrogen for the methanation reaction,

$$3H_2 + CO \rightleftharpoons CH_4 + H_2O. \tag{31.28}$$

The sulfur in the coal is converted primarily to H_2S in the gasification stage, and this may be converted to sulfur in a Claus process,

$$SO_2 + 2H_2S \rightleftharpoons 2H_2O + 3S. \tag{31.29}$$

In the open-cycle coal gasification system the hot gas is sent directly to a gas turbine, avoiding the boiler altogether. However, turbine temperatures of 1400°C are required, whereas current gas turbines are operating around 1100°C. Removal efficiency for SO_2 is greater than 95%.

31.3.1.b. Fluidized Bed Combustion

Fluidized bed combustion is one of the emerging sulfur removal technologies that appear most attractive because of its simplicity and low operating costs. Fluidization is achieved by using air to suspend a bed of crushed coal mixed with limestone ($CaCO_3$) at high temperature. Oxygen in the air reacts with the coal particles and liberates heat. The boiler tubes are submerged in the fluidized bed, allowing higher heat transfer rates and lower combustion temperatures than in conventional boilers, hence lowering the amount of NO_x formed. The SO_2 removal efficiencies are 80–95%.

The limestone is calcined,

$$CaCO_3 \rightarrow CaO + CO_2 \tag{31.30}$$

and the oxide reacts with SO_2 to produce gypsum,

$$CaO + SO_2 + \tfrac{1}{2}O_2 \rightarrow CaSO_4. \tag{31.31}$$

This product can be regenerated at about 1050°C,

$$CaSO_4 + CO \rightarrow CO_2 + SO_2 + CaO \tag{31.32}$$

yielding a stream concentrated in SO_2, which permits recovery of elemental sulfur.

Factors affecting SO_2 removal efficiencies are the porosity and size of the crushed particles, temperature, contact time, and calcium content in the bed.

31.3.1.c. Flue Gas Desulfurization

Two types of flue gas desulfurization that are currently available and capable of reducing SO_2 emissions to comply with EPA standards are limestone scrubbing and sodium sulfite scrubbing. Several different scrubbing systems have been utilized; these include spray chambers, packed columns, and Venturi scrubbers.

In the limestone process (Figure 31.4), a limestone slurry reacts with the SO_2 in a wet scrubber, producing an insoluble sludge of $CaSO_3/CaSO_4$:

$$CaCO_3 + CO_2 + H_2O \rightarrow Ca(HCO_3)_2 \tag{31.33}$$

$$Ca(HCO_3)_2 + SO_2 + H_2O \rightarrow CaSO_3 \cdot 2H_2O \downarrow + 2CO_2 \tag{31.34}$$

$$CaSO_3 \cdot 2H_2O + \tfrac{1}{2}O_2 \rightarrow CaSO_4 \cdot 2H_2O \downarrow . \tag{31.35}$$

The main advantages of the limestone scrubbing approach are the relative ease with which equipment can be added to existing power plants, and the relative availability and low cost of limestone.

Aqueous solution of sodium sulfite is a strong absorbent of SO_2. The absorbed SO_2 forms sodium bisulfite, which when cooled is precipitated as pyrosulfite ($S_2O_5^{2-}$). This is then heated to release SO_2 and regenerate sulfite:

$$SO_2 + SO_3^{2-} + H_2O \rightleftharpoons 2HSO_3^- \tag{31.36}$$

$$2HSO_3^- \rightarrow S_2O_5^{2-} \downarrow + H_2O \tag{31.37}$$

$$S_2O_5^{2-} \rightarrow SO_2 + SO_3^{2-}. \tag{31.38}$$

The SO_2-rich gas is processed for recovery as sulfuric acid.

The main disadvantage to wet scrubbing is that the flue gas is cooled and must be reheated to achieve necessary stack temperatures for plume buoyancy. Wet scrubbing also poses serious corrosion problems that can only be overcome by the use of high-quality steel equipment. The sodium sulfite process offers one advantage over limestone scrubbing in that the final product, sulfuric acid, is salable, whereas calcium sulfate is, until the market improves, still a throwaway item.

31.3.2. Nitrogen Oxides

Two forms of NO_x, NO and NO_2, exist at concentrations of 0.25 ppm and higher in large cities. These compounds play a key role in the formation of photochemical smog. The NO_x reduce the brightness and contrast of distant objects and produce a yellow-brown hue in the sky at the horizon.

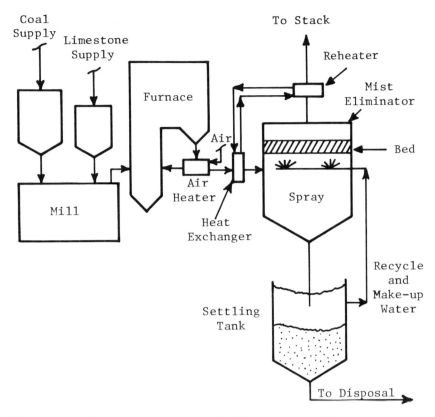

Figure 31.4 Combustion engineering SO_2 limestone scrubbing process.

31.3.2.a. Thermodynamics in Combustion Processes

Nitric oxide is produced in the combustion of fuel when oxygen and nitrogen, present in the air, react at high temperatures:

$$N_2 + O_2 \rightleftharpoons 2NO. \tag{31.39}$$

For most stationary combustion processes, residence times are too short for the oxidation of NO to NO_2. Furthermore, NO is favored thermodynamically at high temperatures; therefore, combustion gas NO_x are 90–95% NO.

31.3.2.b. Nitrogen Oxide Control

Modifications of combustion conditions are the primary control measures, at present, for reduction of NO_x emissions. The main factors affecting NO_x concentrations are temperature, residence time, air-to-fuel ratio, combustion zone cooling, and furnace configuration.

The rates of NO formation and decay are highly temperature dependent. Data from full-scale boiler tests demonstrate a threefold increase in NO_x emissions if combustion air is preheated from 27 to 315°C. Flue gas recirculation can lower this peak flame temperature, and is effective when about 10–15% of the gas is mixed with the primary air prior to combustion. Injection of low-temperature water or steam will also reduce the flame temperature.

The reduction of excess air has a marked effect on NO_x emissions. In one case NO_x decreased from about 560 ppm at 25% excess air to about 175 ppm at 1.4%. The accompanying decrease in combustion efficiency was from 99.5% to around 92%.

High heat release rates increase NO_x concentrations because of the effect on flame temperatures. Therefore, measures to reduce heat removal rates counter-balance this effect. The use of two-stage combustion has been successful in this regard. Here the NO_x concentration in the first stage is limited by incomplete combustion with low amounts of oxygen. Secondary air is injected downstream, where the resulting CO and HC are consumed in the second stage. The combination of flue gas recirculation with two-stage combustion can reduce the NO_x emissions by as much as 50%.

31.3.3. Hydrocarbon and Carbon Monoxide Control

Atmospheric HC are made up of dozens of different compounds. Methane is the most prevalent, with a background level, due to natural sources, of 1.5 ppm. It is not considered to be an air pollutant because it is relatively inert and its main source is natural. Other HC in contaminated air usually contain five or fewer carbon–hydrogen groups. There are three major classes of HC: saturated, unsaturated, and aromatic. In the saturated class are ethane, propane, and higher straight-chain HC. In the unsaturated class are olefins and acetylenes. In the aromatic class are benzene, toluene, and m-xylene. The individual concentrations reflect their volatility and source of emission (mostly petroleum and natural gas). The HC are not, by themselves, a hazard, but the products of their reactions with NO_x and sunlight produce photochemical smog.

In the HC combustion process, in addition to unoxidized HC, CO, and CO_2, are reaction products in varying ratios depending on the efficiency of combustion. It is believed that CO_2 is formed in a two-step reaction:

$$HCO + OH \rightleftharpoons CO + H_2O \tag{31.40}$$

$$CO + OH \rightleftharpoons CO_2 + H. \tag{31.41}$$

Flames from HC combustion are known to contain considerable quantities of OH, possibly from the reaction

$$H + H_2O \rightleftharpoons OH + H_2 \tag{31.42}$$

which shifts heavily to the right at elevated temperatures.

The source of CO in the combustion effluent is thus the first reaction, and since the second reaction is about 10 times slower than the first, it is the rate-controlling step. Therefore, combustion processes that do not allow the second step to go to completion will produce an effluent high in CO. The most abundant and widely distributed air pollutant is CO, mainly due to mobile sources (63% of the man-made sources).

Both HC and CO pollution are a result of incomplete or inefficient combustion and can usually be controlled by further oxidation, adsorption, condensation, and absorption.

Afterburners are incineration chambers in which unburned HC, CO, smoke, and other objectionable gases issuing from a process are oxidized to CO_2 and water vapor. The combustion may be via direct or indirect flame or by catalysis. If a direct flame is used, the waste gas must have sufficient heating value to fuel its own combustion, and this must be at a steady rate. Indirect heating of thermal incinerators involves burning natural gas or propane and mixing the waste gas streams with the hot combustion products at 650–815°C; CO oxidation requires temperatures in the 675–790°C range, whereas HC oxidation is completed at 510–760°C. Therefore, if both gases are to be oxidized the design temperature must take this into account.

Catalytic afterburners have been primarily used to control organic vapor emissions. The waste gases are preheated by a natural gas burner to the temperature needed for catalytic combustion. Some dilution air may be required to avoid explosions.

Adsorption by activated carbon is used because it is selective in removing organic vapors at very low concentrations. The use of carbon is limited to low temperatures and is susceptible to fouling by PM.

If the waste gas stream contains a large amount of condensables, such as water vapor and organic compounds, condensation of the steam will remove much of the organic material. The volume of the emissions is reduced and the high molecular weight fats and oils may be recovered.

Organic pollutants can be removed by wet scrubbing if solutions of oxidizing agents are used to oxidize the organics to water-soluble aldehydes, acids, and CO_2. The waste water must then be treated before disposal.

Suggested Reading

Crawford, M. Air Pollution Control Theory. New York: McGraw-Hill, 1976.

Friedlander, S. K. Smoke, Dust and Haze. New York: Wiley, 1976.

Liptak, B. G. (Ed.). Environmental Engineers Handbook, Vol. 2, Air Pollution. Radnor, Pa.: Chilton, 1974.

Seinfeld, J. H. Air Pollution, Physical and Chemical Fundamentals. New York: McGraw-Hill, 1975.

Wark, K., Warner, C. F. Air Pollution, Its Origin and Control. Hagerstown, Md.: Harper & Row, 1976.

Steven H. Cadle
George J. Nebel

32

Control of Automotive Emissions

32.1. Introduction

Automotive emission control technology has been directed toward modifying automotive design in a way that will eliminate or reduce emissions and at the same time not impair the automobile's basic function. This goal has been largely accomplished. In this chapter the technical aspects of automotive emission control systems will be briefly discussed, as well as the magnitude, measurement, and composition of regulated and unregulated emissions. The primary emphasis is on exhaust gases, but other vehicle emissions such as fuel evaporation, crankcase gases, and tire and brake wear products are also discussed. Only the conventional gasoline-powered automobile is considered.

32.2. Regulated Emissions

The Clean Air Act of 1967 and subsequent amendments in 1970 and 1977 have established emission standards for motor vehicles that must be met before the vehicle can be sold in the United States. This act, which is administered by the EPA, regulates three categories of emissions. The first and most familiar category is the exhaust emissions, consisting of total HC, CO, and NO_x. For light-duty vehicles, HC and CO have been regulated since 1968, and NO_x since 1973. The light-duty standards for various model years are listed in Table 32.1 along with the best estimates of the emissions in 1960, the baseline year before any emissions controls were instituted. It is apparent from Table 32.1 that exhaust emissions have been reduced substantially during the last decade and will continue to be reduced as older cars are scrapped and as the more stringent 1980 and 1981 standards become effective.

The second category is the evaporative emissions. These are the low molecular weight HC that evaporate from gasoline in the fuel tank and carburetor, both when the car is driven and when it is parked with the engine off (soaked).

Table 32.1   Federal Exhaust Emission Standards for Light-Duty Vehicles[a]

Model year	Maximum allowable emission[b] (g/mile)		
	HC	CO	NO_x
1960 (baseline)	10.6	84	4.1
1968–1969	6.3	51	—[c]
1970–1971	4.1	34	—[c]
1972	3.0	28	—[c]
1973–1974	3.0	28	3.1
1975–1976	1.5	15	3.1
1977–1979	1.5	15	2.0
1980	0.41	7	2.0
1981	0.41	3.4[d]	1.0[e]

[a]Less than 6000 lb.

[b]Adjusted to be equivalent to 1975 federal test procedure before 1975 model year.

[c]Not regulated.

[d]Possible waiver to 7.0 g/mile under specified conditions.

[e]Possible waiver to 1.5 g/mile for innovative technology under specified conditions.

Evaporative emissions have been regulated since 1971. The present standard is 6.0 g/test, but will be reduced to 2.0 g in 1981.

The third category is the crankcase, or blowby, emissions. These are the gases (primarily unburned air–fuel mixture) that leak past the piston rings and into the crankcase and escape, if not controlled, to the atmosphere. Crankcase emissions have been regulated in California since 1961 and nationwide since 1963. The law requires that crankcase emissions be eliminated completely. There is no test procedure as such, but compliance is determined on the basis of the engineering features of each system.

The Clean Air Act allows the state of California to set emission standards that in aggregate are at least as restrictive as the federal standards. California has exercised this right and in 1978 adopted exhaust standards (in g/mile) of 0.41 HC, 9.0 CO, and 1.5 NO_x and will adopt an evaporative standard of 2.0 g in 1980. According to the 1977 Amendments to the Clean Air Act, other states have the option of adopting the California standards under certain conditions.

The Clean Air Act also requires that all cars be certified at both low and high altitudes (over 4000 ft) beginning in 1984. In general, HC, CO, and evaporative emissions tend to increase with altitude. High-altitude engine options to reduce emissions and improve drivability are available on new cars in some areas.

32.3. Emission Control Technology

32.3.1. Exhaust

HC and CO are present in exhaust gases because of incomplete fuel combustion, whereas NO and NO_2 are formed in a reaction between nitrogen and oxygen at high temperatures in the combustion chamber. Different control methods are usually required for these two classes of pollutants.

Before 1975, HC and CO were controlled by engine modifications and, on some cars, the injection of air into the exhaust manifold to promote oxidation. Since 1975, most cars have relied on the oxidation catalytic converter to reduce HC and CO emissions. The active metal in automotive oxidation catalysts is platinum, or a mixture of platinum and palladium, and is deposited on a high surface area alumina substrate. The physical form of the catalyst is either pelleted or monolithic honeycomb. The catalyst housing is fabricated of a high-temperature, corrosion-resistant steel. Some systems also inject extra air upstream from the catalyst to promote more complete oxidation.

The oxidation catalytic converter has little effect on NO_x emissions. To date, NO_x has been controlled primarily by exhaust gas recirculation (EGR), in which a portion of the exhaust is recirculated back into the intake manifold. This reduces the combustion temperature and, consequently, the formation of NO_x. The amount of exhaust recirculated is generally limited to 10–15% to avoid poor drivability, and should be reduced to zero at idle and wide open throttle to ensure an acceptable idle and adequate power for passing and emergencies. In general, the engine conditions most favorable for efficient fuel utilization produce the largest amount of NO_x.

The NO_x emissions can also be controlled catalytically. One experimental approach uses "dual" catalysts in series, the first to reduce NO_x and the second to oxidize HC and CO. Another approach uses a "three-way" catalyst that destroys HC, CO, and NO_x in a single converter. Three-way systems are installed on some 1978 model cars sold in California. The three-way system differs from the present oxidation system in the composition of the catalyst and in the need for precise air–fuel ratio control. Three-way catalysts contain rhodium to catalyze the reduction of NO_x, as well as platinum (or platinum and palladium) to catalyze the oxidation of HC and CO. The oxidation and reduction reactions will take place simultaneously only when the air–fuel ratio is within a narrow band centered on the stoichiometric or chemically correct ratio. Precise air–fuel ratio control is achieved by means of a closed-loop carburetor that utilizes an exhaust oxygen sensor located between the engine and the catalyst. The three-way catalytic converter substantially reduces the emissions of all three pollutants under the proper operating conditions.

It should be emphasized that exhaust emissions, fuel economy, and drivability are all interrelated. Selecting the optimum emission control system invariably requires some compromise. Sound design and engineering are essential to make this compromise acceptable to the motoring public.

32.3.2. Fuel Evaporation

Before they were controlled, most evaporative emissions escaped through the fuel tank and carburetor vents, although there were other less significant sources. Today, almost all cars are equipped with the activated carbon canister system to control evaporative emissions. The canister, fuel tank, and carburetor are interconnected in such a way that the activated carbon traps fuel vapors during "hot soak" and "diurnal" periods when the engine is not running. When the engine is running, the canister is backflushed and the trapped HC are stripped off the carbon and inducted into the carburetor along with any vapors from the fuel tank. Again, the system must be carefully engineered to obtain the proper balance between effective vapor recovery and minimum interaction or interference with vehicle operation.

The carbon canister system controls about 85% of the running and soak losses from the vehicle itself. It does not control refueling losses, that is, the HC vapors displaced by gasoline being pumped into the tank. Refueling emissions are regulated in some California communities, but not nationwide, although the EPA is considering such regulations. Refueling emissions can be controlled by either on-board or on-station systems. The on-board system uses an enlarged carbon canister on the car to capture displaced vapors. The on-station system uses return hoses on the service station pumps to route the vapors back to the underground storage tanks. Some of these proposed systems require a leak-tight seal between the filler pipe and the pump nozzle, which raises the question of their compatability with older cars.

32.3.3. Blowby

It is ironical that blowby was the last automotive pollutant source to be identified and the first to be controlled. (It was well known that a little gas escaped from the crankcase, but its high HC concentration was not recognized). The solution was simple and effective: remove the breather tube and reroute the crankcase effluent back into the intake manifold so that the HC could be burned in the engine instead of discharged to the atmosphere. This is the positive crankcase ventilation (PCV) system. In the closed PCV system (now mandatory), air to purge the crankcase is withdrawn from inside the air cleaner. Careful design is required to ensure that none of the vapors escape and that carburetion is not upset, lest the car drive poorly. The PCV system also requires periodic maintenance for continued efficient operation. The overall efficiency, which includes the lack of maintenance of some vehicles in use, has been estimated to be at least 98%.

A sketch of a complete emission control system is shown in Figure 32.1. The key features discussed in the preceding paragraphs are identified.

32.3.4. Gasoline Composition

The most important gasoline property from an emission control standpoint is whether or not lead alkyl antiknock compounds are present. Typical leaded gasoline contains about 2 g lead/gal, enough to deactivate precious metal catalysts rather quickly. To ensure that unleaded gasoline is used in catalyst cars, the EPA has required that the filler neck on the gas tank of catalyst cars be smaller in diameter than the standard service station pump nozzle and be able to accept only the smaller nozzle from pumps dispensing unleaded gasoline. This strategy has worked fairly well, although there are periodic reports of leaded gasoline use in catalyst-equipped cars.

Unleaded gasoline is permitted to contain up to 0.05 g lead/gal because of the residual lead from storage tanks, tank trucks, etc. Some unleaded gasoline contained methylcyclopentadienyl manganese tricarbonyl (MMT) as an anti-knock substitute for lead. However, because there were reports of catalyst plugging and increased emissions with MMT, the EPA prohibited its use late in 1978.

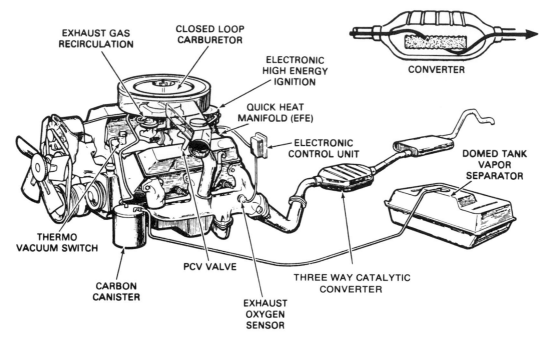

Figure 32.1 Emission control system utilizing the three-way catalytic converter.

Gasoline composition also affects some of the unregulated exhaust emissions such as individual HC and sulfur compounds; these will be discussed in Section 32.5.

32.4. Emission Test Procedures

In the 1950s and early 1960s, automotive emissions were measured directly on the road. Today, almost all emission testing is done on chassis dynamometers, with more repeatable results. In the present federal test procedure (FTP), evaporative and exhaust emissions are measured sequentially following a rigidly prescribed protocol. The preparatory steps include fueling the car with the test gasoline, preconditioning (driving) it on the dynamometer, and soaking the vehicle at room temperature for 12–24 hr. The diurnal evaporative emissions, which simulate the breathing losses of the fuel system, are measured first. The fuel tank is electrically heated from 60 to 84°F as the car is parked in a "sealed housing for evaporative determination" (SHED). The HC concentration inside the SHED is monitored for 1 hr, and the diurnal emissions (in grams per test) are calculated from the increase in the HC concentration.

The car is pushed out of the SHED and onto the chassis dynamometer for the measurement of exhaust emissions. There, the car is driven through a 41-min test cycle that simulates typical urban driving. The exhaust is directed into a constant volume sampler (CVS), where it is diluted with a large excess of air, and samples of the diluted exhaust and of the background air are collected continuously in plastic bags. One set of samples is collected during the first 505 sec of the test; a second set during the next 867 sec; and a third set as the first 505 sec of the cycle is rerun after a 10-min soak. This complex procedure is supposed to account for the number of cold-start and hot-start trips of the average motorist. After the test, the six bag samples are analyzed for total HC, CO, CO_2, and NO_x by conventional gas analyzers, and the emissions and fuel economy are calculated.

The hot soak evaporative emissions are measured last. The car is driven off the dynamometer back into the SHED. As the engine heat warms the carburetor and the fuel lines, the gasoline in them tends to evaporate. Any vapors escaping from the charcoal canister or other leakage points are measured in the same way as the diurnal losses. The evaporative emission system is designed to prevent any vapors from escaping when the engine is running, so the measurement of running losses is not required.

It should be emphasized that the official federal test procedure is a unique test and that attempts to develop short-cut exhaust emission tests that correlate with it have not been successful.

32.5. Unregulated Exhaust Emissions

There are some minor constituents of automobile exhaust that are considered air pollutants, or potential air pollutants, but are not regulated by law. All of them are present in very low concentration.

32.5.1. Individual Hydrocarbons

Auto exhaust contains more than 100 different HC, many of them formed during combustion and not present in the fuel. Although these individual HC vary widely in photochemical reactivity and air pollution potential, only the total HC emission is regulated. There have been proposals to account for the reactivity differences between HC in setting exhaust emission standards, but they have not been accepted for various reasons. The only exception is California's nonmethane HC standard, which allows the use of a correction factor to account for the difference in the exhaust methane content of catalyst and noncatalyst (baseline) cars. This is a scientifically sound approach since methane is generally not considered to be an air pollutant. Methane is a prominent natural constituent of the atmosphere and is not involved in the photochemical processes involved in smog formation.

Methane constitutes about 15% by weight of the exhaust HC from catalyst cars and about 5% from noncatalyst cars. Methane is enriched in catalytically treated exhaust, relative to other HC, because it is the most difficult HC to oxidize catalytically.

Benzene is another individual HC of interest because of its toxicity. Benzene emissions are reduced by 80–90% by the catalytic converter. The benzene fraction is about 3% by weight for catalyst cars and about 4% for noncatalyst cars. Both these exhaust concentrations are higher than the 1–2% of benzene in typical gasoline because the engine produces a small amount of benzene by dealkylating other aromatic HC.

The 12 predominant HC in the exhaust from catalyst-equipped vehicles are listed below, in order of decreasing weight fraction:

1. Methane
2. Toluene
3. Trimethylpentane(s)
4. Ethylene
5. *i*-Pentane
6. *n*-Butane

7. Xylene(s)
8. Benzene
9. Propylene
10. Ethane
11. Acetylene
12. l-Butene.

Typically, these 12 HC constitute about 65% of the total HC by weight. Four of the 12 (methane, benzene, ethane, and acetylene) are of very low reactivity in photochemical smog formation.

32.5.2. Oxygenates

Oxygenates are organic compounds containing oxygen and include aldehydes, alcohols, ketones, organic acids, ethers, and phenols. They are formed in the engine by the incomplete combustion of the fuel. Most of the oxygenates in auto exhaust are aldehydes.

There has been speculation that catalytic converters might increase aldehyde emissions; however, all the available evidence indicates that the catalytic converter oxidizes HC completely to CO_2 and H_2O, if at all, and that aldehydes are oxidized much more efficiently than HC or CO. Typical aldehyde emissions, as measured by the standard 3-methyl-2-benzothiazolone hydrazone (MBTH) method, are 10–20 mg/mile for catalyst cars and 100–200 mg/mile for noncatalyst cars. As a rule of thumb, aldehyde emissions are an order of magnitude lower than HC emissions.

Formaldehyde is the major aldehyde in automobile exhaust. Smaller amounts of acetaldehyde, propionaldehyde, and benzaldehyde, and still smaller amounts of acrolein, butyraldehyde, valeraldehyde, and the tolualdehydes are also present. There is not enough information to tell whether the distribution of individual aldehydes is affected by catalytic converters. There is also very little information about nonaldehyde exhaust oxygenates, although methanol, acetone, methyl ethyl ketone, propylene oxide, and nitromethane were detected in the exhaust from a prototype catalyst car in one study.

32.5.3. Sulfur Compounds

Gasoline contains small quantities of organosulfur compounds that are oxidized almost exclusively to SO_2 when the gasoline is burned. However, since gasoline contains relatively little sulfur (about 0.03% by weight) compared to other fuels, automobile exhaust is not a major SO_2 source. It contributes about 1% of the total SO_2 nationwide and perhaps 4% in urban areas with high traffic density. Thus, automotive sulfur emissions were of little concern until 1975, when catalytic converters were installed on most new U.S. automobiles.

The catalytic converter complicates the sulfur compound emission picture because SO_2 can react over the catalyst. Under some conditions a small amount of the SO_2 forms SO_3, which quickly combines with water to form H_2SO_4. The H_2SO_4 condenses at about 120°C and is discharged from the tailpipe as fine droplets or mist. (These particulate "sulfate" emissions are discussed in Section 32.5.5.)

Occasionally, some of the sulfur is emitted as H_2S or carbonyl sulfide (COS). These sulfides impart a characteristic rotten egg odor to the exhaust. Since H_2S has one of the lowest odor thresholds known, about 1 ppb, the odor can be detected when the emission rate is extremely low. Four conditions seem to favor sulfide emission: (a) a low oxygen concentration in the exhaust; (b) a relatively high concentration of reducing species (H_2, CO, HC); (c) a hot catalyst; and (d) a relatively long contact time of the exhaust over the catalyst. The combination of these requirements makes sulfide emissions sporadic, but they are most likely to occur when the car idles after having been driven at high speeds. Sulfides are also likely to be formed when the car is started, particularly when the ambient temperature is low. This is illustrated in Figure 32.2. Because this particular test was a deliberate attempt to form sulfides, the H_2S and COS concentrations were relatively high, up to 7 ppm. More typically, sulfide concentrations are in the parts per hundred million range. Since exhaust is rapidly diluted by 1000-fold in the atmosphere, pedestrians rarely detect the sulfide odor. Three-way catalyst systems may also form H_2S and COS, particularly if the air–fuel mixture is enriched in fuel by a malfunction of the closed-loop fuel system.

The emission rates of the various sulfur compounds are highly variable and difficult to reproduce in the laboratory because SO_2 (or perhaps SO_3) reacts with the alumina substrate of the catalyst, forming an unstable sulfur–oxygen–alumina complex. The complex subsequently decomposes and releases the sulfur as SO_2, SO_3, H_2S, or COS. Thus, sometimes the catalyst removes sulfur from the exhaust, whereas at other times it adds sulfur. This storage-and-release phenomenon makes sulfur emissions erratic. Some of the factors known to affect

Figure 32.2 H_2S and COS emissions from a rich malfunctioning car. Car soaked at −29°C before start.

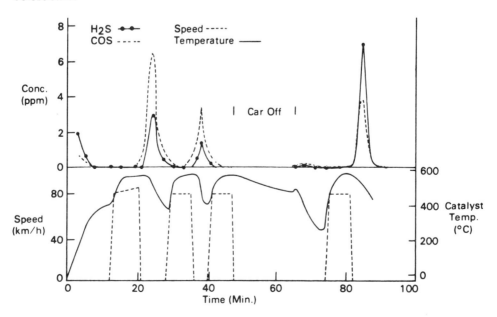

sulfur emissions are the exhaust oxygen concentration, the engine air–fuel ratio, the catalyst temperature, the fuel sulfur content, and the immediate-past driving history of the car. The last factor probably reflects the extent of sulfur storage on the catalyst. Sulfur storage is greater with pelleted catalysts than with monolith catalysts, presumably because pelleted catalysts contain more alumina.

32.5.4. Nitrogen Compounds

Most of the fixed nitrogen in automobile exhaust is in the form of NO and NO_2, the regulated emissions. Much smaller amounts of N_2O, NH_3, HCN, and possibly traces of organic nitrogen compounds such as amines and nitriles are also formed during engine combustion. There is little information on N_2O in exhaust since it is unreactive and of little interest as an air pollutant. (Natural biological action in soil produces enough N_2O to maintain a constant atmospheric concentration of 0.3 ppm.) Similarly, there has been little interest in the NH_3 and HCN emissions of noncatalyst cars.

The main effect of the oxidation catalytic converter on fixed nitrogen compounds is to reduce a small percentage of the NO_x to N_2. Normally, it also destroys most of the HCN formed in the engine, but does not affect the NH_3 significantly. The catalyst does not oxidize NO and NO_2 to HNO_3, as it does SO_2 to H_2SO_4. Only traces of HNO_3 (or nitrates) have been found in automobile exhaust (with or without a catalytic converter). However, both oxidation and three-way catalysts will form NH_3 if the air–fuel mixture becomes excessively fuel rich. This can happen if the fuel system malfunctions. HCN may also be formed under rich conditions over a three-way catalyst, but not in as large amounts as NH_3. Some typical NH_3 and HCN emission rates illustrating these points are given in Table 32.2. The EPA has established an emission criterion of 300 mg/mile for HCN that must not be exceeded under any test conditions. There is no criterion for NH_3.

The presence of ammonia in exhaust gases suggests that alkyl amines may also be present. Although they are only moderately toxic themselves, these amines may be atmospheric precursors of nitrosamines, which are known carcinogens. However, the little evidence available indicates that amine emissions are very low. Nitrosamines have never been detected in automobile exhaust.

32.5.5. Particulates

Particulate emissions from automobiles depend primarily on the gasoline used (whether leaded or unleaded) and the emission control system. Some typical exhaust particulate data are shown in Table 32.3. The emission rate is highest for noncatalyst cars burning leaded gasoline, most of the particulate being lead in the form of complex oxyhalides. With leaded gasoline, there is a moderate amount of carbonaceous matter, including polynuclear aromatic hydrocarbons (PNAs), and small amounts of sulfur, iron, and other metals. The sulfur is probably combined with the lead. When unleaded gasoline is burned in noncatalyst cars, the lead emission is reduced by about 99%, proportional to the reduction of lead in the gasoline, and most of the particulate is carbonaceous matter and iron.

Table 32.2   Typical Ammonia and Hydrogen Cyanide Exhaust Emissions (mg/mile)

Emission system	NH_3	HCN
Noncatalytic	3	12
Oxidation catalyst	4	1
Three-way catalyst (normal)	7	3
Three-way catalyst (rich malfunction)	200	50

Table 32.3   Typical Properties of Automobile Exhaust Particulate Emissions

Emission system	Gasoline	Emission (mg/km)	Approximate Composition (wt %)			
			Lead	Sulfate	Carbon	Other[a]
Noncatalytic	Leaded	150	75	1	10	14
Noncatalytic	Unleaded	25	4	4	70	22
Oxidation catalyst	Unleaded	10[b]	10	35	10	45[c]
Oxidation catalyst plus air pump	Unleaded	30[b]	3	45	2	50[c]

[a]Iron, zinc, manganese, aluminum, nickel, bromine, and/or chlorine.

[b]These emissions are for low-mileage catalysts. The particulate sulfate will decrease substantially with mileage.

[c]Including water bound with H_2SO_4.

The lead emissions from catalyst cars are also very low, since they must use unleaded gasoline. The catalyst destroys 80–90% of the carbonaceous matter formed in the engine, including the PNAs such as benzo[a]pyrene. As mentioned above, it also oxidizes some of the SO_2 to SO_3, which is hydrated and discharged as fine H_2SO_4 mist. Sulfate emissions from catalyst cars are difficult to characterize because they vary greatly under supposedly identical test conditions as well as from one test (driving) condition to the next. This is particularly true with pelleted catalysts. Nevertheless, we do know that sulfate emissions are relatively low during low-speed cyclic driving and relatively high during high-speed, steady-state operation, that the use of a secondary air pump increases sulfate emissions, and that three-way catalyst systems produce very little sulfate. These effects have been explained on the basis of the oxidizing properties of the exhaust.

The concern about automotive sulfate emissions was that drivers, pedestrians, and others living or working near heavily traveled roadways might receive excessive exposures. The congested freeway is considered to be the most critical case. There have been two large-scale studies to evaluate the sulfate exposures near freeways. The first, conducted at the General Motors Proving Ground at Milford, Michigan, in 1975, was a simulated study involving all catalyst-equipped vehicles on a large test road. The second was the Los Angeles Catalyst Study conducted by the EPA and its contractors alongside the San Diego

Freeway in Los Angeles, California, between 1974 and 1978. These studies have shown that automotive sulfate emissions disperse more rapidly than predicted by simple models because of vehicle-induced turbulence and that sulfate levels approach background levels within a few meters of the freeway. In addition, it has been determined that sulfate emissions decrease with increasing mileage. Therefore, it was concluded that public exposure to automotive sulfates would not be excessive even if all cars were equipped with catalytic converters.

It has been suggested that a small amount of material that contains platinum and palladium can be worn from the catalyst. Due to the extremely low emission rates of this material, only limited data are available. In one investigation that used a sensitive radiometric technique, the attrition rate of a commercial pelleted catalyst was 1.2–3.1 mg/km and the platinum emission rate was 0.8–1.9 μg/km, depending upon how the car was driven. Over 80% of the emitted platinum was attached to particles larger than 125 μm, less than 10% of the platinum was water soluble, and the fraction of platinum in the abraded material was the same as in the original pellets. Other studies using less sensitive methods have failed to detect platinum emissions. It is expected that palladium and rhodium emissions will be lower than platinum emissions because their concentration in the catalyst is smaller.

32.6. Tire-Wear Emissions

The amount of rubber worn off automobile tires has been estimated from vehicle registrations and tire sales to be about 360 mg/km/car. This is greater than the exhaust particulate emission rate with leaded gasoline, so it is not surprising that tire-wear emissions have been implicated as potential air pollutants. To decide whether they are, it is necessary to know the size distribution of the particles worn off tires and whether any gaseous products are formed. Tire-wear emissions have been studied in both indoor tests, in which a tire is run against a simulated road surface inside a closed chamber, and outdoor tests. The outdoor tests were conducted in highway tunnels and alongside roadways; particulate samples were collected and analyzed for styrene–butadiene rubber, the major constituent of tire tread rubber.

Both the indoor and outdoor tests have shown that most of the tire-wear debris consists of large, nonsuspendable particles. Some of these particles are 1 mm or more in diameter, although the average diameter is probably a few hundredths of a millimeter. The composition of the particles is essentially the same as the tread material (polymer, extender oil, carbon black, and additives), although as much as 40% of the polymer may be degraded to lower molecular weight materials by the wear process. Since these large particles settle within 30 m of the roadway and slowly degrade or wash away, they do not appear to cause any environmental problems.

The indoor tests have shown that the airborne particulate fraction is less than 10% of the total wear rate under all conditions and less than 1% under high-wear conditions; 75% of these airborne particles are (by mass) larger than 7 μm. Similarly, in one outdoor study, the mass median diameter of the airborne rubber particles was greater than 20 μm. Thus, the available evidence, although limited, indicates that airborne tire-wear particulates are mostly relatively large, nonrespirable particles.

The indoor tests have also shown that the gases formed during tire wear are mostly HC. The identified gases include HC monomers such as butadiene, isoprene, and styrene, and traces of SO_2, COS, and CS_2. The total HC emission rate was estimated at 2.4 mg/km/car, or less than 1% of the total wear rate, and was surprisingly independent of the total wear rate. Gaseous emissions from tires appear to be negligible compared to other sources of these pollutants.

32.7. Brake-Wear Emissions

Brake-wear emissions have been estimated to be about 20 mg/km/car from the weight loss and mileage of brake linings. Asbestos emissions are of primary concern, since brake linings contain 45–70% chrysotile asbestos plus phenolic resin binder and inorganic fillers. A few cars use metallic brake linings, but they will not be considered here.

Like tires, brake lining wear products can be divided into three categories: gases, airborne particulates, and retained dust. Brake-wear emissions have been studied primarily in the laboratory. The gaseous emissions (CO_2, CO, and HC) are derived from the oxidation of the binder and account for about 40% of the weight of material lost. Another 40% of the wear products are airborne particulates of a wide size range, some as large as 50 μm. Most of the airborne particulate is inorganic matter (silicon, magnesium, calcium, and iron) of irregular shape. Only about 0.01% is asbestos, and most of that is small fibrils rather than the original large fibers. It is apparent that almost all of the asbestos is converted to a nonfibrous (nonasbestos) material by the high temperatures and stresses at the braking interface. Therefore, it appears that brake wear contributes a negligible amount of asbestos to the atmosphere compared to other sources.

The remaining 20% or so of the material is retained in the brake housing and wheel hub. This dust has essentially the same composition and asbestos content as the airborne material.

Suggested Reading

Anderson, A. E., Gealer, R. L., McCune, R. C., et al. Asbestos emissions from brake dynamometer tests (Paper 730549). Soc. Automotive Eng. 82:1832–1841, 1973.

Anderson, E. V. Phasing lead out of gasoline: Hard knocks for lead alkyls producers. Chem. Eng. News, Feb. 6, 1978.

Black, F., High, L. Automotive hydrocarbon emissions patterns in the measurement of nonmethane hydrocarbon emission rates. Paper 770144, presented at the Society of Automotive Engineers International Automotive Engineering Congress, Detroit, March 1977.

Bradow, R. L., Stump, F. D. Unregulated emissions from three-way catalyst cars. Paper 770369, presented at the Society of Automotive Engineers International Automotive Engineering Congress, Detroit, March 1977.

Cadle, S. H., Williams, R. L. Gas and particle emissions from automobile tires in laboratory and field studies. J. Air Pollut. Control Assoc. 28:502, 1978.

Heywood, J. B. Pollutant formation and control in spark-ignition engines. In Chigier, N. A. (Ed.). Pollution Formation and Destruction in Flames. New York: Pergamon Press, 1976, pp. 135–164.

McConnell, W. A. Auto certification testing. Environ. Sci. Technol. 12:393, 1978.

Pierson, W. R., Brachaczek, W. W., Hammerle, R. H., et al. Sulfate emissions from vehicles on the road. J. Air Pollut. Control Assoc. 28:123, 1978.

Seizinger, D. E. Oxygenates in Exhaust Gases Subjected to Catalytic or Thermal Conversion. USERDA Report BERC/RI-75/1. Bartlesville, Oklahoma: Bartlesville Energy Research Center, 1975.

Starkman, E. S., Bowditch, F. W. Vehicular emission control. In Pitts, J. N., Metcalf, R. L. (Eds.). Advances in Environmental Science and Technology, Vol. 7. New York: Wiley, pp. 55–73, 1977.

Stork, E. D. The federal statutory automobile emission standards. In Pitts, J. N., Metcalf, R. L. (Eds.). Advances in Environmental Science and Technology, Vol. 7. New York: Wiley, pp. 29–54, 1977.

A. F. Gaudy, Jr.

33

Waste Water Treatment

33.1. Introduction

Serious students of environmental toxicology are already familiar with the general workings of the environment, which, when stripped of all its important but nonessential trappings, is the life support system: air–water–food. A goal shared alike by environmental toxicologists and environmental engineers is the successful care and control of the life support system. The brief coverage given it here is intended simply to help the reader position the technological subcycle within the great life supporting cycles—the hydrologic cycle and the carbon–oxygen cycle—which make our existence possible. Some familiarization with the work and areas of expertise of environmental engineers is as useful to environmental toxicologists as is knowledge of the toxicologists' work to environmental engineers. Thus the information provided in this chapter is intended more as an introduction to the unit processes and operations (the technological subcycle) employed by engineers to control the life support system than as a compilation of ways to treat or remove environmental toxicants. The latter type of information would indeed be useful but is beyond the scope of this chapter. In any event there would be many void spaces in such a broad narration because there are large gaps in our knowledge regarding removal and ultimate environmental fate of various toxicants. Detailed information on some of these is given in other chapters in this text. In this chapter we shall be more involved with the control of a general category of materials, waste organic matter, which can produce a variety of toxic effects when allowed to enter the environment without the necessary technological control.

Some, possibly many, toxic compounds are removed from water supplies and from waste waters, along with other contaminating materials, by the standard methods of treatment described below. Toxic compounds that are not removed by these methods should obviously be prevented from reaching the water resource. Where such compounds do appear in waste waters, additional treatments (tertiary or advanced) must be designed for removal of the specific compounds in a particular effluent before its discharge to the water resource is permitted. Testing for the presence of toxic compounds represents an additional and very large expense to the taxpayer which may be expected to increase the cost of water supplies to the consumer in the future.

33.2. Carbon–Oxygen Cycle

Figure 33.1 is a simplified diagram of the carbon–oxygen cycle. This important cycle is represented by the large circle. The upper portion of the circle is the synthetic leg of the cycle, and it is this photosynthetic portion that receives and captures the sun's energy and results in the fixation of inorganic carbon into organic compounds (the food supply) and release of a by-product, oxygen (the air supply), which permits aerobic heterotrophic life. The bottom half of the circle represents the decay leg of the carbon–oxygen cycle. For the cycle to be balanced, aerobic metabolism must govern in the decay leg. It is the control of this leg of the carbon–oxygen cycle that is of most vital overall concern to environmental technologists, and it is the determination not to discharge sufficient amounts of waste organic matter to create environmental pockets of

Figure 33.1 Carbon–oxygen–water cycle. Water supply and waste treatment comprise the major elements of the technological subcycle within the decay leg of the natural cycle.

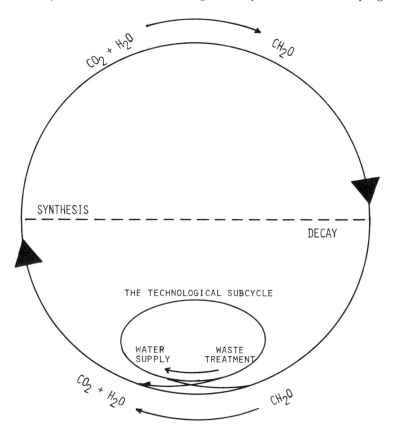

anaerobiosis that is the basic philosophy of PL 92-500, the law passed by Congress in 1972 in response to a public aroused and concerned over increasing water pollution.

What has water to do with the carbon–oxygen cycle? The cycle is biological in nature, and all of the vital biochemical reactions of life take place in an aqueous environment; this necessity for water makes it one of the triumvirate of the life support system. All of the other necessities of modern human life style, such as shelter, energy, education, health care, transportation, and recreation, are like icing on the cake compared to food, air, and water. Water is often the most critical ingredient because it is more scarce than the air supply. It is well known that we all live on the shore of a great sea of air (with some highly polluted local bays). Water is often the key factor in the development of an adequate food supply. Thus, it is for the most part the weak link in the life support system chain, and the protection from pollution of that supply which is available is of vital concern.

While control of air pollution is important, solution of air pollution problems is often best obtained through dispersal of the pollutant in the atmospheric ocean. Dilution is a useful solution to pollution in this case, but, because of the narrower confines of the liquid portion of the life support system, such a solution has not been possible except for some coastal cities where the continental shelf falls away sharply to the ocean depths. There is a relationship between air and water pollution because gaseous pollutants (toxic and nontoxic) can be transferred to atmospheric water and retained in the liquid, and thus be recycled by another natural cycle, the hydrologic cycle.

33.3. Hydrologic Cycle

All of the water in the world is subjected to purification and recycling by the physical processes of evaporation and condensation. This cycle not only provides a supply of pure water and a means of carrying away wastes but also serves to temper climatic conditions on the earth through capture and redistribution of solar energy. Each year approximately 120,000 cubic miles of water are evaporated, mostly over the equatorial regions. For each gram of water evaporated, 600 calories of solar energy are absorbed (1000 btu/lb water). The moisture-laden air rises and migrates toward the poles, and, as the atmosphere cools, the water condenses, releasing the heat (over 10^{20} kg-cal/year) back to the atmosphere. This process is largely responsible for creation of the temperate zones, and the condensation of the water provides a water supply with which to maintain the carbon–oxygen cycle.

It should be understood that transfer of other elements essential to life also occurs in cycles involving physical and biological phenomena. Cycling of nitrogen, sulfur, and phosphorus is vital to the maintenance of the life cycle. Nitrogen and sulfur participate in cycles involving the liquid and gaseous phases of the hydrologic cycle and are distributed through the processes of evaporation and condensation because they can exist in gaseous as well as liquid forms. Phosphorus is restrained from free participation in this recycling scheme because there are no gaseous forms of phosphorus. The reader should refresh his or her knowledge of the ways in which these other vitally important elements are cycled.

33.4. Technological Subcycle

Mankind, through social and technological activity, has become a major factor, for better or for worse, in the function of the great natural cycles of water and the elements essential to life. For reasons given earlier, we shall be more concerned with technology as it affects the water supply, although we must also be aware of the long-term effects of social and technological activity on atmospheric and climatic quality. The technological subcycle is a result of the sociological development of mankind. It should be remembered that as soon as the first small band of humans came together for reasons of common benefit (a social occurrence), some form of technology and management of the society was born, and it was originated in order to sustain the community life with respect to food and water; that is, technology at an ever-increasing level of knowledge has become a part of the life of mankind.

Figure 33.2 presents a more detailed look at the interior loop shown in Figure 33.1. The technological cycle as shown in this figure operates essentially in the decay leg of the carbon–oxygen cycle and is intimately associated with the hydrosphere. Beginning with the left half of the cycle, water obtained from ground or surface supplies originates from two sources: first, water delivered by

Figure 33.2 Technological subcycle. Toxicants can enter at any place in the cycle but some major points of entry are runoff from agricultural applications and some industrial effluents.

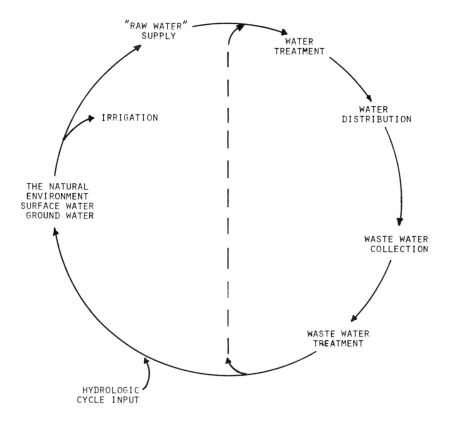

the hydrologic cycle, which has been purified by evaporation and condensation, and, second, water delivered to the natural environment as used water, which has been purified by natural processes and by technological processes that have been placed in the path of the return flow for the express purpose of removing unwanted material. In different localities, the proportions of the water supply derived from the two sources vary over a broad range. The most important of the unwanted constituents in water returned to the environment is excess organic matter, which is removed in order to prevent that portion of the decay leg which takes place in an aqueous environment from becoming anaerobic. On the left-hand side of the figure, water is removed from the environment for support of food production, crops, forage, fish, and game and for direct use as municipal and industrial water supplies. Most of the water resource is used for purposes other than to support human life. That portion used for this purpose must be highly purified, and a raw water supply is seldom in such condition.

There are two major reasons for the increasing cost of treating water. First, the water supply in many locations contains increasing amounts of contaminants that are deleterious and/or undesirable for human ingestion. This comes about because an increasing fraction of the water supply is made up of return flow (used water). Second, increasing human activity and expanding knowledge produce, on the one hand, more pollutants (toxicants) and, on the other, more concern over the potential health hazard. This turnabout is familiar to toxicologists who, on the one hand, may be involved in producing toxicants for a specific beneficial purpose, such as the production of pesticides to enhance the food supply, and, on the other hand, are involved in assessing the fate and effect of these materials on other segments of the life support system such as the air and water supply.

The reader can readily appreciate the many possible points of entry of toxic materials to the water subcycle shown in Figure 33.2. Various toxicants can invade the cycle from sources such as manufacturing, mining, and agricultural, commercial, and household activities or even natural sources (e.g., salts and minerals). Neither water nor waste water treatment systems have traditionally been designed for removal of toxic materials (except in specific cases of treatment of known toxic waste streams). Monitoring of such materials has not been generally performed. We have attempted to obtain uncontaminated water supplies and to prevent their contamination, and we have usually not tested water supplies (or treated waste waters) for specific toxic compounds.

It can be argued that one does not need to prepare all the water supply used by a community for human ingestion. There are two general arguments against this, however. First, one would need a multiple distribution system, and this would be extremely costly in view of the fact that the cost to the public of the distribution system is much more than the cost of treating the water. Second, even though most of the treated water that is delivered to the consumer is not used directly for drinking, a good deal of it comes in direct or indirect contact with humans (cleaning and preparing food, bathing, etc.). The possibility of contamination with disease-causing microorganisms or with toxic or harmful materials makes it highly desirable to ensure that the supply that is delivered to the tap is suitable for human ingestion. A large proportion of the water used in households, and in businesses and industry as well, is used for carrying away unwanted matter suspended or dissolved in the water.

33.4.1. Water Treatment and Distribution

With the need for treatment of the raw water supply firmly established, it is important to become familiar with some of the contaminants and the processes used for removing them.

33.4.1.a. Raw Water Reservoir

The treatment, as well as the pollution, of the water supply begins in the reservoir, ground or surface, into which the raw water is gathered naturally or by technological intervention. Usually water is benefited by long detention in a surface reservoir. Natural biological activity and sedimentation usually bring about considerable purification if the watershed and the immediate area of the reservoir are subject to close monitoring and surveillance and are well managed. The fact that water is a multipurpose resource is brought into sharp focus because many raw water supply reservoirs are also employed for recreational purposes, camping, swimming, boating, fishing, etc., and can be contaminated by those using them. Ground water reservoirs are equally in need of technological surveillance and monitoring because they cover a wide area underlying both public and private lands. They can be easily subjected to pollution due to contaminants seeping through the soil to the ground water table. Thus it is clear that the relatively pure water delivered by the hydrologic cycle is, after its collection in some type of reservoir, generally no longer in ideal condition for use at the tap. Some of the constituents removed from raw waters and the processes employed for their treatment are discussed below.

33.4.1.b. Removal of Calcium and Magnesium

Excessive amounts of calcium and magnesium are responsible for a water characteristic referred to as "hard" water. Such waters form suds poorly with normal household soaps (potassium and sodium salts of certain fatty acids). Calcium and magnesium form complexes with the fatty acids of soap; these are insoluble and form scums that not only prevent the use of the soap as a cleanser but contribute extra material to be removed. There are various options that may be employed when the raw water is hard. It can be treated to remove the hardness; this can be accomplished by precipitating the calcium and magnesium as hydroxides. Various procedures for addition of either lime or lime and soda ash are commonly employed, depending upon the anions that are associated with the calcium and magnesium cations. Ion exchange is another chemical process commonly used to soften water. The offending cations are exchanged for those that do not interfere with the sudsing and cleansing action of soaps, e.g., sodium and, in some cases, hydrogen.

As another alternative, one can switch to cleansers that do not form insoluble soaps with calcium and magnesium. This alternative was largely responsible for the wide usage of detergents (which do not form insoluble salts of calcium and magnesium). However, the detergents themselves became an environmental issue because many were nonbiodegradable organic compounds, and the persistence of the detergent in the environment caused foaming in public water supplies. Today the problem of hard water, i.e., water of greater than 75 mg/liter hardness expressed as calcium carbonate, is handled by a combination of softening and the use of biodegradable detergent compounds.

33.4.1.c. Removal of Iron and Manganese

Excessive amounts of iron and manganese are sometimes found in both surface and ground waters, but they are more commonly a problem in ground water supplies. In reduced form Fe^{2+} and Mn^{2+} are colorless, but upon exposure to oxygen they are oxidized to Fe^{3+} and Mn^{3+}, which exist as highly colored precipitates and discolor or stain plumbing fixtures. Ground waters are usually devoid of oxygen; therefore, when these waters are oxygenated, the precipitates are formed. Formation of such precipitates by aeration at the water treatment plant is much more desirable than their formation at the consumer's tap. Thus aeration is a common treatment for removal of iron and manganese in water supplies.

33.4.1.d. Removal of Turbidity

Many surface waters contain various amounts of colloidal organic and inorganic matter that, in very low concentrations, is apparent to the naked eye when light strikes the water. The suspended matter may be largely inorganic (e.g., clay), organic (e.g., decaying vegetation), or a combination of both. The colloids generally carry a negative surface charge, and they can be incorporated into larger particles formed as a precipitate upon addition of various chemicals. Ferric chloride and lime or alum are often added, resulting in the formation of insoluble hydroxides that attract and entrap the negatively charged colloidal materials. Care must be taken to provide rapid ("flash") mixing followed by slow mixing to allow the flocculated particles to build in size and weight; this is followed by a period of quiescent settling to allow subsidence of the precipitate.

33.4.1.e. Filtration

Following the treatments previously described, most waters are passed through a bed of specially graded sand or other suitable medium in order to entrap bits of suspended particles not removed by flocculation and subsidence. The granules of the filter medium also serve as surfaces for adsorption of suspended solids and as surfaces of attachment for microorganisms that can extract soluble pollutants from the waters.

33.4.1.f. Disinfection

The processes of precipitation and filtration described above are responsible for removal of most of the organisms that may be present in a water supply. However, there is no guarantee that the water will be essentially free of disease-causing organisms until it is disinfected. Chemicals are by far the most widely used means of disinfecting water supplies.

Chlorine is by far the most widely used chemical disinfectant. Chlorine is a potent oxidizer of organic matter and probably destroys living cells in many ways, not the least of which is the oxidation of microbial enzymes that are active only in the reduced state. However, chlorine combines with many other types of organic matter, and the formation of certain chlorinated organic compounds has recently been linked to cancer. If the water has been purified to a high degree prior to chlorination, there should be little organic matter to form chloroorganic compounds, and chlorination should serve as an excellent safeguard against disease-causing organisms. However, chlorination has, for many years, been employed at water treatment plants for purposes other than the final polishing treatment. Chlorination of waters prior to rapid sand filtration has often been practiced as a means of extending the time between backwashing operations. Furthermore, depending on the degree of contamination of the raw water supply, prechlorination has been practiced. These practices have recently been shown to be a major source of chloroorganic compounds. Where disinfection or oxidation of organic matter prior to or during treatment is desirable, substitutes for chlorination that do not produce harmful by-products are needed so that postchlorination can be used to protect the water in the distribution system. One of the most frequently used substitutes for chlorine is ozone.

Ozone is an even more potent oxidizing agent than chlorine. It has an overriding disadvantage in comparison to chlorine in that it leaves no residual disinfecting power as the finished water moves through the distribution system to the consumer. One advantage that has been claimed for it is that it does not produce organic by-products known to be harmful to humans. Such an advantage looms large in view of recent findings regarding chloroorganic compounds. In point of fact, little is known about the nature of organic by-products of ozonation or their effects in the human system. The lack of residual killing power and the cost of ozone-generating equipment are usually cited as the reasons it has not competed well with chlorine for use in the United States. It is rather widely employed in Europe, especially in France, and may become more popular in other locations due to fears over possible hazards of chlorination.

33.4.2. Waste Water Collection

After its preparation in the water treatment plant and its distribution and use by various types of consumers, water performs one of its most important functions. It removes unwanted material by serving as the universal solvent and carrier of suspended matter. The collection system differs from the distribution system in a number of ways. First, flow in sewers is usually by gravity rather than by pressure flow, as in the distribution system. Second, disinfection of waste water prior to entry into the collection system is not generally practiced. Microorganisms can proliferate in sewers, which often leads to problems because, even though the sewer is vented approximately every 300 ft and the sewer pipe does not flow full, there is often insufficient aeration to permit aerobic metabolism. If the grade of the sewer is rather low and the time of travel to the outfall rather long, anaerobiosis develops in the sewage, leading to the production of hydrogen sulfide, which volatilizes and condenses in the aqueous film covering the sewer pipe above the water line. Here aerobic autotrophic microorganisms can oxidize the hydrogen sulfide to sulfuric acid, which destroys the concrete (the material of which most large sewers are made), leading ultimately to structural failure of the sewer.

The cost of building the collection systems far outweighs the cost of building the waste water treatment plants into which the sewered material is channeled.

Thus, efforts are sometimes made along the collection system, either "in-line" or "on-line," to enhance aerobic conditions in the liquid or to avert microbial metabolism. Injection of ozone into the sewage may be a useful practice since its disinfecting power should slow the metabolism of organic matter, and the breakdown product, oxygen, dissolves in the water to encourage aerobic metabolism by the cells that are not inhibited or killed by the ozone. The installation of aeration stations along the route can also help to prevent odors and structural problems in the sewers due to acid production.

33.4.3. Waste Water Treatment

Waste water treatment may be subdivided into four categories, three of which pertain to the removal of organic pollutants. These are primary, secondary, and tertiary treatment. The fourth category pertains to removal of other materials such as nitrogen, phosphorus, and other inorganic ions or salts; this is referred to as advanced waste treatment. There are differences of opinion among pollution control engineers and scientists regarding the definition of each category, and the reader must be careful to discern an author's meaning in regard to these terms. The distinction made above is probably that used by the majority of practicing professionals.

We may distinguish another category of treatment as pretreatment. This term is acquiring a rather specific meaning as that treatment which may be required for various industrial wastes before their discharge to a publicly owned collection and treatment system is allowed. Such pretreatment may be required to bring the concentration of a biologically available carbon source to that generally considered representative of municipal wastes in the particular locale, or to remove or reduce concentrations of specific toxic or hazardous compounds. The latter objective is assuming great significance not only because of the general potential environmental hazard but because such compounds can hamper the effectiveness of the municipal plants, which are, under public law (PL) 92-500, underwritten for up to 75% of their cost by federal tax monies. Industrial and/or commercial wastes that are not sewered to a public system may be subjected individually to primary, secondary, tertiary, or advanced treatment as dictated by the nature of the waste and the stringency of the effluent standards imposed. Figure 33.3 shows a general layout of the various categories of treatment for a municipal sewage treatment plant providing relatively "complete" treatment.

33.4.3.a. Primary Treatment

The purpose of primary treatment is to remove settleable or screenable organic material that has been held in suspension in the waste water during transit in the sewer. Primary treatment is usually carried out under quiescent conditions in a settling basin or tank with a mean hydraulic retention time of 1–3 hr. The heavy organic solids settle to the bottom, where they are collected by a scraper mechanism. Solids with a specific gravity less than that of the liquid (e.g., fatty materials) "float" to the top, where they are skimmed and collected.

The collected solid materials are a waste product of treatment that must be disposed of in some way. These materials are often treated by an anaerobic biological process (digestion), wherein a significant fraction of the organic matter is converted to carbon dioxide, methane, and low molecular weight organic

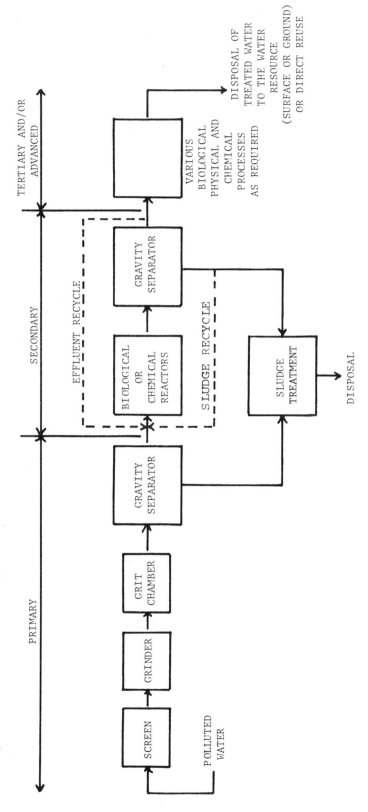

Figure 33.3 Generalized flow diagram for a municipal sewage treatment plant showing primary, secondary, tertiary, and advanced treatment. This figure shows the usual sequence in which the various unit operations and processes mentioned in the text are assembled. This should not be considered a typical flow diagram; modern design dictates assembling the unit processes and operations according to the specific character of specific waste waters.

acids. The solid material remaining after anaerobic digestion contains little putrescible organic matter and can be disposed of on land or buried. Other widely practiced disposal methods are drying and incineration of the sludge and aerobic digestion.

In some waste waters, notably municipal wastes, rather dense inorganic sand and grit particles are carried along in the sewer. These are usually removed in settling basins (grit chambers) before reaching the primary settling tank. Detention times of 1–3 min suffice to "drop out" the grit while leaving the organic particles in suspension for later removal in the primary settling tank. Thus inorganic and organic particles are "classified" due to their different settling velocities. The grit is nonputrescible and can be disposed of easily on land. Sometimes the waste water is channeled to a shredder prior to entry to the primary settling tank. The shredder functions essentially as a large garbage grinder. The plant equipment is usually protected by placement of a bar screen or a rack in front of the shredder and grit chamber.

Primary treatment can be accomplished by flotation as well as by settling. Particles that settle slowly can often be separated from the liquid more easily by enhancing their flotation rather than their subsidence. Particles more dense than the bulk density of the liquid can be floated due to their attachment to finely divided air bubbles. Often a more concentrated sludge can be produced by flotation than by subsidence. The density of the sludge produced during settling can be increased by addition of a flocculating chemical prior to entry into the primary tank. This is not usually done since the colloidal organic matter passing the primary settling tank can be removed by secondary treatment.

The effectiveness of primary treatment in removing pollution-causing organic matter is in direct proportion to the fraction of the putrescible organic matter that may be termed settleable solids, i.e., the portion that is removable in the mean hydraulic retention time allowed for primary settling. For municipal wastes this may amount to 25–40% of the BOD of the waste. The BOD is actually a measure of the amount of oxygen consumed during growth and autodigestion of the biomass using a specific amount of the waste water in a standard incubation time. The standard incubation time usually employed is 5 days, and the term BOD_5 has come into wide usage. The use of this bioassay procedure has become a very controversial issue in the water pollution control field. The interested reader should consult some of the references listed at the end of this chapter for further discussion of this important subject.

33.4.3.b. Secondary Treatment

The purpose of secondary treatment is to remove nonsettleable putrescible organic matter, i.e., colloidal and soluble BOD. The most successful of the secondary processes are biological in nature; that is, the organic matter that causes the BOD is removed by microorganisms that use it as substrate for growth. Rather than having this organic matter removed biologically in the natural reactor—the receiving stream, in which there would be biological utilization of dissolved oxygen—it is removed in engineered growth reactors on shore prior to entry of the waste water into the water resource. As stated earlier, technology is "inserted" into the path of the return flow to the natural conduits and biological reactors in order that these natural reactors do not become stressed beyond their capacity to assimilate the organic substrate. Not all secondary treatment processes are biological in nature. Some involve chemical and physical processes.

33.4.3.c. Chemical–Physical Treatment

In the past, chemical treatment similar to that used for water supplies has been employed in certain instances in which the organic matter not removed in the primary process was mostly colloidal material. Two disadvantages militate against wide adoption of this process: (a) usually this treatment process will not yield the needed amount of organic removal, and (b) large amounts of highly putrescible sludge are produced.

Recently the use of activated carbon following precipitation of the colloids and chemical floc has been shown to be rather effective as a means of improving the efficiency of removal of organic matter. The percent removal for chemical treatment followed by activated carbon, i.e., chemical–physical treatment, depends on the amount of soluble organic material in the waste water that is adsorbable on activated carbon. This will vary from waste to waste. It should also be remembered that the bed of activated carbon over which the water is passed after chemical coagulation and settling of the precipitates acts as an attachment surface for microorganisms that could metabolize nonadsorbable organic matter as it passes through the bed of activated carbon. However, such beds are not well-aerated and may become anaerobic; also large amounts of growth on the carbon particles can cause serious clogging problems in the bed and can destroy the adsorbing power of the carbon surfaces. The cost of chemical treatment and replacement or regeneration of the activated carbon, coupled with the development of copious amounts of highly putrescible sludge, as well as sometimes erratic results, have recently led to decreased use of such chemical–physical treatment.

33.4.3.d. Biological Treatment Processes

Biological processes have the advantage of being "nature's way," but in a speeded up and controlled (i.e., engineered) manner. However, they have a disadvantage in that we are largely trying to control and speed up processes that we do not fully understand. It seems clear that biological ecosystems in nature as well as those under engineering control perform at their best and are most stable when they are characterized by slow growth and maturity, which imparts great diversity of species. Such systems have considerable internal stability when the inputs from the external environment, such as nutrient materials, contribute a small fraction of the overall food material and effect only small changes in the ecological balance of the system. Thus, the aim in biological treatment processes is to strive for rapid removal of the external carbon source while allowing for fairly slow growth in the feeding population. One can accomplish this by maintaining the biomass concentration at a high level in relation to the amount of food material. To do this one must provide for retention of the biomass in the system. There are two ways in which to accomplish this, and they involve the two major categories of biological treatment processes, the fluidized aeration tank (activated sludge processes) and the fixed bed reactors (e.g., trickling filters).

There are many variations of activated sludge processes, but in all of them the waste water flows into a growth reactor containing a heterogeneous microbial population. The liquid and the cells are mixed, and the cells are held in suspension by rapid agitation and/or diffused aeration. Either the mixing or the aeration provides the metabolic oxygen required for aerobiosis. A high concentration of the feeding population is maintained by returning to the reactor cells that have settled in a secondary settling tank, into which the effluent from the aerated reactor (activated sludge tank) flows. The overflow supernatant from the secondary clarifier or sedimentation tank is the purified waste water. The portion of the underflow sludge not recycled to the aeration tank is excess sludge and is subject to disposal in various ways, just as is the primary sludge.

In processes using fixed bed reactors, or biological contactors, the waste water is caused to flow through or over a fixed inert medium such as rock, ceramic, or plastic materials of various configurations. Microbial cells become attached to the surfaces and proliferate due to the assimilation of the organic nutrients flowing by them. Generally, a very large amount of biomass attaches to the surfaces. Due to hydraulic forces and to the weight of the microbial growth, continued build-up of the biomass on the medium surface is limited and eventually a "sloughing" of biomass occurs. Sloughing may occur continuously or periodically, depending largely on the rate of flow through the medium. The waste water "trickles" downward over and through the medium. The common term "trickling filter" is often used to describe such processes but is more descriptive of the rock beds of large diameter and shallow depth than of the more recently developed tower configurations using various types of plastic media. The contact bed treatment is followed by passage through a secondary clarifier. Sometimes the effluent, and less often the underflow, is recycled to the contact bed. The loading of waste water to the bed must be controlled so as not to clog the medium with growth or to so overload it that air that passes through the bed is insufficient to provide for aerobic metabolism.

Recently, another type of fixed bed reactor has come into usage. The medium consists of a series of rotating discs spaced 1–2 in. apart, mounted on a central axle positioned longitudinally in an open trough. The waste water is allowed to flow through the trough. The depth of flow is such that less than one-half of the disc is submerged. As the discs rotate they are continually wetted with waste water (submerged portion), and the thin film of liquid is lifted into the gaseous phase and aerated as the previously submerged portion of the disc emerges from the liquid. Copious biological slimes develop on the rotating discs and these are responsible for metabolism of the organic matter as it flows through the trough. The fluid is channeled through a secondary settling tank where sloughed material and suspended growth may be removed.

Any of the secondary biological treatment processes can remove 85–99% of the influent putrescible organic matter. The problems of accurate prediction of performance (the process design) and of reliable delivery of the performance predicted by the design after the process is "on stream" (operations) are of great concern in the pollution control field and are worthy of much more discussion than can be presented here. Biological treatment is the core of water pollution control, and interested readers are encouraged to delve into the voluminous literature on the subject (see the Suggested Reading list at the end of this chapter).

33.4.3.e. Tertiary Treatment

There are circumstances in which secondary treatment, even when performing at a high efficiency, cannot reliably deliver a sufficiently high degree of removal of organic matter. One of the most common problems involves the loss of some suspended solids, largely microbial cells, in the secondary clarifier effluent. It must be remembered that the individual microbial cells are of such low density and small size that they do not settle. If the separation process to be used is quiescent settling of mixed liquor or sloughed materials, the cells must exist in flocculated or clumped biological communities consisting of billions of cells. The mechanisms by which autoflocculation of various species of microorganisms, bacteria, protozoa, and fungi occurs and formation of readily settled floc particles comes about is not fully understood. However, it may be stated that it is generally observed to occur in older (slower growing) biomasses. There are times when the ecological make-up of the heterogeneous population, perhaps the predator–prey relationship of protozoa and bacteria, can become disordered, leading to excessive amounts of nonflocculated, suspended cells, which exit in the effluent. Standby sand filters may be used to remove the suspended solids that did not settle in the secondary clarifier. Since the cells were developed from the carbon source in the original waste water, this third line of defense, which backs up secondary treatment, is aptly termed tertiary treatment. Chemical flocculation of turbid secondary effluent also represents a form of standby tertiary treatment. A turbid effluent not only is unsightly, but the autodigestion of the cells requires oxygen, thereby imparting a BOD to the effluent.

Sometimes there may be excessive amounts of soluble organic matter (soluble BOD) in the effluent, and the waste water may be channeled to a polishing pond for fairly long-term detention. Shallow ponds (oxidation ponds) may be employed for this purpose, although there is danger here that the effluent from the oxidation pond may contain more organic matter than did the influent. Oxidation ponds are aerated biologically by algae; they are, in a sense, the carbon–oxygen cycle of Figure 33.1 in microcosm. Thus the carbon dioxide produced by bacterial metabolism of the organic matter in the inflowing waste is reconstituted into algal organic matter. The "trade-off" in organic matter does not constitute biological waste treatment unless the algae are removed before the effluent is discharged. Ponds with free discharge of effluent and no provision for removal of suspended solids were formerly considered a valid form of secondary treatment, but now they are only permitted as secondary treatment in areas where the evaporation rate is greater than the inflow rate to the pond (thus eliminating discharge to a receiving stream) or where provision is made to remove suspended solids. Oxidation ponds are also being employed as secondary treatment where ultimate disposal of the effluent on or through soil is technologically and economically feasible.

In summary, tertiary treatment is sometimes needed as a backup to secondary treatment to remove organic matter residual to the secondary processes. It may consist of chemical, physical, or biological processes.

33.4.3.f. Advanced Treatment

The purpose of advanced waste treatment is to remove material, other than organic material, that can cause stress to the natural body of water into which the waste must eventually pass. Among the constituents commonly in need of removal from municipal sewage are nitrogen and phosphorus. These are vital nutrients for biological growth and are removed to some extent during secondary treatment, but municipal sewage contains concentrations of nitrogen and phosphorus in excess of those needed for metabolism of the carbon sources they contain. The excess may pass into the receiving body, where it can encourage growth of photoautotrophs, e.g., algae, thus contributing to eutrophication of the receiving body. Nitrogen in reduced form (NH_3-N), actually exerts a BOD. The autotrophic nitrifying bacteria, (e.g., *Nitrosomonas* and *Nitrobacter*) use ammonia as an electron donor in energy-producing oxidation–reduction reactions for which oxygen is the final electron acceptor—just as it is for aerobic organotrophic metabolism. For this reason wastes containing excessive amounts of ammonia are often aerated beyond the carbonaceous stage; that is, nitrification is permitted to occur on shore at the treatment plant site rather than permitting this nitrogenous BOD to be exerted in the receiving stream.

In general, this is a good practice; it can be accomplished as an add-on process or it may be caused to take place in the secondary treatment reactor by slowing the growth rate beyond that needed to remove carbonaceous substrates. This usually requires extended holding times and/or reduced organic loadings to the secondary processes. Although nitrogen in the form of nitrate is less harmful to the receiving stream than is nitrogen in the form of ammonia, the nitrates are available for algal growth, and it is often necessary to remove this form of nitrogen as well. This may also be accomplished using biological processing. In the absence of dissolved oxygen, some organisms can use nitrate as an electron acceptor (the denitrifying organisms) thus reducing it to the gaseous form, N_2, wherein it escapes to the atmosphere. Some organisms, notably the blue-green bacteria, can fix N_2, so the nitrogen problem may not be entirely solved by nitrification–denitrification processes, but the course of eutrophication is certainly impeded by removal of excess nitrogen from waste waters.

Phosphorus is a critical nutrient because it is a vital element that is needed in only small concentrations. Its removal from waste waters certainly can impede the course of eutrophication, but in some agricultural areas phosphorus from fertilized soil finds its way to the receiving body. Some phosphorus is removed during the growth of microorganisms in secondary processes, and certain organisms can store rather significant amounts of phosphorus, providing some basis for biological treatment to remove this element. However, there are problems with maintenance of the required species in the biomass as well as problems of release of stored phosphorus, so that the method usually employed for removal of phosphorus is alkaline precipitation, i.e., addition of lime and formation of insoluble calcium phosphate.

Treatment to remove various inorganic salts and specific compounds may also be required, depending upon the waste water and the ultimate disposition of the effluent. Such processes as adsorption on activated carbon, chemical precipitation, ion exchange, and reverse osmosis are available. Another process is chemical oxidation of the organic and inorganic materials that may be present in the secondary or tertiary effluents. Disinfection, although usually considered a part of secondary treatment, is in a sense a form of advanced waste treatment because, if one uses chlorine or ozone to disinfect the waste, these general oxidants also oxidize a considerable amount of soluble and insoluble inorganic matter present in the effluent. This oxidation may be beneficial or harmful; we do not really know as yet. The addition of such chemical oxidants can have a definite impact on the aqueous environment.

33.4.3.g. Disposal and Utilization of Treatment Plant Effluents

It can be seen in Figure 33.2 that the technological subcycle within the carbon–oxygen–water cycle depicted in Figure 33.1 is essentially a closed loop. Advanced waste treatment interfaces with water supply treatment, with the natural receiving streams linking them together. The receiving streams may be looked upon as a form of advanced, slow treatment for the relatively pure water leaving the waste water treatment plant. Alternatively, the natural receiving streams may be looked upon as natural reservoirs for pure water. Although the goals of PL 92-500 favor the latter view, it most probably will be the former view which will, with considerable effort and public patience and perseverance, become the mode of successful operation and management of the aqueous environment.

It seems to this author that there is really no need to deny to the public the use of the natural purification capacity of the receiving streams at the expense of needed monies for education, transportation, energy development, etc. in order to achieve "zero" pollutant discharge. The amendments made in 1977 appear to reinforce this point of view. It must be emphasized, however, that use of the natural assimilation capacity of the water resource requires close technological monitoring and control of the aqueous environment. It must also be borne in mind that disposal of partially treated waste water on land rather than into a receiving stream can impregnate far-reaching ground water reservoirs with toxic materials. The needed monitoring of ground and surface waters will require the services of many environmental engineers and scientists skilled in water, waste water, stream, and ground water quality management, and also of scientists skilled in toxicology and assessment of the environmental fate of the vast numbers of new (and old) compounds entering the life support system.

Suggested Reading

American Water Works Association. Water Quality and Treatment, third edition. New York: McGraw-Hill, 1971.

Culp, R. L., Culp, G. L. Advanced Wastewater Treatment. New York: Van Nostrand Reinhold, 1971.

Gaudy, A. F., Jr., Gaudy, E. T. Biological Concepts for Design and Operation of the Activated Sludge Process. EPA Report 17090 FQJ 09/71. Washington, D.C.: U.S. Government Printing Office, 1971.

Leh, F. K. V., Lak, R. K. C. Environment and Pollution. Springfield, Ill.: Thomas, 1974.

Mackenthun, K. M. The Practice of Water Pollution Biology. Washington, D.C.: U.S. Department of the Interior, 1969.

Metcalf & Eddy, Inc. Wastewater Engineering. New York: McGraw-Hill, 1972.

Mitchell, R. (Ed.). Water Pollution Microbiology. New York: Wiley, 1972.

National Academy of Sciences. Principles for Evaluating Chemicals in the Environment. Washington, D.C., 1975.

Nemerow, N. L. Liquid Waste of Industry. Reading, Mass.: Addison-Wesley, 1971.

The Biosphere. Sci. Am. Vol. 223, 1970.

J. Robie Vestal

34

Pollution Effects
of Storm-Related Runoff

34.1. Introduction

Storm water is the direct response of atmospheric precipitation in the form of rain, snow, sleet, etc. The runoff from storm water can solubilize and/or transport many different types of organic and inorganic chemicals and particulate matter to a receiving water (stream, river, lake, estuary, or ocean). If these components impair the natural quality of the receiving water, they can be considered as pollutants. In this chapter the sources of pollution carried by storm water runoff and the effect of pollutants on receiving water quality are discussed. "Clean" water is essential for all life forms but is particularly important to humans for drinking, recreational use, industry, etc.

When it rains, the water impinges on either pervious (soil, lawns, etc.) or impervious (streets, roofs, parking lots, etc.) surfaces. The water is usually absorbed by the pervious surface until it becomes saturated. Continued rain will cause the water to pool or flow across the surface. If water strikes an impervious surface, it flows or pools immediately. Any debris containing chemicals will thus be washed away in the water. This effect holds true for solid water (snow or ice) as it melts due to increasing temperature. The runoff water becomes a vector for any component caught in its flow.

Depending on the urban area, storm-water runoff usually flows in a storm sewer, combined sewer, or no sewer. Storm sewers, found in about 38.3% of the urban areas in the United States, are separate sewer lines that collect the storm-water runoff from impervious areas. The water is carried, usually by gravity, directly to the receiving water, where it is expelled without treatment. Combined sewers, found in about 14.4% of urban areas, consist of storm sewer lines connected to sanitary sewer lines. When stormwater is present, it is usually treated through the sanitary sewage treatment process. This process, however, is constructed such that when the maximum flow for the sewage treatment plant is reached, any overflow is expelled into the receiving water directly. If the storm-water runoff is overflowing during a storm, any sanitary sewage also overflows, thus expelling raw sewage into the receiving water. About 47.3% of urban areas have no sewered storm drainage.

In the following discussion the sources of pollutants found in stormwater runoff are considered, but no distinction is made between combined and separate storm-water sewers; the reader should keep the distinction in mind when considering urban runoff.

34.2. Urban Runoff

In the United States, about 70% of the total human population is concentrated into urban areas covering about 3% of the land surface. The density is, on the average, 5.1 people/acre (12.6 people/ha). The daily activities of such a dense population require the use of many natural resources. This use produces waste (personal, commercial, or industrial) that eventually is discharged into the atmosphere, land, or natural waters. These wastes can be toxic to the normal biota. During storms, a significant amount of the air-borne pollutants and land-dispersed pollutants can be solubilized by the water to contribute to water pollution.

In the urban setting, pervious areas are rapidly being changed to impervious areas (e.g., streets, houses, parking lots, and buildings). Impervious areas cause the production of more runoff during a storm. Thus, storm-water runoff pollution is increased by more urbanization.

There are four types of land use in the urban setting: construction, industry, streets and highways, and residential. The process of construction involves site preparation and then the actual construction of the building, road, sewer, etc. During site preparation, the normal, pervious soil is removed. When a storm occurs, the subsoil erodes and the runoff contains a large amount of sediment. With the sediment, toxic compounds and inorganic nutrients are often leached. During site preparation dust is generated that can be widely dispersed. During the initial phases of a storm, this dust becomes water borne and is eventually washed away in the runoff. Associated with construction are common industrial pollutants such as oils used as machinery lubricants, metals and inorganic chemicals leached or corroded from various building materials, and organic waste associated with litter and food.

Contributions to storm-water runoff pollution from industry occur through leaching from stockpiles of materials, the handling of materials, leakage from corroded pipes or storage facilities, and dissolving of other pollutants on exposed surfaces. Process gases, which can become water borne as dustfall or washout, can have a detrimental effect due to toxicity, pH, heavy metals, oils, etc.

Streets and highways carry people and commerce. Pollutants accumulate in the air as exhaust emissions and dust and on the street surface as rubber, oil, lead compounds, asbestos, etc. Most streets are either concrete or asphalt, which are highly impervious materials. Erosion of particulates and asphaltic materials from these surfaces is also carried in storm-water runoff. The initial movement of water across an impervious area at the beginning of a storm event, which picks up these pollutants, is referred to as the first flush. This action can initially perturb a receiving water drastically due to the accumulation of pollutants. It is followed by a dilution effect. As the period of time between storms increases, the amount of pollutants accumulating on impervious surfaces also increases. After a long dry period, a storm could release a drastic pollutional load in the first flush. Typical amounts of various pollutants that can accumulate on impervious surfaces as a result of industrial, commercial, and residential traffic are listed in Table 34.1. It is obvious that a first flush runoff will not only carry large amounts of solid materials, but also significant amounts of inorganic nutrients (contributing to eutrophication), toxic heavy metals, and carcinogenic chemicals. Clearly, storm-water runoff can be the source of considerable water pollution.

During the winter, in the latitudes that have significant snowfall, air-borne pollutants can be adsorbed to snow. Typical levels of various pollutants associated with snow deposits are presented in Table 34.2. During the spring thaw, a major pollutional load is released.

Another significant source of inorganic chemicals that are detrimental to water quality is the practice of ice and snow control on roadways. In addition to sand

Table 34.1   Rates of Accumulation of Roadway Materials as a Result of Traffic (Washington, D.C., Metropolitan Area)

Parameter	Rate[a]	
	lb/axle-mile	g/axle-mile
Dry weight	2.38×10^{-3}	6.71×10^{-4}
Volatile solids	1.21×10^{-4}	3.41×10^{-5}
BOD	5.43×10^{-6}	1.53×10^{-6}
COD	1.28×10^{-4}	3.61×10^{-5}
Grease	1.52×10^{-5}	4.28×10^{-6}
Total phosphate-P	1.44×10^{-6}	4.06×10^{-7}
Orthophosphate-P	4.31×10^{-8}	1.21×10^{-8}
Nitrate-N	1.89×10^{-7}	5.33×10^{-8}
Nitrite-N	2.26×10^{-8}	6.37×10^{-9}
Kjeldahl-N	3.72×10^{-7}	1.05×10^{-7}
Chloride	2.20×10^{-6}	$6.2 \ \times 10^{-7}$
Petroleum	8.52×10^{-6}	$2.4 \ \times 10^{-6}$
n-Paraffins	5.99×10^{-6}	1.69×10^{-6}
Asbestos	3.86×10^{5b}	2.39×10^{5b}
Rubber	1.24×10^{-5}	3.49×10^{-6}
Lead	2.79×10^{-5}	7.86×10^{-6}
Chromium	1.85×10^{-7}	5.21×10^{-8}
Copper	2.84×10^{-7}	8.00×10^{-8}
Nickel	4.40×10^{-7}	1.24×10^{-7}
Zinc	3.50×10^{-6}	9.86×10^{-7}
Cadmium	3.11×10^{-8}	8.76×10^{-9}
Magnetic fraction	1.26×10^{-4}	3.55×10^{-5}
PCBs	$1.0 \ \times 10^{-9}$	2.82×10^{-10}
Litter dry weight	1.69×10^{-4}	4.76×10^{-5}
Litter BOD	3.49×10^{-7}	9.84×10^{-3}

Source: Shaheen, D.G. Contributions of Urban Roadway Usage to Water Pollution. EPA-600/2-75-004 (NTIS No. PB 245 854), Environmental Protection Agency, 1975.

[a]An axle-mile is the length traversed for each axle of a vehicle. Hence in traveling 1 mile, a two-axle vehicle will contribute 2 axle-miles.

[b]In fibers/axle-mile and fibers/axle-km.

and cinders, chemical preparations (e.g., NaCl, $CaCl_2$, NH_4NO_3, marine salt, urea, Prussian blue) are used. During an early thaw, these compounds become dissolved in the runoff and can have drastic effects on a receiving water by affecting pH and ionic strength.

The quantity of pollutants generated in residential areas generally depends on the population density, although standard of living and amount of open space can have an effect. The common pollutants collected by storm-water runoff include organic materials, (pesticides, leaf litter, grass cuttings, etc.), bacteria (from human and animal excreta), and inorganic nutrients (from fertilizers). Significant amounts of asphaltic materials from roofs can also be associated with storm-water runoff. The same types of pollutants associated with dustfall due to traffic can be found in residential streets.

Table 34.2 Levels of Pollutants Found in Snow Deposits

Pollutant and location	Windows adjacent to street (mg/kg)	Snow disposal sites (mg/kg)
Suspended solids		
Arterial street	3570	—
Collectors	1920–4020	—
Local	1215–2530	—
Parking lot	1620	—
BOD		108[a,b]
Arterial street	16.6	—
Collectors	13.2	—
Local	5.5	—
Parking lot	5.5	—
Chlorides	0–4500	175–2250
Oils	28.6[a]	28.6[a]
Greases	19.6[a]	19.6[a]
Phosphates		1.5[a]
Arterial street	0.032[a]	—
Collectors	0.087[a]	—
Local	0.065[a]	—
Lead		0.9–9.5
Residential	2[a]	—
Industrial	4.7[a]	—
Commercial	3.7[a]	—
Highway	102.0	—
Cadmium	—	<0.05
Barium	—	<0.50
Zinc	—	0.6
Copper	—	0.19
Iron	—	30.0
Chromium	—	<0.02
Arsenic	—	<0.02

Source: J.L. Richards and Associates, Ltd., and Labrecque, Verina and Associates. Snow Disposal Study for the National Capital Area Technical Discussion. Report for the Committee on Snow Disposal, Ottawa, Ont., Canada, 1973.

[a]Mean concentration at all sites.

[b]In mg/liter.

As noted in the preceding discussion, dustfall and its components generated in the urban setting contribute significantly to the pollution of urban runoff. These pollutants can severely affect water quality. Typical daily accumulations of pollutants are listed in Table 34.3

34.3. Agricultural Runoff

The land area of the United States is about 2264×10^6 acres. Of this total, 47% (1064×10^6 acres) is classified as farm land. This includes croplands, grasslands and pastures, and feed lots. Croplands and pastures comprise about 36% and 51% of the total, respectively. Consequently, there is a great amount of land that can contribute to runoff pollution.

Croplands produce large amounts of sediment, inorganic and organic nutrients, and pesticides. Often cropland is plowed after fall harvest, which allows the land to be exposed to fall rains. The erosion of cropland, in addition to contributing pollutants, also removes significant amounts of fertile soil. As a result, more fertilizers have to be placed in the soil in order to grow crops during the next growing season. Fertilizers, containing nitrogen, phosphorus, and potassium, when washed into receiving waters, can cause eutrophication of the water. Herbicides and insecticides in addition to being a source of toxic compounds, can also contribute to the BOD and COD of the receiving waters. The stubble from crops after harvesting also contributes to the BOD and COD of receiving waters after storm-water runoff.

Grasslands and pastures are not normally disturbed by cultivation; thus their permanent cover is seldom removed. Storm-water runoff from these pervious areas is not a major source of pollution, although animal wastes can lower the quality of receiving waters.

Animal feed lots are relatively small areas in which large numbers of animals are fed before being slaughtered. Consequently, there is a large build-up of animal waste in a small area in a short time. Storm-water discharges from feed lots are very high in soluble organic compounds, solids, nitrogen, and especially bacteria. Cattle produce about 6.5 times as much excrement as humans.

34.4. Mining Runoff

Although a small percentage of the total land area of the United States is affected by mining operations (0.5%), the runoff from mining operations can cause pollution of usually pristine receiving waters. A classic example is acid mine drainage, which is associated with pyritic coal strata in, for example, the Appalachian coal region. The reduced iron and sulfur are oxidized chemically, and biologically by bacteria of the genus *Thiobacillus*, to produce ferric hydroxide precipitates and sulfuric acid. The final pH of most acid drainages is 2.5–4.0. There are numerous accounts of the first flush introducing great amounts of acid into recreational lakes, resulting in serious fish kills. Many municipalities whose drinking water must come from acid-contaminated streams must use large amounts of limestone to neutralize the water and precipitate the salts before the water is potable. As acid mine drainage percolates over or through strata containing heavy metals (e.g., arsenic, uranium, and copper), these metals can be solubilized and contribute to lowered water quality.

Table 34.3 Average Daily Dust and Dirt Accumulation and Related Pollutant
Concentrations for Residential (Single and Multiple Family), Commercial,
and Industrial Sites

| Location | Dust and Dirt Accumulation (lb/curb-mile/day) | | N^a |
	Mean	Range	
Chicago	$158(44)^b$	$19–536(5–15)^b$	334
Washington	134(38)	36–365(10–103)	22
Multicity	175(49)	3–1,500(1–423)	44

| Pollutant | Accumulation (mg/kg/day) | | N |
	Mean	Range	
BOD	5030	1,288–14,540	292
COD	46,120	18,300–498,410	292
Total N	480	323–480	270
Kjeldahl-N	640	230–1,790	22
NO_3-N	24	10–35	21
NO_2-N	15	0	15
Total PO_4	170	90–340	21
PO_4-P	53	0–142	291
Chlorides	220	100–370	22
Asbestos	57.2×10^{6c}	$0–172.5 \times 10^{6c}$	16
Ag	200	0–600	3
As	0	0	3
Ba	38	0–80	8
Cd	3.1	0–11.0	57
Cr	180	10–430	65
Cu	90	25–810	65
Fe	21,220	5,000–48,000	45
Hg	0.02	0–0.1	6
Mn	410	160–700	45
Ni	62	1–170	65
Pb	1,970	0–7,600	64
Sb	54	50–60	3
Se	0	0	3
Sn	17	0–50	3
Sr	21	0–110	45
Zn	470	90–3,040	65
Fecal streptococci	370^d	$44–2,420^e$	17
Fecal E. coli	$94,700^d$	$26–1,000,000^e$	287
Total E. coli	$1,070,000^d$	$18,000–5,600,000^e$	290

Source: Manning, M.J., et. al. Nationwide Evaluation of Combined Sewer Overflows and Urban Stormwater Discharges Vol. 3: Characterization of Discharges. EPA-600/2-77-604C, Environmental Protection Agency, 1977.

[a]Number of observations.

[b]Value in parentheses is in kg/curb-km/day.

[c]In fibers/lb; in fibers/kg, mean 126×10^6, range $0–380 \times 10^6$.

[d]Geometric mean in number/g.

[e]In number/g.

34.5. Runoff from Forests and Woodlands

Storm-water runoff from forests and woodlands usually does not contribute significantly to water pollution. The soil is very pervious and absorbs rainfall well. Sometimes organisms from decaying leaf-litter and nutrients from the soil can be washed away after soil saturation due to heavy precipitation. Pollution associated with forests mainly occurs when they are disturbed by logging operations, particularly clear-cutting. This allows for sediment, organic compounds, inorganic nutrients, and soil bacteria to be washed into receiving waters during storms.

34.6. Summary

Storm-water is a serious source of water pollution. While precipitation can "cleanse" the environment, its runoff can serve as a vector for many toxic and nontoxic pollutants that add to the deterioration of the quality of natural waters. The first flush carries vast quantities of pollutants that have accumulated primarily due to human activities. The largest storm-water problem is associated with urban areas.

Abatement and control of storm-water pollution are difficult to accomplish due to the probabilistic nature of precipitation. The amount, duration, volume, and type of precipitation all affect the runoff, which makes prediction of pollution effects difficult. The topography and perviousness of the area, which are unique to each locale, also affect pollution abatement or treatment procedures. Qualitative studies have led to predictive modeling, but quantitative data are difficult to obtain because every storm is different. The problems introduced in this chapter demand careful consideration if ways of controlling or treating this type of water pollution are to be found.

Suggested Reading

Bartlett, R.E. Surface Water Sewerage. New York: Wiley, 1976.

Field, R., Olivieri, V.P., Davis, E.M., et al. Proceedings of Workshop of Microorganisms in Urban Stormwater. EPA-600/2-76-244, Cincinnati, 1976.

Heaney, J.P., Huber, W.C., Medina, M.A., et al. Nationwide Evaluation of Combined Sewer Overflows and Urban Stormwater Discharges, Vol. 2: Cost Assessment and Impacts. EPA-600/2-77-064b, Cincinnati, 1977.

Manning, M.J., Sullivan, R.H., Kipp, T.M. Nationwide Evaluation of Combined Sewer Overflows and Urban Stormwater Discharges, Vol. 3: Characterization of Discharges. EPA-600/2-/77-064c. Cincinnati, 1977.

Mitchell, R. (Ed.). Water Pollution Microbiology. New York:, Wiley, 1972.

Overton, D.E., Meadows, M.E. Stormwater Modeling. New York: Academic Press, 1976.

Sullivan, R.H., Manning, M.J., Heaney, J.P., et al. Nationwide Evaluation of Combined Sewer Overflows and Urban Stormwater Discharges, Vol. 1: Executive Summary. EPA-600/2-77-064a, Cincinnati, 1977.

Wanielista, M.P. (Ed.). Storm-water Management Workshop: Proceedings. Orlando, Fla.: Florida Technical University, 1975.

Wullschleger, R.E., Zanoi, A.E., Hansen, C.A. Methodology for the Study of Urban Storm Generated Pollution and Control. EPA-600/2-76-145, Cincinnati, 1976.

Thomas J. Schoenbaum
Donald Huisingh
Patricia E. McDonald

35

Legal Considerations

35.1. Introduction

Throughout this text the several authors have presented a diversity of perspectives on one toxicological problem or another. Many referred to governmental regulations and controls that have been or are being enacted and implemented with varying degrees of impact. In this chapter we provide a more detailed view of the historical development of the various legislative and regulatory approaches that have been or are being utilized to help protect human beings and the environment as a whole from undue stresses from toxic substances.

Three stages may be distinguished in the history of governmental attitudes toward the use of toxic and hazardous substances in the human environment. The first was a policy of laissez faire liberalism. In the 19th and early 20th centuries, the problem of hazardous substances was perceived not as a societal problem, but only as a matter of liability and duty between private individuals. A person or industry was free of governmental constraints in the use of potentially toxic substances but was liable for injury caused to other individuals under the private law system.

With the increasingly greater use of toxic pollutants and their introduction into the environment in the 20th century, it was recognized that protection of individuals could no longer be left to private law. Laws were passed and agencies were created, especially on the federal level, to regulate the use of these substances. Governmental intervention was piecemeal, however, responding only when the general public perceived a problem, such as occurred with respect to pesticides after publication of *Silent Spring* by Rachel Carson. The result was a patchwork of uncoordinated federal laws administered by dozens of governmental agencies; most of this legislation is still on the statute books.

The third stage in the evolution of governmental regulation of toxic substances, comprehensive administrative control, began with the passage of the Federal Toxic Substances Control Act of 1976. This law, which has yet to be fully implemented, gives the government broad authority to control the production, distribution, and use of all potentially hazardous chemicals and, in the words of one commentator, converts the chemical industry into a regulated industry. The effectiveness of this new law will depend upon how its complex provisions are administered by the EPA.

35.2. Private Law System

Under the private law system, the incentive to avoid activities that cause harm to other persons arises from the fact that the person causing injury or damage is liable to pay the value of the harm inflicted. Liability for injury to the person or to property is today for the most part based upon some moral or social fault, expressed in legal terms as a breach of duty owed to the plaintiff in a lawsuit. Our system of justice in general does not compensate people for injury suffered if the person causing the injury was not at fault in some way or guilty of at least negligent conduct.

A very early development of the common law that is still applied today, however, is that persons who engage in very hazardous activities or who use highly dangerous substances may be liable for injury caused to others irrespective of fault or negligence. This principle was established in the common law by the case of *Rylands v. Fletcher*, decided in England in 1868. The defendants in this case, mill owners in Lancashire, constructed a reservoir that broke, flooding the plaintiff's adjacent mine. The defendants were held liable despite the fact that they were free from any personal blame. The general rule evolved by the courts in England and later by a majority of U.S. jurisdictions is that where one person damages another by a thing or activity that is unduly dangerous and inappropriate to the place where it occurs or is maintained, there is "strict liability" for damages—which means the person injured can recover without proving negligence or fault on the part of the defendant.

This rule of private law has been applied to cases involving injury through the use of toxic substances such as pesticides. For example, in a 1949 case decided by the Supreme Court of Arkansas, *Chapman Chemical Company v. Taylor* [222 S.W.2d 820], the chemical company that supplied 2-4-D to a farmer who sprayed his rice crop was held liable without fault to a neighboring cotton farmer whose crop was damaged by the herbicide.

Despite this rule of strict liability, it is obvious that the private law system is grossly inadequate to protect people and society against the consequences of the widespread use of toxic substances that characterizes our economy today. First, the rule of liability does not prevent or regulate the use of such substances. Anyone is free to introduce any material into the environment as long as he is willing to risk potential liability. Second, the common law rule does not define those substances or activities that will be considered to invoke the principle of strict liability. This definition can only be developed on a case-by-case basis in the courts. Third, liability will be imposed only where the chain of causation is immediate and direct. We know, however, that in most cases threats to health and the environment from toxic materials are indirect or not evident until after many years and in many instances at locations distant from the point of discharge. The recognition of these defects of the private law system soon led to the passage by Congress of laws to deal with the most acute problems of the use of hazardous substances.

35.3. Regulation of Particular Target Problems

Over a period of many years, each time Congress perceived a particular difficulty with the use of toxic substances, it passed a law to deal with the narrow situation involved. The result is an uncoordinated series of legislative initatives aimed at solving immediate problems.

35.3.1. Radiation and Nuclear Materials

Since 1946, the federal government has exercised control over the production and use of atomic energy through the Atomic Energy Commission, which was reorganized in 1974 and replaced by the Nuclear Regulatory Commission (NRC) and the Energy Research and Development Administration (ERDA). Under the Atomic Energy Act of 1954, private parties are permitted to engage in the production of atomic energy for industrial and commercial purposes if they obtain a license issued by the NRC.

Due to early recognition of the danger of radioactive materials, the comprehensive scheme of regulation under the Atomic Energy Act includes source material, special nuclear material that is enriched for use in nuclear reactors, and by-product material that is generated as waste or by exposure to radiation. The NRC is authorized by law to enforce standards sufficient "to protect health or to minimize danger to life and property," and it has established maximum permissible releases by elements and isotopes of all types of radioactive materials. In addition, licensees of the NRC are asked to make every reasonable effort to maintain releases as far below the legal limits as possible. The standards developed by the NRC represent a judgment that certain levels of exposure to radiation are not harmful to humans. This has been the subject of controversy, but the NRC's authority in this area has been upheld in the courts. Neither an individual state nor another federal agency such as the EPA can require stricter standards.

Other federal agencies do regulate certain aspects of public protection against radiation hazards, however. The transportation of radioactive materials is under the jurisdiction of the Department of Transportation, the Federal Aviation Administration, the Postal Service, and the Coast Guard. These agencies have established standards for packaging and shipping radioactive materials. Workers in uranium mines are protected by regulations developed by the Department of Labor. The emission of radiation from electronic products is controlled by the Department of Health, Education and Welfare, which has established a Technical Electronic Products Radiation Safety Standards Committee to develop standards on a product-by-product basis. In addition, under the Marine Protection, Research, and Sanctuaries Act of 1972, no person is permitted to dump any radiological agent or high-level radioactive waste into the oceans.

35.3.2. Pesticides

Pesticides have long been regulated by the federal government. The Food, Drug and Cosmetic Act of 1938, as amended in 1954, gave the administrator of the FDA the power to establish tolerance limits for pesticide residues on raw agricultural commodities and processed foods. In addition, the Federal Insecticide, Fungicide and Rodenticide Act (FIFRA), passed in 1947, required the registration of all pesticides with the Department of Agriculture and the correct labeling of such products. FIFRA proved inadequate to deal with the problem, however, and in 1972 this law was overhauled and strengthened by Congress.

Under the amendments of 1972, FIFRA requires that any pesticide distributed or sold must first be registered with the EPA. Four criteria established by law must be met before any product can be registered: (a) "its composition is such as to warrant the proposed claims for it," (b) "its labeling and other material required to be submitted comply with the requirements of this Act," (c) "it will perform its intended function without unreasonable adverse effects on the environment," and (d) "when used in accordance with widespread and commonly recognized practice it will not generally cause unreasonable adverse effects on the environment."

In order to register a product, the applicant must submit data on its chemistry, potential hazards to humans and the environment, and its effectiveness. The EPA administratively invokes a "rebuttable presumption" against registration if the data submitted suggest high risk to humans or the environment. The burden of proof is then on the applicant to show that the economic, social, and environmental benefits outweigh the risk of use. The EPA has the power to register the pesticide for either general or restricted use only by certified applicators. In 1975, Congress provided a 2-year period to October 1977, for the reregistration of all pesticide products now in use. The requirement to consider some 46,000 pesticide products within 2 years proved to be an insurmountable task, however, and the EPA failed to meet this deadline. The EPA has also been slowed in its task of reexamining all pesticide products by the inadequacy of toxicological data submitted by pesticide manufacturers.

A registered pesticide must be sold under a label that states ingredient information, warning and caution statements, and directions for use and proper application. This information must be phrased in such a way as to be understandable by the layman and potential user. A manufacturer not complying with these requirements is subject to penalties for false and misleading labeling.

FIFRA also contains exceptions that allow the use of a pesticide without prior registration. First, the EPA is authorized to issue an experimental use permit to allow field testing of products before registration. Second, registration and labeling can be dispensed with in the event of an emergency, such as a pest outbreak, with the concurrence of the EPA. Third, states can register pesticides for "special local needs" and permit their use before federal registration has been accomplished. The EPA has 90 days to veto any state-registered use.

The EPA is also empowered by FIFRA to cancel the registration of any pesticide if it appears that the product or its labeling does not comply with the requirements of the law or causes "unreasonable adverse effects on the environment." The invocation of a cancellation proceeding does not in itself prevent the sale or distribution of the product involved; however, a hearing, which may go on for many years, must first be held to determine whether this step should be taken. If there is an "imminent hazard" from continued use of the pesticide, the EPA can take the more drastic action of registration suspension, which stops the sale and use immediately. The EPA is required to prepare an "economic impact analysis" at least 60 days before any notice to cancel or suspend a pesticide registration. This gives the Department of Agriculture an opportunity to comment on the decision. The most well-known cancellation and suspension decisions occurred between 1972 and 1975, when most applications of the persistent insecticides (DDT, aldrin, dieldrin, chlordane, and heptachlor) were discontinued.

Under present law, tolerance limits for pesticide residues on raw agricultural commodities and processed foods are established by the EPA. The FDA now only has the authority to enforce—by seizure of the products if necessary—the limits established by the EPA. A tolerance is the maximum permissible quantity (expressed in parts per million) of a particular substance in a particular food product. The EPA has generally rejected setting zero tolerances and has taken the view that permitting some level of pesticide residue is consistent with protection of the public health. The EPA also has the power to exempt any pesticide chemical from the tolerance requirement if the particular standard is not necessary to protect the public health.

Any person who distributes or sells an adulterated, mislabeled, or unregistered pesticide is guilty of a violation of law. It is also prohibited for any person to use a registered pesticide in a way different than permitted according to the label, although this requirement is difficult to enforce. Penalties against violators may include (a) criminal sanctions including fines and imprisonment for willful violators, (b) civil fines, (c) an administrative order issued by the EPA to forbid further distribution of a product, and (d) seizure and destruction of the offending product.

35.3.3. Toxic Air Pollutants

The major federal law to combat air pollution is the Clean Air Act of 1970. This complex legislation employs several different regulatory techniques for hazardous and toxic air pollutants. However, the EPA has been slow to exercise the full extent of its authority under the act.

First, the principal method of controlling stationary source pollution is to designate those air pollutants that have an adverse effect on health and come from numerous sources so that criteria for maximum permissible amounts in the ambient air can be set. These are known as "criteria pollutants" because a criteria document for each one is issued by the EPA. Thus far seven criteria pollutants have been designated: sulfur dioxide, particulate matter, carbon monoxide, photochemical oxidants, hydrocarbons, nitrogen oxide, and lead. Lead was added to the list by court order after a citizen suit in 1976. Once standards for criteria pollutants have been set by the EPA, individual states, through regional implementation plans, are required to take action against offenders to attain the level of the standards. The primary ambient air standards, setting maximum concentrations to safeguard the public health, were supposed to have been met by 1975; however, due to delay in implementation, levels of pollution exceed the standards in many regions of the country.

Second, the EPA has authority to set emission standards for certain noncriteria hazardous pollutants emitted by both new and existing stationary sources. By law, the emission standards must provide an ample margin of safety to protect the public health. The EPA has been slow to exercise this authority, however. The initial listing of hazardous air pollutants, in 1971, included only beryllium, mercury, and asbestos: vinyl chloride was added in 1975 and benzene in 1976.

Third, the primary regulatory mechanism to control hazardous pollutants emitted by mobil sources of pollution (cars, buses, trucks and other vehicles) is directed toward emission limitations directly and is binding on manufacturers. Standards have been developed for hydrocarbons, carbon monoxide, and nitrogen oxide. In addition, the content of lead in fuel has been regulated by the EPA. Oil producers and refiners were required to market at least one grade of lead-free gasoline after July 1, 1974. Other motor vehicle gasoline had to achieve a phased reduction of lead content, attaining a level of 0.5 g/gal by 1979.

These measures have succeeded in allieviating some problems of toxic substances in the air. However, the EPA never adopted a broad program to control these emissions but only reacted to particular problems after they developed. Moreover, the motor vehicle performance standards alone do not solve the problem of increasing numbers of trucks, cars, and buses in city areas, so that nonattainment of minimally acceptable air quality is common despite the achievement of increasingly strict emission controls. This and similar situations suggest that the purely technological approach to toxic substance control is insufficient and that other approaches, such as "alternative life styles," should also be explored.

35.3.4. Toxic Water Pollutants

During the past few years the problem of toxic pollutants in the nation's waters has been well publicized. The James River Estuary in Virginia has been polluted by chordecone (Kepone), asbestos tailings have posed a problem in Lake Superior, the Hudson River has been contaminated by PCBs, and the Lower Mississippi River has been found to be polluted by numerous chemical and metallic substances. During the summer of 1978, 211 miles of North Carolina highway roadsides and the adjacent areas were contaminated by the wilful dumping of thousands of gallons of PCBs. These problems have persisted despite the provision of the Federal Water Pollution Control Act (FWPCA) that sets as "national policy" that "the discharge of toxic pollutants in toxic amounts be prohibited."

Since 1972, the FWPCA has contained a specific provision to control toxic effluents into the nation's waters. The EPA is given authority to list toxic pollutants that it intends to regulate and to adopt either standards or discharge prohibitions for the listed substances. The agency did not give high priority to implementing this provision, however, until in 1976 it settled a lawsuit brought by the National Resources Defense Fund by agreeing to develop and promulgate standards for some 65 toxic pollutants. It appears that the designated watchdog, the EPA, is propelled into action to fulfill its mandated role only if pressure is brought to bear from the outside. In 1976, stringent effluent standards were proposed for aldrin, dieldrin, DDT, endrin, toxaphene, benzidene and PCBs. Over the next several years, the EPA intends to continue developing standards for other toxic pollutants.

Other provisions of the FWPCA have also been used to regulate toxic substances. The EPA has developed effluent standards on an industry-by-industry basis for almost all polluting industries. These are uniform numerical pollution limits by industrial category. This is the principal authority under which the EPA has acted to regulate chemical and metallic discharges. In addition, water quality limits (stream standards) have been developed and are supposed to be enforced by individual states subject to the approval of the EPA, which specifies maximum permissible quantities of toxic pollutants for various categories of streams. The EPA also regulates these substances through regulations promulgated for controlling pollution from storm sewers and nonpoint sources of pollution such as fertilizer and pesticide runoff from croplands. Standards for a wide variety of toxic pollutants have been promulgated by the EPA for treated drinking water from all public water supplies under the Safe Drinking Water Act of 1974. Acid drainage into streams from active and abandoned mining operations has been a significant problem and is now regulated under the Federal Strip Mining Act of 1977 as well as strip mining legislation in effect in many states.

The FWPCA contains a special provision to deal with the problem of accidental spills of oil and other hazardous substances. This is directed especially to spills from vessels in ocean and coastal waters, although it is applicable more broadly to any accidental spillage. Discharges of oil or hazardous substances entails a civil fine and owners and operators of vessels and facilities must reimburse the federal government for cleanup costs. A notable loophole in this legislation is the lack of any liability or compensation for damages, and in 1978 legislation was introduced in Congress to establish such liability and a liability fund to pay for damages. The intentional dumping of toxic or hazardous substances into the oceans requires a permit and is regulated by the EPA under the Marine Protection, Research and Sanctuaries Act of 1972.

In 1978, Congress amended the FWPCA to provide further controls on toxic substances. First, the EPA is given virtually complete authority to add any chemical to the toxic substances list: its decision can be reversed only in the event of arbitrariness. Second, the EPA is free to establish strict standards down to zero discharge where necessary. Third, industry will not be able to obtain any waiver of compliance with any toxic substance discharge standard.

35.3.5. Safeguards for Workers

Under the 1970 Occupational Safety and Health Act (OSHA), the Department of Labor is required to adopt workplace standards for toxic substances to protect the health of workers. Three types of standards are envisioned. First, "consensus standards" are set, reflecting the existing guidelines and practices of industry. These are basically maximum 8-hr average atmospheric concentration standards (i.e., time limit values, TLVs) for the specified substances. Second, more stringent permanent standards can be developed on an individual basis. Third, emergency standards can be promulgated where necessary.

Over 400 consensus standards have been promulgated under OSHA since 1971. The difficulty of following an intricate set of procedural steps and lack of basic research have inhibited the setting of permanent standards, however. For example, some 1500–2000 agents have been identified by the National Institute for Occupational Safety and Health (NIOSH) as being "suspect carcinogens," which means that they have been found to cause cancer in human or animal populations. However, OSHA has set regulatory standards on only 17 since 1971.

On October 4, 1977, the Department of Labor proposed to adopt general rules applicable to all carcinogens. Substances identified as carcinogenic are to be listed and exposure limits are to be set as low as feasible (category I). If there are suitable substitutes that pose less hazard to workers, no exposure will be permitted (category II). If further data are needed before any regulatory activity, a substance is listed in category III. Finally, those toxic substances that are not yet found in U.S. workplaces are put into category IV. The advantage of this categorization is that it will permit comprehensive regulation of toxic substances in the workplace, replacing the present ad hoc approach.

Adequate enforcement has also been a major problem in implementing OSHA standards. The average U.S. workplace can be inspected only once every few decades with present manpower. In the permanent standards adopted under OSHA, therefore, employers are required to make medical examinations available to workers on a regular basis, to monitor levels of hazardous substances, and to report any standards violations to employees. In practice this is often equivalent to the fox guarding the chicken house!

35.3.6. Consumers and Hazardous Substances

The Food, Drug and Cosmetic Act and the Public Health Act require manufacturers of consumer food and consumer products to demonstrate the safety and efficacy of their products. A major problem in the regulation of consumer goods has been that the industry-sponsored tests are inaccurate or deficient. The FDA has proposed more stringent testing standards to compensate for this lack.

The Delaney amendment to the Food, Drug and Cosmetic Act has adopted a strict approach to food additives that have been found to cause cancer when ingested by either humans or animals. These food additives must be banned under current law, although the FDA has suffered a spate of adverse publicity when it has acted under this authority to ban well-known products.

The FDA has also experienced difficulty in requiring labeling to disclose the ingredients used in food and cosmetic products. Only after a 2-year court fight was the FDA successful in requiring cosmetic product labels to list each ingredient in decreasing order of volume.

The Consumer Product Safety Commission also cooperates with the FDA and the EPA in regulating unsafe consumer products. Regulations adopted in 1977 phase out all nonessential uses of fluorocarbons, used principally as refrigerants and aerosol can propellants, because there is evidence that these compounds deplete the stratospheric ozone layer that protects the earth's surface against the sun's UV radiation. Increased amounts of UV have been linked to an increased incidence of human skin cancer. The Consumer Products Safety Commission has also acted to ban the flame retardant chemical TRIS, a carcinogen used in children's clothing.

35.4. Toxic Substances Control Act of 1976

The Toxic Substances Control Act of 1976 (TSCA) represents the first attempt to provide comprehensive regulation of potentially dangerous chemical substances. The EPA is given the power to control the introduction, production, distribution, and commercial use of any chemical compound that presents an "unreasonable risk of injury to health or the environment." In addition to its basic regulatory authority, EPA may require testing of substances, premarket notification, and reports and records.

TSCA is written very broadly to cover a wide variety of substances and manufacturers' activities. Chemical substances are defined as "any organic or inorganic substance of a particular molecular identity, including—(i) any combination of such substances occurring in whole or part as a result of a chemical reaction or occurring in nature, and (ii) any element in 'uncombined radical'." This definition encompasses naturally occurring substances when produced commercially and the end products from chemical reactions. "Mixture" is defined as a combination of chemical substances not occurring in nature and not the result of chemical reactions. The chemical processes subject to TSCA requirements include both primary production and the intermediate use of chemicals in manufacturing. The effect of these broad definitions is that TSCA can be applied to almost any substance (excluding the specified exceptions) at all stages of manufacture. Pesticides (regulated under FIFRA), tobacco, nuclear material, firearms and ammunition, food, food additives, drugs, and cosmetics, are exempt from TSCA.

35.4.1. Regulation of Hazardous Chemical Substances and Mixtures

The core provisions of TSCA are contained in Section 6, the Regulation of Hazardous Chemical Substances and Mixtures. The Administrator of the EPA is given the authority to prohibit or limit the manufacture, processing, labeling, distribution in commerce, use, or disposal of any chemical substance or mixture if these activities pose an unreasonable risk to health or the environment. The informal hearing is the forum used by the EPA Administrator for making findings and promulgating rules under this section. There are provisions for notice of proposed rules and opportunity for interested persons to participate in the hearings.

The critical issue in the regulatory scheme is whether there is a finding of "unreasonable risk of injury to health or the environment." TSCA clearly envisions a balancing process in which both the benefits and risks of a chemical substance or mixture are weighed. Congress recognized that a risk-free society is impossible and directed the EPA Administrator to consider the environmental, economic, and social impacts of his/her decisions. In making a judgment on the presence of an unreasonable risk posed by a chemical, the EPA Administrator must address and publish a statement on the following issues:

1. The effects of such substance or mixture on health and the magnitude of the exposure of human beings to such substance or mixture.

2. The effects of such substance or mixture on the environment and the magnitude of the exposure of the environment to such substance or mixture.
3. The benefits of such substance or mixture for various uses and the availability of substitutes for such uses.
4. The reasonably ascertainable economic consequences of the rule, after consideration of the effect on the national economy, small business, technological innovation, the environment, and public health.

Federal regulations make it clear that human health or environmental effects need not be demonstrated conclusively, as long as evidence links the chemical substance or mixture to the effects. Risks to human health include the following:

1. Any instance of cancer, genetic mutation, birth defects, or toxicity that results in death or serious or prolonged incapacitation.
2. Any pattern of effects or evidence that reasonably supports the conclusion that the chemical substance or mixture produces cancer, genetic mutations, birth defects, or toxicity effects resulting in death or serious or prolonged incapacitation.

Adverse environmental effects include the following:

1. Extreme persistence of a chemical substance not occurring naturally or occurring in greater than natural concentrations as a result of commerce.
2. Pronounced bioaccumulation.
3. Interference with critical biogeochemical cycles, including toxicity to key organisms in the cycles.
4. Excessive stimulation of primary producers in aquatic ecosystems, resulting in nutrient enrichment, or eutrophication, of aquatic ecosystems.
5. Any ecologically significant effects on nonhuman organisms due to acute or chronic toxicity, such as cancer, mutation, birth defects, or serious or prolonged incapacitation.
6. Facile transformation or degradation to a chemical having an unacceptable risk as defined above.

35.4.2. Testing of Chemical Substances or Mixtures

The EPA Administrator may take regulatory action to control the chemical manufacturers and processors to test a chemical substance or mixture if it may present an unreasonable risk of injury to health or the environment. This section establishes a much lower threshold finding before the EPA Administrator can take action than pertains in regulatory Section 6. The basis for requiring *testing* is a finding that the chemical *may* present an unreasonable risk, as opposed to a requirement that there *is* an unreasonable risk before *regulatory* sanctions can be applied. Alternatively, the EPA Administrator may order testing if the chemical substance or mixture will be produced "in substantial quantities," and it will either enter the environment in substantial quantities or there will be a significant exposure to humans.

The testing is meant to reveal health and environmental effects such as carcinogenesis, mutagensis, teratogenesis, behavioral disorders, cumulative or synergistic, or other effects that present a risk. Acceptable methodologies for testing include epidemiological studies, serial or hierarchical tests, in vitro tests, and whole animal tests. A committee is established to recommend a priority list for testing of chemical substances and mixtures. The quantity of the chemical, the level of human exposure, the effects from closely related chemicals, and the availability of facilities for testing are factors considered by the committee. There are provisions for the EPA Administrator to spread the cost of testing among all persons who benefit from previous tests conducted and paid for by other individuals.

35.4.3. Manufacturing and Processing Notification

Manufacturers of chemicals are required to give premarket notification to the EPA before the manufacture of a new chemical substance or the manufacture or processing of a chemical for a significant new use. The difference between chemical substances and mixtures is important; users of mixtures do not have to give notice unless the mixture involves a significant new use. As one commentator has noted, this provision reflects a strong proenvironmentalist bias that all new products should be reviewed before they cause environmental damage and attract investments. These provisions are intended to provide time for the EPA Administrator to review and evaluate information concerning the health and environmental effects of the chemical substance or mixture. If there is either insufficient data to evaluate or an unreasonable risk to health or environment, the EPA Administrator may take regulatory action to control the chemical substance or mixture.

The notification process begins with a list compiled by the EPA Administrator of chemicals manufactured or processed in the United States for at least 3 years prior to the TSCA effective date. The manufacturer is required to give notice at least 90 days before production or use begins if the chemical substance is not on this inventory list. The EPA Administrator determines if there is a significant new use according to (a) the predicted volume of manufacturing and processing, (b) the extent to which the use alters the type or the duration of exposure to humans or to the environment, and (c) the methods of use and disposal. Unless notice of the chemical is published along with detailed health information and testing results, manufacturing and use of the chemical are prohibited. In certain cases, the EPA must give reasons for failing to act within the notice time period before the chemical can be produced.

If the EPA Administrator determines there are insufficient data or the anticipated cases may present an unreasonable risk to human health or may adversely affect the environment, he/she may issue a proposed order to "prohibit or limit the manufacturing, processing, distribution in commerce, use, or disposal" of the chemical substance or mixture. Depending on the severity of restriction and formal objections from the manufacturer or processor, the EPA Administrator may be forced to obtain an injunction from a federal court. After taking these administrative steps, the EPA may invoke Section 6 of TSCA and issue a restrictive rule to control the chemical substance or mixture.

35.4.4. Emergency Powers, Record Keeping Requirements, and Other Provisions

For chemical substances or mixtures that pose an imminent hazard to human health or the environment, the EPA Administrator may ask a court to enforce seizure or any other relief necessary to protect health and the environment. An imminently hazardous chemical substance or mixture is one that presents an immediate and unreasonable risk of serious or widespread injury to health or the environment. The emergency power is meant to be used if the injury would take place before the EPA Administrator could promulgate regulations under the formal procedure of Section 6.

Other provisions of TSCA give the EPA Administrator authority to require manufacturers and processors of chemical substances or mixtures to submit reports and maintain records. The information required to be reported concerns the chemical identity and molecular structure, the categories of use, the total amount to be manufactured or used, and a description of by-products resulting from the manufacture, use, or disposal of the chemical, in addition to all existing data on health and environmental effects and the number of individuals exposed to the chemical at their places of employment. Records must be kept detailing any significant adverse health or environmental reactions attributable to a chemical substance or mixture. Other provisions of TSCA call for expanded research activities on the effects of chemical substances and mixtures, address the relationship of this law to other laws, and to provide for citizen civil suits and petitions to enforce TSCA.

The EPA Administrator can only regulate exports if the chemical substances or mixtures present an unreasonable risk to health or environment in the United States. Imported chemical substances, mixtures, or articles containing such items will only be admitted into the country if they conform to rules and regulations promulgated under TSCA. Miscellaneous sections protect the confidentiality of information reported under TSCA and give the power to the EPA to inspect business premises and to impose civil and criminal penalties for violations. TSCA specifically prohibits the manufacturing and processing of PCBs after January 1979, and all distribution of PCBs in commerce after July 1979. The harmful effects from PCBs illustrate the dangers presented by certain chemicals and provided some of the impetus for passing this legislation. It is appropriate that PCBs were targeted for special restrictions.

The full impact of TSCA has yet to be felt. The EPA is completing the process of establishing the procedures that will be used to collect and evaluate the information received from manufacturers and processors. The inventory of existing chemical substances and mixtures, published in April 1977, contained 30,000–40,000 chemical agents. It has been continually updated to include new chemical substances and mixtures. TSCA has the potential to be a far reaching, comprehensive measure that will reduce human and environmental exposure to dangerous chemical substances and mixtures. It will be extremely difficult to administer and apply.

35.5. Benefit–Risk Analysis

In addition to difficulties in administration, once agreed-upon standards have been established, there is increasingly strong pressure for the performance of risk–benefit analyses (RBA). These analyses are designed to evaluate the proposed alternatives by comparing the risks and the benefits of each. Since many human, natural, and economic resources are involved in every major decision, it is only fitting that good RBAs be performed. The performance of good RBAs requires quantification of all factors of a particular case. Some aspects are readily quantifiable but others, such as esthetics, clean air, clean water, freedom from undue noise, and the long-term maintenance of ecosystem viability, are essentially nonquantifiable.

While repeated attempts have been made to develop satisfactory quality of life indicators to be used in the performance of RBAs, comparatively little progress has been made to date. As a consequence, many of the qualitative environmental factors are often given inadequate weight in the CBA process.

If we are to address the issues raised by the enactment and enforcement of laws such as the Clean Air Act, the Clean Water Act, and TSCA, we must make progress in developing acceptable RBAs that emphasize all short term and long term risks and benefits fairly.

Suggested Reading

Council on Environmental Quality, Washington, D.C. Eighth Annual Report. 1977.

Hall, K. The control of toxic pollutants under the federal Water Pollution Control Act Amendments of 1972. Iowa Law Rev. 53:329, 1978.

Lawrance, W. W. Of Acceptable Risk: Science and the Determination of Safety. Los Altos, Calif.: Kaufmann, 1976.

Rodgers, W. H. Environmental Law. New York: West, 1977.

Zener, R. V. The Toxic Substances Control Act: Federal regulation of commercial chemicals. Business Lawyer, 32:1682, 1977.

Index